Higher-Order Differential Equations and Elasticity

Mathematics and Physics for Science and Technology

Series Editor: L.M.B.C. Campos
Director of the Center for Aeronautical
and Space Science and Technology
Lisbon University

Volumes in the series:

Topic A – Theory of Functions and Potential Problems

**Volume I (Book 1) – Complex Analysis with Applications to Flows
and Fields**
L.M.B.C. Campos

**Volume II (Book 2) – Elementary Transcendentals with Applications
to Solids and Fluids**
L.M.B.C. Campos

**Volume III (Book 3) – Generalized Calculus with Applications to Matter
and Forces**
L.M.B.C. Campos

Topic B – Boundary and Initial-Value Problems

**Volume IV – Ordinary Differential Equations with Applications
to Trajectories and Vibrations**
L.M.B.C. Campos

Book 4 – Linear Differential Equations and Oscillators
L.M.B.C. Campos

Book 5 – Non-Linear Differential Equations and Dynamical Systems
L.M.B.C. Campos

Book 6 – Higher-Order Differential Equations and Elasticity
L.M.B.C. Campos

**Book 7 – Simultaneous Differential Equations and Multi-Dimensional
Vibrations**
L.M.B.C. Campos

Book 8 – Singular Differential Equations and Special Functions
L.M.B.C. Campos

**Book 9 – Classification and Examples of Differential Equations and
their Applications**
L.M.B.C. Campos

For more information about this series, please visit: https://www.crcpress.
com/Mathematics-and-Physics-for-Science-and-Technology/book-series/
CRCMATPHYSCI

Mathematics and Physics for Science and Technology

Volume IV

Ordinary Differential Equations with Applications to Trajectories and Vibrations

Book 6

Higher-Order Differential Equations and Elasticity

By

L.M.B.C. CAMPOS

*Director of the Center for Aeronautical
and Space Science and Technology
Lisbon University*

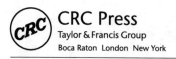

CRC Press
Taylor & Francis Group
Boca Raton London New York

CRC Press is an imprint of the
Taylor & Francis Group, an **informa** business

CRC Press
Taylor & Francis Group
6000 Broken Sound Parkway NW, Suite 300
Boca Raton, FL 334 87-2742

International Standard Book Number-13: 978-0-367-13720-5 (Hardback)

DOI: 10.1201/9780429029691

Visit the Taylor & Francis Web site at
http://www.taylorandfrancis.com

and the CRC Press Web site at
http://www.crcpress.com

to Leonor Campos

Contents

Diagrams, Lists, Notes, and Tables

Diagrams

Lists

Notes

Tables

Preface

Volume IV (*"Ordinary Differential Equations with Applications to Trajectories and Oscillations"*) is organized like the preceding three volumes of the series *Mathematics and Physics for Science and Technology*: volume I, *Complex Analysis with Applications to Flows and Fields*; volume II, *Elementary Transcendentals with Applications to Solids and Fluids*; and volume III, *Generalized Calculus with Applications to Matter and Forces*. Volume IV consists of ten chapters: (i) the odd numbered chapters present mathematical developments; (ii) the even numbered chapters contain physical and engineering applications; (iii) the last chapter is a set of 20 detailed examples of (i) and (ii). The first book, *Linear Differential Equations and Oscillators*, and second book, *Non-linear Differential Equations and Dynamical Systems*, of volume IV correspond respectively to books 4 and 5 of the series and consist of chapters 1 to 4 of volume IV. The present book, *Higher-Order Differential Equations and Elasticity*, is the third of volume IV, corresponds to the sixth of the series, and consists of chapters 5 and 6 of volume IV.

Chapter 1 begins with linear differential equations of any order with constant or homogeneous power coefficients and chapter 3 concerns non-linear differential equations of the first order, including variable coefficients. Chapter 5 continues with non-linear differential equations of the second and higher orders. It also includes special differential equations, whose solutions include, besides the general integral, special integrals not included in the general integral for any choice of constants of integration. The methods presented include dual variables and differentials, related by Legendre transforms, which have application in thermodynamics.

Chapters 2 and 4 concern respectively linear and non-linear oscillators, including damping/amplification, forcing, and ordinary/parametric/non-linear resonance as examples of dynamical systems, all leading to second-order differential equations. Chapter 6 concerns deformations of one(two)-dimensional elastic bodies that are specified by differential equations of: (i) the second-order for non-stiff bodies like elastic strings (membranes); and (ii) the fourth-order for stiff bodies like elastic beams (plates). The differential equations are linear for small deformations and gradients and non-linear otherwise. The deformations for beams include bending by transverse loads and buckling by axial loads. Buckling and bending couple non-linearly for plates. The deformations depend on material properties; for example, isotropic or anisotropic elastic plates, with intermediate cases such as orthotropic or pseudo-isotropic.

Organization of the Book

The chapters are divided into sections and subsections; for example, chapter 5, section 5.1, and subsection 5.1.1. The formulas are numbered by chapters in curved brackets; for example, (6.2) is equation 2 of chapter 6. When referring to volume I, the symbol I is inserted at the beginning; for example, chapter I.36, section I.36.1, subsection I.36.1.2, equation (I.36.33a). The final part of each chapter includes: (i) a conclusion referring to the figures as a kind of visual summary; (ii) the note(s), list(s), table(s), diagram(s), and classification(s) as additional support. The latter (ii) apply at the end of each chapter, and are numbered within the chapter (for example, diagram 6.1, List 6.3, note 5.9, table 5.2); if there are more than one they are numbered sequentially (for example, notes 5.1 to 5.20). The chapter starts with an introductory preview, and related topics may be mentioned in the notes at the end. The "Series Preface," and "Mathematical Symbols" from the first book of volume IV are not repeated, and the "Physical Quantities," "References," and "Index" focus on the contents of the present third book of volume IV.

Acknowledgments

The fourth volume of the series justifies renewing some of the acknowledgments also made in the first three volumes, to those who contributed more directly to the final form of the volume: Ms. Ana Moura, L. Sousa, and S. Pernadas for help with the manuscripts; Mr. J. Coelho for all the drawings; and at last, but not least, to my wife as my companion in preparing this work.

About the Author

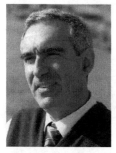

L.M.B.C. Campos was born on March 28, 1950, in Lisbon, Portugal. He graduated in 1972 as a mechanical engineer from the Instituto Superior Tecnico (IST) of Lisbon Technical University. The tutorials as a student (1970) were followed by a career at the same institution (IST) through all levels: assistant (1972), assistant with tenure (1974), assistant professor (1978), associate professor (1982), chair of Applied Mathematics and Mechanics (1985). He has served as the coordinator of undergraduate and postgraduate degrees in Aerospace Engineering since the creation of the programs in 1991. He is the coordinator of the Scientific Area of Applied and Aerospace Mechanics in the Department of Mechanical Engineering. He is also the director and founder of the Center for Aeronautical and Space Science and Technology.

In 1977, Campos received his doctorate on "waves in fluids" from the Engineering Department of Cambridge University, England. Afterwards, he received a Senior Rouse Ball Scholarship to study at Trinity College, while on leave from IST. In 1984, his first sabbatical was as a Senior Visitor at the Department of Applied Mathematics and Theoretical Physics of Cambridge University, England. In 1991, he spent a second sabbatical as an Alexander von Humboldt scholar at the Max-Planck Institut fur Aeronomic in Katlenburg-Lindau, Germany. Further sabbaticals abroad were excluded by major commitments at the home institution. The latter were always compatible with extensive professional travel related to participation in scientific meetings, individual or national representation in international institutions, and collaborative research projects.

Campos received the von Karman medal from the Advisory Group for Aerospace Research and Development (AGARD) and Research and Technology Organization (RTO). Participation in AGARD/RTO included serving as a vice-chairman of the System Concepts and Integration Panel, and chairman of the Flight Mechanics Panel and of the Flight Vehicle Integration Panel. He was also a member of the Flight Test Techniques Working Group. Here he was involved in the creation of an independent flight test capability, active in Portugal during the last 30 years, which has been used in national and international projects, including Eurocontrol and the European Space Agency. The participation in the European Space Agency (ESA) has afforded Campos the opportunity to serve on various program boards at the levels of national representative and Council of Ministers.

His participation in activities sponsored by the European Union (EU) has included: (i) 27 research projects with industry, research, and academic institutions; (ii) membership of various Committees, including Vice-Chairman of the Aeronautical Science and Technology Advisory Committee; (iii) participation on the Space Advisory Panel on the future role of EU in space. Campos has been a member of the Space Science Committee of the European Science Foundation, which works with the Space Science Board of the National Science Foundation of the United States. He has been a member of the Committee for Peaceful Uses of Outer Space (COPUOS) of the United Nations. He has served as a consultant and advisor on behalf of these organizations and other institutions. His participation in professional societies includes member and vice-chairman of the Portuguese Academy of Engineering, fellow of the Royal Aeronautical Society, Astronomical Society and Cambridge Philosophical Society, associate fellow of the American Institute of Aeronautics and Astronautics, and founding and life member of the European Astronomical Society.

Campos has published and worked on numerous books and articles. His publications include 10 books as a single author, one as an editor, and one as a co-editor. He has published 152 papers (82 as the single author, including 12 reviews) in 60 journals, and 254 communications to symposia. He has served as reviewer for 40 different journals, in addition to 23 reviews published in *Mathematics Reviews*. He is or has been member of the editorial boards of several journals, including *Progress in Aerospace Sciences*, *International Journal of Aeroacoustics*, *International Journal of Sound and Vibration*, and *Air & Space Europe*.

Campos's areas of research focus on four topics: acoustics, magnetohydrodynamics, special functions, and flight dynamics. His work on acoustics has concerned the generation, propagation, and refraction of sound in flows with mostly aeronautical applications. His work on magnetohydrodynamics has concerned magneto-acoustic-gravity-inertial waves in solar-terrestrial and stellar physics. His developments on special functions have used differintegration operators, generalizing the ordinary derivative and primitive to complex order; they have led to the introduction of new special functions. His work on flight dynamics has concerned aircraft and rockets, including trajectory optimization, performance, stability, control, and atmospheric disturbances.

The range of topics from mathematics to physics and engineering fits with the aims and contents of the present series. Campos's experience in university teaching and scientific and industrial research has enhanced his ability to make the series valuable to students from undergraduate level to research level.

Campos's professional activities on the technical side are balanced by other cultural and humanistic interests. Complementary non-technical interests include classical music (mostly orchestral and choral), plastic arts (painting, sculpture, architecture), social sciences (psychology and biography), history (classical, renaissance and overseas expansion) and technology (automotive, photo, audio). Campos is listed in various biographical publications, including *Who's Who in the World* since 1986, *Who's Who in Science and Technology* since 1994, and *Who's Who in America* since 2011.

Physical Quantities

The location of first appearance is indicated, for example "2.7" means "section 2.7," "6.8.4" means "subsection 6.8.4," "N8.8" means "note 8.8," and "E10.13.1" means "example 10.13.1."

1 Small Arabic Letters

a_i — acceleration vector: 6.8.3

b — stiffness dispersion parameter of an elastic bar: N6.12

$\bar{b}$ — stiffness dispersion parameter for an elastic plate: N6.10

c — phase speed of waves: N5.13, N6.14

c_1, c_2 — speed of transversal waves in the directions of principal stress of an anisotropic elastic membrane: N6.7

c_e — speed of transversal waves in an elastic string: N6.3

— speed of transversal waves in an isotropic elastic membrane: N6.4

c_ℓ — speed of longitudinal waves in an elastic rod: N6.6

c_r — isothermal sound speed: 5.5.25

c_s — adiabatic sound speed: 5.5.14

c_t — speed of torsional waves along an elastic rod: N6.5

e_{ijk} — three-dimensional permutation symbol: 6.8.4

$\vec{f}$ — force vector per unit area: 6.5.4

f_i — force vector per unit volume: 6.8.3

g — acceleration of gravity: 6.3.14

h — thickness of a plate: 6.5.4

k — Boltzmann constant: 5.5.16

— transversal wavenumber: N5.14

— curvature: 6.1.11

k' — differential resilience of a distributed spring: 6.3.1

$\bar{k}$ — resilience of a point rotational spring: 6.2.6

k_1, k_2 — principal curvatures: 6.7.2

k_{ij} — matrix of curvatures and cross-curvatures: 6.7

n — number of degrees of freedom of a molecule: 5.5.22

$\vec{n}$ — unit vector normal to a curve: 6.9.7

p — pressure: 5.5.4, 6.5.1

— buckling parameter: 6.1.2

s — arc length: 6.1.1

u — longitudinal displacement of a bar: 6.4.1

$\vec{u}$ — displacement vector: 6.4.1, 6.8.5

$\vec{v}$ — velocity vector: 5.2.1

w — group velocity: N6.16

x — independent variable in ordinary differential equation: 5.1.1

— Cartesian coordinate: 6.1.1

y — dependent variable in ordinary differential equation: 5.1.1

— Cartesian coordinate: 6.1.1

z — Cartesian coordinate: 6.5.1

2 Capital Arabic Letters

A — Avogadro number: 5.5.17

A_{ab} — elastic compliance matrix: 6.8.10

C — torsional stiffness of an elastic rod: N6.4

$\vec{C}$ — bending vector: 6.7.8

C_p — specific heat at constant pressure: 5.5.12

C_v — specific heat at constant volume: 5.5.12

C_{ab} — elastic stiffness matrix: 6.8.7

$C_{ijk\ell}$ — elastic stiffness tensor: 6.8.6

D — bending stiffness of an elastic plate: 6.7.2

— generalized bending stiffness: 6.8.14

D_2 — relative area change: 6.5.5

D_3 — relative volume change: 6.5.1

E — Young modulus of elasticity: 6.4.1, 6.5.1

E_0, E_1 — coefficients in the non-uniform Young modulus: 6.4.4

$\bar{E}_b$ — elastic energy per unit area of in-plane deformation: 6.9.4

$\bar{\bar{E}}_b$ — total elastic energy of in-plane deformation: 6.9.5

E_c — elastic energy per unit area for the deflection of an elastic membrane: 6.6.2

$\bar{E}_c$ — total elastic energy of deflection for a membrane: 6.6.2

$\bar{\bar{E}}_c$ — total elastic energy of deflection for a plate: 6.9.5

E_d — elastic energy per unit volume for a plate: 6.7.8

$\bar{\bar{E}}_d$ — total elastic energy for a plate: 6.7.8

$\tilde{E}_d$ — elastic energy per unit length along the boundary of a plate: 6.8.16

E_v — kinetic energy: 6.8.5

F — free energy: 5.5.8

    — longitudinal force in a bar: 6.4.1

$\vec{F}$ — force vector: 6.5.4

G — free enthalpy: 5.5.8

H — enthalpy: 5.5.8

$\bar{I}$ — deformation vector: 6.7.9

J — electric current: 4.7.1

    — heat flux: 6.4.2

K — longitudinal wavenumber: N5.14

    — curvature quadratic form: 6.7.3

L — lengthscale of variation of wave speed: N5.19

M — molecular mass: 5.5.17

    — moment of the inertia force: N6.4

$\vec{M}$ — moment of forces: 6.8.4

M_1, M_2 — principal bending moments: 6.7.2

M_a — applied axial moment: N6.4

M_n — normal stress couple: 6.8.16

M_x, M_y — stress couples: 6.7.4

M_{xy} — twist couple: 6.7.4

N — number of particles: 5.5.17

$\vec{N}$ — unit outer normal to a surface: 5.5.1

    — turning moment: 6.7.6

N_n — normal turning moment: 6.8.16

$\bar{N}_n$ — augmented normal turning moment: 6.9.5

N_x, N_y — turning moments: 6.7.6

Q — heat source: 6.4.2

R — perfect gas constant: 5.5.17

    — radius of curvature: 6.1.1

S — strain: 6.4.1

    — surface adsorption coefficient: N7.48

S_a — row of components of the strain tensor: 6.8.7
S_{ij} — strain tensor: 6.5.1, 6.8.8
T — tangential tension along an elastic string: 6.1.1
$\bar{T}$ — effective axial tension: 6.3.12
$\vec{T}$ — stress vector: 6.6.2, 6.8.3
T_a — row of components of the stress tensor: 6.8.7
T_{ij} — stress tensor: 6.5.1, 6.8.3
$\overset{o}{T}_{ij}$ — residual stresses: 6.8.6
U — internal energy: 5.5.4
V — specific volume: 5.5.4
W — work: 5.5.4
W_b — work of deformation: 6.8.5
W_v — work of the inertia force: 6.8.5

3 Small Greek Letters

χ — thermal conductivity: 6.4.2
— stiffness ratio parameter: 6.8.16
— damping parameter: 6.8.14
δ_{ij} — identity matrix: 6.5.1, 6.8.4
$\varphi_\pm$ — phase of waves propagating in opposite directions: N6.14
γ — adiabatic exponent: 5.5.12
μ — kinematic friction coefficient: N6.10
ν — number of particles per unit volume: 5.5.17
— resilience of distributed translational spring: N6.10
θ — angle of inclination of a string or a beam: 6.1.11
— temperature: 6.4.2
ρ — mass density per unit volume: 5.8.11
ρ_1 — mass density per unit length: N6.3
ρ_2 — mass density per unit area: N6.4
σ — Poisson ratio: 6.5.1
τ — twist: 6.7.13
— torsion: N6.5
ω_1 — fundamental natural frequency: N6.13

ω_n — natural frequency of harmonics: N6.13

$\bar{\omega}_n$ — oscillation frequency of harmonics: N6.17

ω_r — natural frequency for rotary spring: N6.10

ω_t — natural frequency for rotary translational spring: N6.10

ω_{r1}, ω_{r2} — natural frequencies for a vector rotary spring: N6.10

ζ — transverse deflection of a string, beam, membrane, or plate: 6.1.1

4 Capital Greek Letters

ϑ — resilience of a rotary spring in one dimension: N6.10

$\vec{\vartheta}$ — resilience vector of a rotary spring in two dimensions: N6.10

Θ — stress function: 6.5.5

Ω_{ij} — rotation bivector: 6.8.6

5

Special, Second, and Higher-Order Equations

There are two distinct concepts of singularities in connection with differential equations: one relating to points and one relating to integrals. At a singular point of a differential equation, the highest order derivative either is not defined or takes multiple values; for example, it corresponds to a stagnation point of a flow (sections 4.1–4.2). The singular integral of a differential equation is a particular solution that is not contained in the general integral; that is, it cannot be obtained by any choice of arbitrary constants, and it has been designated a special integral (subsections 1.1.4–1.1.7) to avoid using the word "singular" with two meanings, by restricting it to singular points of a differential equation. The consideration of special integrals is simplest for first-order differential equations (sections 5.1–5.4) and complements the preceding account on general integrals (section 1.1). The preceding account (chapter 3), of the solution of several types of first-order differential equations by a variety of methods, concentrated on obtaining the general integral involving one constant of integration and representing a family of regular integral curves. If these curves have an envelope (subsections 1.1.4–1.1.7), the tangents to the latter coincide, at the points of contact, with the tangents to the former, and thus the envelope is a solution of the differential equation. This is called a special integral, since it is a solution of the differential equation involving no arbitrary constants, and it is not a particular case of the general integral; that is, the envelope is a special (or singular), not a regular integral curve (section 5.1).

Conversely, the family of integral curves may specify sets of singular or special points that form lines such as the tac, cusp, and node loci (section 5.2); these curves may (or may not) be solutions of the differential equation; that is, correspond (do not correspond) to special integrals. Certain types of first-order differential equations, namely Clairaut's and D'Alembert's forms, always have special as well as general integrals (section 5.3). Most types of differential equations do not have singular integrals, if the integral curves have no envelope. The integral curves may have special points; such as: (i) double or multiple points, where it crosses itself; (ii) cusps, where it forms an edge because the right and left tangents exist but do not coincide; and (iii) nodes, where different curves of the family touch. If the special points lie along a curve, they form respectively a node (i), cusp (ii), or tac (iii) locus. These loci are generally not a special integral of the differential equation, unless the integral curves are tangent to them.

The solution of first-order differential equations, whether or not they have special integrals, is facilitated if the equation can be solved for the slope, or for one of the variables (section 5.4). If a first-order differential equation is not solvable, it may happen that its dual equation is simpler (section 5.5). A second-order differential equation, in which one of the variables or the slope is missing, can always be reduced to a first order differential equation (section 5.6). An ordinary differential equation of order more than two may, in some cases, be reduced to a first-order equation; more often, it may be possible to depress the order of a differential equation (section 5.7), for example if it is an exact differential, or can be factorized (section 5.8), or is homogeneous (section 5.9). The homogeneous differential equation of order N is a generalization of the homogeneous first-order type; in the linear case, it reduces to Euler's equation with power coefficients and homogeneous derivatives (sections 1.6–1.8), that together with the case of constant coefficients (sections 1.3–1.5) is a generally solvable class of differential equations of N-th order (chapter 1). The non-linear homogeneous differential equation of order N can be transformed into an equation of order $N-1$ by means of a change of variable; this transformation, like others indicated in this section, is only useful if it leads to a differential equation simpler to solve than the original.

5.1 *C*-, *p*-discriminants and Special Curves and Integrals

The general integral of a first-order differential equation specifies a one-parameter family of integral curves (subsections 1.1.3 and 5.1.1); the associated special lines or loci of special points if they exist (subsection 5.1.4) may (may not) be solutions of the differential equation; that is, correspond (do not correspond) to special integrals depending on whether the integral curves are (are not) tangent to a given locus of special points. The special lines, whether or not they correspond to special integrals, satisfy either the C-discriminant (subsection 5.1.2) or the *p*-discriminant (section 5.1.3). The special integrals; that is, solutions of the differential equation that are not included in the general integral for any choice of constant of integration (subsections 1.1.7–1.1.8), exist for differential equations of the first (and higher) order(s) [subsections 5.1.4 (5.1.5)].

5.1.1 General and Special Integrals of a Differential Equation

A first-order ordinary differential equation (5.1b):

$$p \equiv y' \equiv \frac{dy}{dx}: \qquad F(x,y,p) = 0, \qquad f(x,y;C) = 0, \qquad \text{(5.1a–c)}$$

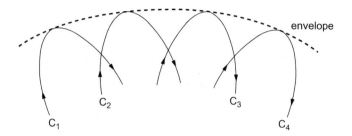

FIGURE 5.1
The general integral (5.1c) of first-order differential equation (5.1a, b) is a family of integral curves, one for each value of the arbitrary constant C, corresponding to a particular integral. The differential equation also has a special integral if there is another solution, not involving an arbitrary constant, which is not contained in the general integral, that is, does not coincide with any particular integral. If the family of integral curves has special curves of the first kind, that is, an envelope, it is always a special integral because: (i) it has the same tangent at the points of contact; (ii) hence it satisfies the differential equation; however, (iii) it does not coincide with any particular integral curve.

has a general integral (5.1c) involving (section 1.1) an arbitrary constant of integration and representing a **family of regular integral curves**; for each value of the constant C one curve of the family is obtained corresponding to a particular integral. Suppose that the family of curves has an **envelope** (Figure 5.1); since the tangents to the envelope coincide with the tangents to the regular integral curves at the points of contact, the envelope is a solution of the differential equation (5.1a, b). Generally the envelope is not a particular integral, obtained by choosing a value for the constant C in the general integral (5.1c). A solution of the differential equation (5.1a, b), that does not involve any constant of integration and is not included in the general integral (5.1c) is called a **special integral** (subsection 1.1.4). Thus, *if a family of integral curves (5.1c) of a first-order differential equation (5.1a, b) has an envelope (distinct from the curves of the family), the (standard XCII) equation of the envelope is a special integral of the differential equation.*

5.1.2 C-discriminant, Envelope, Node, and Cusp Loci

The envelope can exist (Figure 5.1) only if two consecutive curves, with parameters C and $C + \Delta C$, have the same tangent as $\Delta C \to 0$; that is, if the parameter C is a multiple (double or higher) root (5.1d) of the equation (5.1c) of the family:

$$0 = \lim_{\Delta C \to 0} \frac{f(x,y;C+\Delta C) - f(x,y;C)}{\Delta C} = \frac{\partial f(x;y;C)}{\partial C}. \tag{5.1d}$$

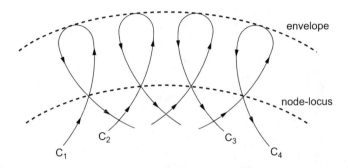

FIGURE 5.2
A second kind of special curves of a first-order differential equation is the node-locus consisting of the multiple points where the integral curves cross themselves, e.g., the double points in Figure 5.2. The node-locus is generally not a special integral of the differential equation unless it is tangent to one of the branches of all integral curves at all multiple points (Figure 5.7).

Elimination of the arbitrary constant C between (5.1c) $\equiv$ *(5.2a) and (5.1d)* $\equiv$ *(5.2b) leads to the* **C-discriminant**:

$$\text{C-discriminant:} \quad f(x,y;C) = 0 = \frac{\partial f(x;y;C)}{\partial C} : \quad \text{roots} \begin{cases} simple : envelope, \\ double : node\text{-}locus, \\ triple : cusp\text{-}locus, \end{cases}$$

$$(5.2a\text{--}e)$$

that specifies (standard XCIII) the **special curves** *of the family (5.1c), leading to three cases: (I) the envelope that is a single root (5.2c) since it touches the integral curves only at one-point (Figure 5.1); (II) the* **node-locus** *that is a double root (5.2d) since it is a line of* **double points** *where the curve crosses itself (Figure 5.2); and (III) the* **cusp-locus** *that is a triple root (5.2e) due to the shrinking of the loops (Figure 5.2) to points (Figure 5.3). The envelope (5.2c) is always a special integral of*

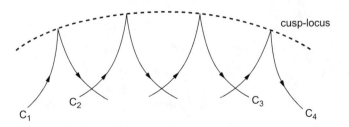

FIGURE 5.3
A third kind of special curve of a first-order differential equation is the cusp-locus, where all integral curves have an angular point; that is, the right and left derivatives exist and may or may not coincide. The cusp-locus is generally not a special integral of the first-order differential equation (Figure 5.3), unless it is tangent to all integral curves (Figure 5.8).

the differential equation (5.1a, b) because it is tangent to the integral curves; the node (5.2d) [cusp (5.2e)] locus is generally not a special integral of the differential equation [Figure 5.2 (5.3)] unless it happens to be tangent to the integral curves.

5.1.3 *p*-discriminant, Envelope, Tac, and Cusp Loci

At the envelope of a family of integral curves (Figure 5.4), the tangents to two consecutive curves $p = y'$ and $p + dp$ coincide as $dp \to 0$, so that the slope p is a multiple (double or higher) root (5.3b) of the differential equation (5.1b) $\equiv$ (5.3a):

$$p\text{-discriminant:} \quad f(x,y,p) = 0 = \frac{\partial f(x,y,p)}{\partial p}: \quad roots \begin{cases} simple : envelope, \\ double : tac\text{-}locus, \\ simple : cusp\text{-}locus, \end{cases}$$

$$(5.3a\text{--}e)$$

*Elimination of (5.1a) between (5.1b) $\equiv$ (5.3a) and (5.3b) leads to a **p-discriminant** that (standard XCIV) has three cases: (I) the envelope is a simple root (5.3c) since there is a single tangent at the points of contact with the integral curves (Figure 5.4); (IV) the **tac-locus** is a double root (5.3d) corresponding to points where two integral curves are tangent with opposite slopes (Figure 5.5); and (III) the **cusp-locus** is a simple root (5.3c) corresponding to points where the integral curves touch with the same tangent (Figure 5.6). The envelope (5.3c) is always [tac and cusp loci (5.3d, c) are generally not] a special integral of the differential equation (5.1a, b) because it is tangent (unless it is tangent) to the integral curves.*

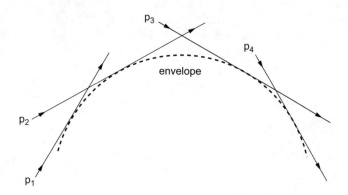

FIGURE 5.4
The only special curve of a first-order differential equation that is always a special integral is the envelope, that is a solution of both the C-discriminant (5.2a–e) [and *p*-discriminant (5.3a–e)] because it is the limit [Figure 5.1(5.4)] of neighboring integral curves as $dC \to 0 (dp \to 0)$.

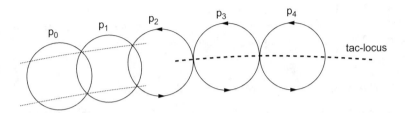

FIGURE 5.5
A fourth kind of special curve of a first-order differential equation is the tac-locus, where distinct integral curves are tangent to each order. The tac-locus is generally not tangent to the integral curves and thus is not a special integral of the differential equation.

5.1.4 Four Special Curves and One Special Integral

The cases I to IV of special lines of a family of curves are summarized in Table 5.1. Table 5.1 is based on geometrical intuition, and is not the result of rigorous analytic proof. Thus it has a purely indicative value, as special cases exist, for example: if the integral curves have triple (M-tuple) points, the node-locus would be a triple root (root of multiplicity M) of the C-discriminant; if the node, tac, or cusp loci happen to coincide with an integral curve or be tangent to the integral curves, they supply a particular integral of the differential equation. *Associated with the differential equation of first order (5.1a, b) and its general integral specifying a family of curves identified by the value of the arbitrary constant, there may be four types of (standard XCV) special curves (Table 5.1) not involving any constant of integration: (I) the envelope is a simple root of both the C-discriminant (5.2b, c) [and p-discriminant (5.3b, c)] that is always a special integral because it touches the integral curves at a single point with a single tangent (Figures 5.1 and 5.4); (II) the node locus where the integral curves cross themselves (Figure 5.2) is a double root of the C-discriminant (5.2b, d) and generally does not satisfy the p-discriminant; (III) the cusp locus where the integral curves have an angular point (Figure 5.3) is a triple root of the C-discriminant (5.2b, c), and may be a simple root of the p-discriminant (5.3b, c) if the right and left tangents coincide (Figure 5.3); and (IV) the tac locus where the integral curves touch each other with*

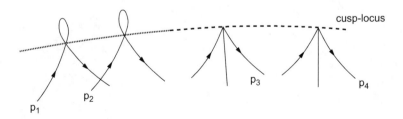

FIGURE 5.6
A special curve could conceivably have more than one kind, if for example it is the node-locus of some integral curves that have double points, and is also the cusp-locus for other integral curves for which the double points reduce to cusps.

TABLE 5.1

Special Lines of Families of Curves

		Root of		
Case	Special Curve	C-discriminant (5.2a, b)	>p-discriminant (5.3a–c)	Figure
I	envelope*	simple	simple	5.1, 5.2, 5.4
II	node-locus**	double	no	5.2, 5.6
III	cusp-locus**	triple	simple	5.3, 5.6
IV	tac-locus**	no	double	5.4

* always a special integral of the differential equation
** generally not a special integral of the differential equation
Note: Four types of special curves of a first-order differential equation that are roots of either the C-discriminant (5.2a–e) or of the p-discriminant (5.3a–e) or of both.

opposite tangents (Figure 5.5) is a double root of the p-discriminant (5.3 b, d) and generally does not satisfy the C-discriminant. The node, cusp, and tac loci are generally not special integrals, unless they happen to be tangent to the integral curves: for example a node (cusp) locus where one (both) branch(es) is (are) tangent to the special curve [Figure 5.7 (5.8)].

5.1.5 Special Integrals of Higher-Order Differential Equations

A differential equation (1.1a, b) ≡ (5.4a) of order N has a general integral (1.3) ≡ (5.4b) that involves N arbitrary constants of integration:

$$0 = f\left(x, y, y', ..., y^{(N)}\right), \qquad f\left(x, y; C_1, ..., C_N\right) = 0. \qquad \text{(5.4a, b)}$$

A **special integral** is:

$$0 \le M < N: \qquad\qquad g\left(x, y; C_1, ..., C_M\right) = 0, \qquad\qquad \text{(5.4 c, d)}$$

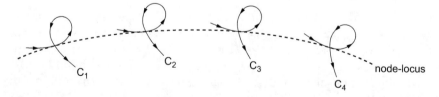

FIGURE 5.7
The node locus (Figure 5.2) is generally not a special integral of the differential equation unless (Figure 5.7) it is tangent to one branch of the integral curves passing through each multiple point; in that case the node-locus will not be tangent to other branches of the integral curves passing through the multiple points. In the case of the tac-locus of double points in Figure 5.7, it is tangent to one branch and not to the other of the integral curve that cuts itself at the double point.

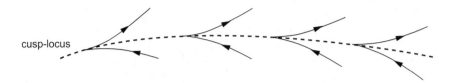

FIGURE 5.8
The envelope, when it exists, is always a special integral of the differential equation (Figure 5.1 and 5.4). The cusp-locus (Figure 5.3) is generally not a special integral unless (Figure 5.8) it is tangent to the integral curves, implying that: (i) the internal (external) angle is $0(2\pi)$ at all angular points; and (ii) at each angular point the right and left hand tangent have the same modulus and opposite signs.

a solution (5.4d) of a differential equation (5.4a) that: (i) involves (5.4c) a number of arbitrary constants of integration less than the order of the differential equation (5.4a); and (ii) is not contained in the general integral (5.4b) for any choice of the N constants of integration. Thus *a differential equation of order* N *could possibility (standard XCVI) have special integrals with 0, 1, … up to* $N-1$ *arbitrary constants of integration.* A first-order differential equation can have special integrals only without constant of integration. The special integral and loci of special points can be illustrated most readily for first-order differential equations. The general discussion of special curves of a first-order differential equation that are or are not special integrals (section 5.1 and Figures 5.1–5.8) is followed by examples arising from the solution (chapter 3) of various types of first-order differential equations (sections 5.2–5.4 and Figures 5.9–5.15).

5.2 Quadratic in the Slope or Arbitrary Constant

In order for a first-order differential equation to have special integrals, it must be of degree higher than the first on the slope so that its roots specify more than one possible slope. The simplest first-order differential with singular integrals is quadratic in the slope (subsection 5.2.1), leading to an immediate determination of the p-discriminant. The C-discriminant requires the general integral of the differential equation (subsections 5.2.2–5.2.4), and three examples are given: (subsection 5.2.2) a family of parabolas with one envelope passing through the vertices, that is, the points of highest curvature (Figure 5.9); (subsection 5.2.3) a family of circles lying between two parallel lines, which are the envelopes, with a tac-locus through the centers (Figure 5.10); and (subsection 5.2.4) a family of lace-like curves with envelope, tac, and node loci (Figure 5.11).

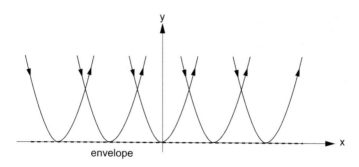

FIGURE 5.9
The family of integral curves consisting of parabolas (5.12a) with vertical axis and vertex on the real axis, has the real axis as envelope, that is a special integral of the differential equation (5.11a).

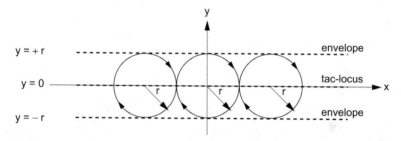

FIGURE 5.10
The family of circles (5.18a) with center on the real axis and the same radius has for special curves two envelopes (plus one tac-locus), namely the horizontal lines of abscissa equal to plus or minus the radius (abscissa zero, that is the real axis), that are (is not a) special integral of the differential equation (5.17a).

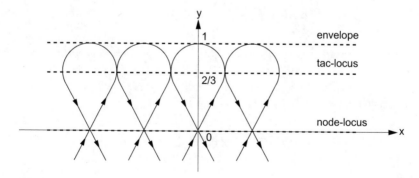

FIGURE 5.11
The family of lace-like curves (5.24a) with double points, one horizontal tangent and two vertical tangents in Figure 5.11 has three special curves, namely: (i) an envelope coincident with the horizontal tangents; (ii–iii) a tac (node)-locus passing through the double points (points with vertical tangents). The former (i) is [latter (ii, iii) are not] special integrals of the differential equation (5.23a).

5.2.1 First-Order Differential Equation—Quadratic in the Slope

A simple case of p-discriminant occurs when the differential equation (5.1a, b) is of degree two (5.5b) not degree one in the slope (5.5a):

$$p \equiv \frac{dy}{dx}: \qquad 0 = F(x,y,p) \equiv L(x,y)\,p^2 + M(x,y)p + N(x,y). \qquad \text{(5.5a, b)}$$

The slopes of the integral curves are the roots of (5.5b):

$$p_{\pm} = \frac{-M \pm \sqrt{M^2 - 4LN}}{2\,L}. \qquad \text{(5.6)}$$

The p-discriminant corresponds to a double root (5.7a):

$$p = -\frac{M}{2\,L}, \qquad\qquad M^2 = 4LN, \qquad \text{(5.7a, b)}$$

and occurs if the condition (5.7b) is met. It can be checked that the condition (5.3b) of a double root, applied to (5.5b), yields:

$$0 = \frac{\partial}{\partial p}\left\{ Lp^2 + Mp + N \right\} = 2Lp + M, \qquad \text{(5.8a)}$$

that coincides with (5.8a) $\equiv$ (5.7a). Also, eliminating p between (5.7a) $\equiv$ (5.8a) and (5.1b) $\equiv$ (5.5b) specifies the p-discriminant:

$$0 = Lp^2 + Mp + N = L\left(-\frac{M}{2L}\right)^2 + M\left(-\frac{M}{2L}\right) + N = -\frac{M^2}{4L} + N, \qquad \text{(5.8b)}$$

that coincides with the condition (5.8b) $\equiv$ (5.7b). *A first-order differential equation (5.1a, b) quadratic (standard XCVII) in the slope (5.5a, b) has p-discriminant (5.3a, b) specified by (5.7a) iff the coefficients satisfy (5.7b).* If the C-discriminant (5.2a, b) is (standard XCVIII) quadratic (5.9) $\equiv$ (5.5b):

$$0 = f(x,y;C) = P(x,y)C^2 + Q(x,y)C + R(x,y), \qquad \text{(5.9)}$$

it is specified:

$$C = -\frac{Q}{2P}, \qquad\qquad Q^2 = 4PR, \qquad \text{(5.10a, b)}$$

by the same conditions (5.10a, b) $\equiv$ (5.7a, b).

5.2.2 A Family of Parabolas with the Real Axis as Envelope

As a first example, consider the differential equation of first-order and degree two (5.11a):

$$y = p^2 \equiv \left(\frac{dy}{dx}\right)^2, \qquad dx = y^{-\frac{1}{2}} dy = 2d(\sqrt{y}), \qquad \text{(5.11a, b)}$$

that is separable (5.11b); it has general integral (5.12a):

$$(x-C)^2 = 4y, \qquad C^2 - 2xC + x^2 - 4y = 0, \qquad \text{(5.12a, b)}$$

that is, quadratic (5.12b) in the arbitrary constant of integration C. The integral curves (5.12a) are a family of parabolas with vertical axis and vertex $x = C$, $y = 0$ (Figure 5.9); their envelope is the x-axis $y = 0$. It can be checked that $y = 0$ is a solution of the differential equation (5.11a); that is, not included in the general integral (5.12a) for any particular choice of C; hence $y = 0$ is a special integral of the differential equation (5.9a) and should specify (Table 5.1) an envelope with zero slope.

Thus the real axis $y = 0$ should be a root of both the p-discriminant and C-discriminant as is checked next: (i) the differential equation (5.11a) ≡ (5.13a) leads (5.13b) to the p-discriminant (5.13c) that is the real axis (5.13d) where the slope (5.13c) is zero:

$$0 = F(x,y,p) = p^2 - y: \qquad 0 = \frac{\partial F}{\partial p} = 2p \Rightarrow p = 0 \Rightarrow y = 0; \qquad \text{(5.13a–d)}$$

$$0 = F(x,y,C) = C^2 - 2xC + x^2 - 4y: \quad 0 = \frac{\partial F}{\partial C} = -2(C-x) \Rightarrow x = C \Rightarrow y = 0 \Rightarrow p = 0,$$
$$\text{(5.14a–e)}$$

and (ii) the general integral (5.12a) ≡ (5.12b) ≡ (5.14a) leads (5.14b) to the C-discriminant (5.14c) that is the real axis (5.14d) corresponding (5.13a) ≡ (5.14e) to zero slope.

The same conclusions can be drawn as a particular case (subsection 5.2.1) of a differential equation (general integral) quadratic in the slope (arbitrary constant of integration): (i) the differential equation (5.11a) ≡ (5.13a) ≡ (5.5b) is quadratic in the slope with coefficients (5.15a), and since (5.15b) is met the real axis (5.15c) is a p-discriminant with zero slope (5.7b) ≡ (5.15d):

$$\{L,M,N\} = \{1,0,-y\}: \qquad 0 = M - 4LN = 4y \Rightarrow y = 0 \Leftarrow 0 = -\frac{M}{2L} = p;$$
$$\text{(5.15a–d)}$$

$$\{P,Q,R\}=\{1,-2x,x^2-4y\}: \quad 0=Q^2-4PR=16y \Rightarrow y=0 \Leftarrow C=-\frac{Q}{2P}=x,$$

$$(5.16a\text{–}d)$$

and (ii) the general integral (5.12a) ≡ (5.12b) ≡ (5.14a) is quadratic in the arbitrary constant of integration (5.9) with coefficients (5.16a), and since (5.10b) ≡ (5.16b) is met the C-discriminant is the real axis (5.16c) corresponding to (5.10a) ≡ (5.16d).

5.2.3 A Family of Circles with Two Envelopes and a Tac-Locus

As a second example, consider the differential equation (5.17a) where r is a constant:

$$\frac{r^2}{y^2}-1=p^2 \equiv \left(\frac{dy}{dx}\right)^2, \qquad dx=\frac{y\,dy}{\sqrt{r^2-y^2}}=-d\left\{\sqrt{r^2-y^2}\right\}, \qquad (5.17a, b)$$

that is separable (5.17b); its general integral (5.18a):

$$(x-C)^2+y^2=r^2, \qquad C^2-2x\,C+x^2+y^2-r^2=0, \qquad (5.18a, b)$$

is a family of circles of radii r, with centers at $x=C, y=0$ on the x-axis (5.18b). The parameter in the differential equation (5.17a) specifies the radius of the circles and the arbitrary constant indicates the abscissa of the center on the x-axis. The special lines are (Figure 5.10) the envelopes at $y=\pm r$ and the tac-locus at $y=0$, all with zero slopes.

As a first check, the differential equation (5.17a) ≡ (5.19a) is quadratic (5.5b) in the slope with coefficients (5.19b):

$$0=F(x,y,p)=p^2y^2+y^2-r^2: \qquad \{L,M,N\}=\{y^2,0,y^2-r^2\}; \qquad (5.19a, b)$$

the slopes (5.7a) ≡ (5.19c) are zero and the condition (5.7b) ≡ (5.19d):

$$p=-\frac{M}{2L}=0; \qquad 0=M-4LN=4y^2\left(r^2-y^2\right): \qquad \left\{\begin{array}{ll} y=\pm r: & envelopes, \\ y=0: & tac\text{-}locus, \end{array}\right.$$

$$(5.19c\text{–}f)$$

leads to: (i) the single roots that are horizontal lines (5.19e) that correspond to envelopes; and (ii) the real axis (5.19f) is a double root specifying a tac-locus.

As a second check the general integral (5.18a) ≡ (5.18b) ≡ (5.20a) is quadratic (5.9) in the constant of integration with coefficients (5.20b):

$$0 = f(x,y;C) = C^2 - 2Cx + x^2 + y^2 - r^2: \quad \{P,Q,R\} = \{1, -2\,x, x^2 + y^2 - r^2\}.$$

(5.20a, b)

The condition (5.10a) ≡ (5.20c) agrees with (5.20a) ≡ (5.20d) and the condition (5.10b) ≡ (4.20d) is met (5.20e) only by the envelope(s):

$$C = -\frac{Q}{2\,P} = x: \qquad 0 = Q^2 - 4\,P\,R = 4(r^2 - y^2) \quad \Rightarrow \quad y = \pm r. \qquad (5.20c\text{--}e)$$

Thus: (i) the envelopes are single roots both of the p-discriminant (5.19e) and of the C-discriminant (5.20e); and (ii) the tac-locus (5.19f) is a double root of the C-discriminant (5.19d) but is not a root of the p-discriminant (5.20d).

A third check is that the envelopes (5.19e) ≡ (5.20e) [tac-locus (5.19f)] do (do not) satisfy the differential equation (5.17a) ≡ (5.19a). The p-discriminant can be obtained (5.21a) from (5.19a) leading to (5.21b) ≡ (5.19f) [(5.21c) ≡ (5.19e)]:

$$0 = \frac{\partial F}{\partial p} = 2py^2: \qquad y = 0 \quad or \quad p = 0 \quad \Leftrightarrow \quad y^2 = r^2; \qquad (5.21a\text{--}c)$$

$$0 = \frac{\partial F}{\partial C} = 2(C - x): \qquad x = C \quad \Leftrightarrow \quad y^2 = r^2 \quad \Leftrightarrow \quad y = \pm r, \qquad (5.22a\text{--}d)$$

the C-discriminant (5.22a) can also be obtained from (5.20a) leading (5.22b) to (5.22c) the envelopes (5.22d) ≡ (5.19e) but not the tac-locus (5.19f).

5.2.4 Integral Curves with Envelope and Node and Tac Loci

As a third and final example, consider the first-order differential equation quadratic in the slope (5.23a) that is separable (5.23b):

$$4\frac{1-y}{(2-3y)^2} = p^2 \equiv \left(\frac{dy}{dx}\right)^2, \qquad dx = \frac{2-3y}{\sqrt{1-y}}\frac{dy}{2} = d\{y\sqrt{1-y}\}; \qquad (5.23a, b)$$

it has general integral (5.24a):

$$(x-C)^2 = y^2(1-y), \qquad C^2 - 2xC + x^2 - y^2(1-y) = 0, \qquad (5.24a, b)$$

that is quadratic (5.24b) in the arbitrary constant of integration C. All the curves of the family (5.24a) have (Figure 5.11): (i) the same maximum, because

$1 - y \geq 0$ in (5.24a), so that $y = 1$ is an envelope ; (ii) two slopes $p^2 = 1$, or $y' = \pm 1$ at $y = 0$ in (5.23a), that is a line of double points or node-locus; and (iii) vertical tangent $p = \infty$ at $y = 2/3$ in (5.23a), where two distinct curves touch, along a tac-locus. It can be checked that the envelope $y = 1$ is a special integral of the differential equation, but the node $y = 0$ and tac $y = 2/3$ loci are not solutions at all.

The differential equation (5.23a) $\equiv$ (5.25a) is quadratic in the slope (5.5b) with coefficients (5.23b):

$$0 = F(x,y,p) = (2 - 3y)^2 p^2 - 4(1 - y): \quad \{L, M, N\} = \left\{ (2 - 3y)^2, 0, 4(y - 1) \right\};$$
(5.25a, b)

the slopes (5.7a) $\equiv$ (5.25c) are zero and the condition (5.7b) $\equiv$ (5.25d):

$$P = -\frac{M}{2L} = 0: \quad 0 = M^2 - 4\,L\,N = 4(1 - y)(2 - 3y)^2: \quad \begin{cases} y = 1: & \textit{envelope,} \\ \\ y = \dfrac{2}{3}: & \textit{tac-locus,} \end{cases}$$
(5.25c–f)

leads to the p-discriminant (5.25d); the envelope (5.25e) is a simple root, the tac-locus (5.25f) a double root, and the node-locus $y = 0$ not a root, in agreement with the Table 5.1. The general integral (5.24a) $\equiv$ (5.24b) $\equiv$ (5.26a) is a quadratic function (5.9) of the constant of integration with coefficients (5.26b):

$$0 = f(x,y;C) = C^2 - 2Cx + x^2 - y^2(1 - y): \quad \{P, Q, R\} = \left\{ 1, -2x, x^2 - y^2(1 - y) \right\};$$
(5.26a, b)

the condition (5.10a) $\equiv$ (5.26c) agrees with (5.26a) $\equiv$ (5.26d) and the condition (5.10b) $\equiv$ (5.26d):

$$C = -\frac{Q}{2P} = x: \quad 0 = Q^2 - 4\,P\,R = 4y^2(1 - y): \quad \begin{cases} y = 1: & \textit{envelope,} \\ y = 0: & \textit{node-locus} \end{cases}$$
(5.26c–f)

leads to C-discriminant (5.26d) consisting of: (i) the envelope (5.26e) $\equiv$ (5.25d) that is a simple root of both the C- and p-discriminants, the node-locus is a (5.26f) a double root, and the tac-locus (5.25f) is not a root, in agreement with the Table 5.1. The C-discriminant can be obtained (5.27a) from (5.26a) and thus (5.27b) consists (5.27c) of the envelope (5.27d) ≡ (5.26e) [node-locus (5.27e) ≡ (5.26f)] as simple (double) roots:

$$0 = \frac{\partial f}{\partial C} = 2(C - x): \qquad x = C \quad \Rightarrow \quad 0 = y^2(1-y) \quad \Rightarrow \quad y = 0 \, or \, y = 1; \quad (5.27a\text{–}e)$$

$$0 = \frac{\partial F}{\partial p} = 2p(2-3y)^2: \qquad y = \frac{2}{3} \quad or \quad p = 0 \quad \Rightarrow \quad y = 1, \qquad (5.28a\text{–}e)$$

the *p*-discriminant (5.28a) can be obtained from (5.25a) and thus consists of the tac-locus (5.28c) ≡ (5.25f) [envelope (5.28d, e) ≡ (5.25e)] as double (single) roots. The method (subsection 5.4.1) for differential equation (general integral) quadratic on the slope (constant of integration) is a particular case of the *p*-discriminant (5.3a–c) [C-discriminant (5.2a–c)], that also applies to other classes of differential equations (special integrals) considered next (sections 5.3–5.4).

5.3 Clairaut (1734) and D'Alembert (1748) Special Equations

A first-order differential equation can have singular integrals even if the slope does not appear algebraically, for example quadratically (section 5.2). Two equations that always have special integrals are the Clairaut (1734) [D'Alembert (1748)] differential equations where the slope appears in the argument of one (two) differentiable functions [subsection 5.3.1 (5.3.3)]; one example is given of each [subsection 5.3.2 (5.3.4)] involving straight lines and parabolas.

5.3.1 Special Integral of Clairaut (1734) Differential Equation

A first-order differential equation that always has special as well as general integrals is (standard XCXI) is the **Clairaut (1734) equation** (5.29b):

$$h \in \mathcal{D}(\,|\,\mathcal{R}): \qquad y = px + h(p), \qquad (5.29a, b)$$

where *h* is an arbitrary differentiable function (5.29a). The Clairaut differential equation is solved (5.30b) by differentiation (5.30a) with regard to *x*:

$$p \equiv \frac{dy}{dx}: \qquad 0 = \frac{d}{dx}[px - y + h(p)] = [x - h'(p)]\frac{dp}{dx}. \qquad (5.30a, b)$$

There are two possible solutions: (i) the first (5.31a) leads to an arbitrary constant slope (5.31b) and to the general integral (5.31c):

$$\frac{dp}{dx} = 0: \qquad\qquad p = C, \qquad y(x;C) = Cx + h(C); \qquad\qquad (5.31a\text{–}c)$$

$$x = h'(p) \quad \wedge \quad h(p) = y - px \quad \Rightarrow \quad y = y(x), \qquad\qquad (5.32a\text{–}c)$$

and (ii) the second (5.32a) allows elimination of the slope from the differential equation (5.29b) ≡ (5.32b) leading to a special integral (5.32c). The special integral is the envelope of the family of straight lines (5.31c) ≡ (5.33a):

$$y(x;C) = Cx + h(C): \qquad\qquad \frac{dy}{dx} = C, \qquad y(0;C) = h(C), \qquad\qquad (5.33a\text{–}c)$$

that have arbitrary slope and ordinate at the origin (5.33c) specified by the function (5.29a) of the slope. It has been *shown that (standard XCIX) the general integral of the Clairaut (1734) equation (5.29a, b), is obtained (5.31c) by replacing $p = y' = C$ by an arbitrary constant of integration C, and represents a family of straight lines; these have an envelope, that is a special integral of the Clairaut equation (5.33c) obtained by eliminating the parameter p between (5.29b) ≡ (5.32b) and (5.32a). This is equivalent to the statement that the curve (5.32c) corresponding to the parametric form (5.32a, b) where (5.29a) is a differentiable function is the envelope of the family of straight lines (5.31c); the envelope (family of straight lines) is the special (general) integral of the Clairaut differential equation (5.29b).*

5.3.2 Parabola as the Envelope of a Family of Straight Lines

As an example, consider the differential equation (5.34a):

$$y = y'x + \frac{a}{y'}: \qquad\qquad y = px + \frac{a}{p}, \qquad h(p) = \frac{a}{p}; \qquad\qquad (5.34a\text{–}c)$$

that is, a Clairaut equation (5.29b) ≡ (5.34b) with the function (5.29a) specified by (5.34c). The general integral (5.35a) is a family of straight lines (5.35b) that have an abscissa at the origin (5.35c) decreasing as the slope increases (Figure 5.12):

$$y = Cx + \frac{a}{C}: \qquad\qquad \frac{dy}{dx} = C, \qquad y(0) = \frac{a}{C}; \qquad\qquad (5.35a\text{–}c)$$

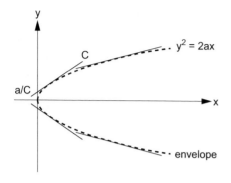

FIGURE 5.12
The family of straight lines (5.35a) with slope C and cutting the y-axis at an abscissa (5.35c) proportional to 1/C has a parabola (5.37a) with horizontal axis and tangent to the vertical axis as the envelope that is a special integral of the differential equation (5.34a).

the slope is infinite $C = \infty$ on the real axis $y(0) = 0$ where tangent is vertical. The envelope of the family of straight lines is obtained by eliminating C between (5.35a) ≡ (5.36a) and (5.2b) ≡ (5.36b):

$$0 = f(x;y;C) = Cx + \frac{a}{C} - y: \qquad\qquad 0 = \frac{\partial f}{\partial C} = x - \frac{a}{C^2}; \qquad (5.36a, b)$$

$$0 = f(x;y;p) = px + \frac{a}{p} - y: \qquad\qquad 0 = \frac{\partial f}{\partial p} = x - \frac{a}{p^2}; \qquad (5.36c, d)$$

this is the same as eliminating p between (5.34b) ≡ (5.36c) and (5.3b) ≡ (5.36d). Thus the C-discriminant (5.36a, b) coincides with the p-discriminant (5.36c, d), and this can only happen for an envelope (Table 5.1); in the present case (5.36b) ≡ (5.36e) substituted in (5.35a) leads to (5.36f):

$$C^2 = \frac{a}{x}: \qquad\qquad y^2 = C^2 x^2 + \frac{a^2}{C^2} + 2ax = ax + ax + 2ax = 4ax. \qquad (5.36e, f)$$

It follows that (Figure 5.12) the parabola (5.36f) ≡ (5.37a) is the envelope of the family of straight lines (5.35a), and a special integral of the differential equation (5.34a) ≡ (5.34b). The latter statement can be confirmed by noting that (5.36f) ≡ (5.37a) is not included in the general integral (5.35a) for any value of C, but:

$$y = 2\sqrt{a\,x}, \qquad\qquad p = y' = \sqrt{\frac{a}{x}}, \qquad (5.37a, b)$$

which satisfies (5.37b) the differential equation (5.34b).

5.3.3 Generalization of the Clairaut to the D'Alembert (1748) Differential Equation

A generalization of the Clairaut equation (5.29a, b) that can be solved by similar methods is (standard C) the **D'Alembert (1748) equation** (5.38c):

$$g, h \in \mathcal{D}(\mathcal{R}): \qquad\qquad y = x g(p) + h(p), \qquad\qquad (5.38a\text{--}c)$$

where g, h are differentiable functions (5.38a, b); the Clairaut's equation (5.29b) is regained for $g(p) = p$. The method of solution is the same; that is to differentiate with regard to x:

$$p = g(p) + \{ x g'(p) + h'(p) \} \frac{dp}{dx}; \qquad \frac{dx}{dp} = \frac{x g'(p)}{p - g(p)} + \frac{h'(p)}{p - g(p)}. \qquad (5.39a, b)$$

If $g(p) = p$ then (5.39a) is no longer decomposed into factors like (5.30a, b); instead use is made of the fact that (5.39a) is a linear differential equation (5.39b) for $x(p)$. The solution (3.27, 3.31a, b; 3.20a) of (5.39b) is:

$$\varphi(p) = \exp \left\{ \int \frac{g'(p)}{p - g(p)} dp \right\}: \qquad x = \varphi(p) \left\{ C + \int \frac{h'(p)}{p - g(p)} \frac{dp}{\varphi(p)} \right\}, \qquad (5.40a, b)$$

is a relation $x(p)$ in (5.40b) involving the function (5.40a). Eliminating p between (5.38c) and (5.40b) supplies a parametric equation of the curves, corresponding to the general integral (5.1c) in implicit form. Hence, *the general integral of the (standard C) D'Alembert (1748) equation (5.38a–c), is obtained by eliminating the parameter* p *with (5.40a, b).*

5.3.4 Family of Parabolas with Envelope Parallel to Diagonals of Quadrants

As an example, consider the D'Alembert equation (5.41c) ≡ (5.38c):

$$\{g, h\} = \left\{ 1, p^2 \left(1 - \frac{2}{3} p \right) \right\}: \qquad y = x + p^2 - \frac{2}{3} p^3, \qquad (5.41a\text{--}c)$$

corresponding to (5.42a, b). Differentiating with regard to x yields (5.422a):

$$0 = 1 - p + (2 p - 2 p^2) \frac{dp}{dx} = (1 - p) \left(1 + 2p \frac{dp}{dx} \right): \quad p = 1 \quad or \quad 2p\, dp + dx = 0,$$

$$(5.42a\text{--}c)$$

that has two possible solutions (5.42b, c). The latter equation (5.42c) has general integral (5.43a), that on substitution in (5.41c) yields (5.43b):

$$x + p^2 = C, \qquad y + \frac{2}{3}p^3 = C; \qquad 4(x-C)^3 = 9(y-C)^2, \qquad (5.43a\text{--}c)$$

thus (5.43a, b) are parametric equations x, y (p; C) of the integral curves; in this case the parameter p can be eliminated showing that the integral curves (5.43c) are a family of semi-cubical parabolas, with vertices at $x = C = y$, along the diagonal $y = x$ (Figure 5.13). These curves have as envelope (5.42b) a straight line (5.44a) parallel to $y = x$, that must be a special integral, that is satisfy (5.41c), leading to (5.44b):

$$y = x + a, \qquad y = x + \frac{1}{3}, \qquad a = \frac{1}{3}; \qquad (5.44a\text{--}c)$$

the envelope (5.44b) is thus a straight line parallel to the diagonal of the odd numbered quadrants where lie the vertices of the parabolas, with ordinate (5.44c) at the origin (Figure 5.13).

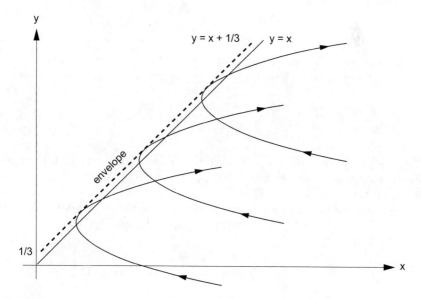

FIGURE 5.13
The family of parabolas (5.43c) with horizontal axis and vertex on the diagonal of the odd quadrants is tangent to a parallel straight line (5.44b) that is thus the envelope and a special integral of the differential equation (5.41c).

5.4 Equations Solvable for the Variables or Slope

Among the singular differential equations (sections 5.1–5.2) of first-order (chapter 3), the Clairaut equation (subsections 5.3.1–5.3.2) is generalized by the D'Alembert equation (subsections 5.3.3–5.3.4). The solution of a special differential equation that has special integrals often involves (sections 5.3–5.4) differentiation of the differential equation with regard to the independent or dependent variable. A further generalization is the first-order differential equations solvable for the dependent (independent) variable, that may also have singular integrals [subsections 5.4.2 (5.4.3)]. Besides the first-order differential equations solvable for the dependent or independent variable (subsections 5.4.1–5.4.3), a third case is solvability for the slope (subsection 5.4.4); an example of the latter is the first-order differential equation of degree N on the slope.

5.4.1 Equation Solvable for the Dependent or Independent Variable

A further generalization of the D'Alembert's equation (5.38a–c), is (Standard CI) a first-order differential equation (5.1b), solvable for the independent variable (5.45b) involving a differentiable function (5.45a):

$$h \in \mathcal{D}(|R^2): \qquad y = h(x,p); \qquad p = \frac{dy}{dx} = \frac{\partial h}{\partial x} + \frac{\partial h}{\partial p}\frac{dp}{dx}, \qquad (5.45a\text{–}c)$$

differentiation of (5.45b) with regard to x yields (5.45c); the latter (5.45c) is a differential equation no longer involving y, that is it is of the form (5.46a):

$$\frac{dp}{dx} = \frac{p - \partial h/\partial x}{\partial h/\partial p} \equiv H(x,p): \qquad\qquad x = x(p;C), \qquad (5.46a, b)$$

whose solution is (5.46b), where C is an arbitrary constant of integration. Eliminating p between (5.45b; 5.46b) specifies the general integral in the implicit form (5.1c).

If, instead, the first-order differential equation (5.1b) is (standard CII) solvable for x in (5.47b) and involves a differentiable function (5.47a):

$$g \in \mathcal{D}(|R^2): \qquad x = g(y,p), \qquad \frac{1}{p} = \frac{dx}{dy} = \frac{\partial g}{\partial y} + \frac{\partial g}{\partial p}\frac{dp}{dy}, \qquad (5.47a\text{–}c)$$

differentiation with regard to y in (5.47c) leads to (5.48a):

$$\frac{dp}{dy} = \frac{1/p - \partial g/\partial y}{\partial g/\partial p} \equiv G(y,p), \qquad y = y(p;C), \qquad (5.48a, b)$$

whose solution is a relation (5.48b) between y and x involving an arbitrary constant of integration C. Taking p as parameter, the general integral is (5.47b; 5.48b).

It has been shown that *a first-order differential equation (1.1b), that is [standard CI (CII)] solvable for the dependent (5.45b) [independent (5.47b)] variable $y(x)$, leads (5.45a) ≡ (5.45c) [(5.47a) ≡ (5.47c)] to a differential equation (5.46a) [(5.48a)] involving only $p \equiv dy/dx$; the general integral of the latter (5.46b) [(5.48b)], together with the original equation, specifies the solution, in parametric form, or eliminating the parameter p, in the implicit form (5.1c).*

5.4.2 Special Integral of Equation Solvable for the Dependent Variable

As an example of equation of the type (5.45a, b) solvable for the dependent variable y, consider (5.49a):

$$3y = 2px - \frac{2p^2}{x}, \qquad 3p = 2p + \frac{2p^2}{x^2} + \left(2x - 4\frac{p}{x}\right)\frac{dp}{dx}, \qquad \text{(5.49a, b)}$$

that, on differentiation with regard to x yields (5.49b); the latter can be split into two factors:

$$0 = p\left(1 - \frac{2p}{x^2}\right) - 2x\left(1 - \frac{2p}{x^2}\right)\frac{dp}{dx} = \left(1 - \frac{2p}{x^2}\right)\left(p - 2x\frac{dp}{dx}\right). \qquad \text{(5.49c)}$$

The second factor of (5.49c) is (5.50a):

$$2\frac{dp}{p} = \frac{dx}{x}, \qquad 2\log p = \log x + \log C, \qquad p^2 = Cx, \qquad \text{(5.50a–c)}$$

which has general integral (5.50b), involving an arbitrary constant C in (5.50c). The latter may be substituted into (5.49a) to yield (5.51a):

$$3y = 2C^{1/2}x^{3/2} - 2C: \qquad \left(3y + 2C\right)^2 = 4Cx^3, \qquad \text{(5.51a, b)}$$

the integral curves (5.51b) with slopes (5.51c):

$$\frac{dy}{dx} = \frac{12\,Cx^2}{6\left(3y + 2C\right)} = \frac{2Cx^2}{2\sqrt{Cx^3}} = C^{1/2}x^{1/2}; \qquad y(0) = -\frac{2C}{3}, \qquad y'(0) = 0,$$

$$\text{(5.51c–e)}$$

this shows that the integral curves (5.51a) ≡ (5.51b) are a family of semi-cubical parabolas (Figure 5.14) with horizontal (5.51c) cusps (5.51d) on the y-axis.

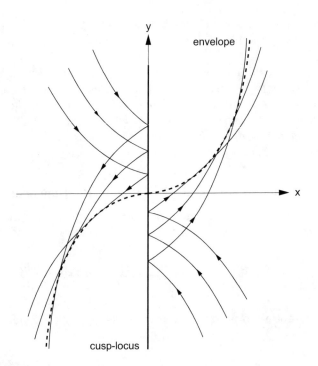

FIGURE 5.14
The double family of cubic parabolas (5.51b) with cusps on the vertical axis and lying to each side of the axis is tangent to the cubic parabola (5.56b) that is thus an envelope and a special integral of the differential equation (5.49a).

The general integral (5.51b) ≡ (5.52a) [differential equation (5.49a) ≡ (5.52c)] is a quadratic (5.9) [(5.5b)] function of the slope (constant of integration) with coefficients (5.52b) [(5.52d)]:

$$0 = f(x,y;C) = 4C^2 + 4C(3y - x^3)C + 9y^2: \quad \{P,Q,R\} = \{4, 4(3y - x^3), 9y^2\},$$
(5.52a, b)

$$0 = F(x,y,p) = 2p^2 - 2px^2 + 3xy: \quad \{L,M,N\} = \{2, -2x^2, 3xy\}.$$
(5.52c, d)

From (5.10a; 5.52b) [(5.7a; 5.52d)] follows the arbitrary constant (5.54a) [slope (5.53b)]:

$$C = -\frac{Q}{2P} = \frac{x^3 - 3y}{2}, \qquad p = -\frac{M}{2L} = \frac{x^2}{2},$$
(5.53a, b)

and from (5.10b; 5.52b) [(5.7b; 5.52d)] follows the C-discriminant (5.54a) [*p*-discriminant (5.54a)]:

$$0 = Q^2 - 4PR = 16\left[(3y - x^3)^2 - 9y^2\right] = 16x^3(x^3 - 6y): \quad \begin{cases} y = \dfrac{x^3}{6}: & \text{envelope,} \\ x^3 = 0: & \text{cusp-locus,} \end{cases}$$

$$\text{(5.54a–c)}$$

$$0 = M^2 - 4LN = 4x^4 - 24xy = 4x(x^3 - 6y): \quad \begin{cases} y = \dfrac{x^3}{6}: & \text{envelope,} \\ x = 0: & \text{cusp-locus.} \end{cases}$$

$$\text{(5.55a–c)}$$

Both the C-discriminant (5.54a) and *p*-discriminant (5.55a) lead to two singular lines: (i) the *y*-axis is the cusp-locus, that is a triple (5.54c) [single (5.55c)] root of the C(*p*)-discriminant, and is not a special integral because it does not satisfy the differential equation (5.49a); and (ii) the cubic parabola that appears as a single root (5.54b) [(5.55b)] both in the C(*p*)-discriminants and is an envelope and a special integral that satisfies the differential equation (5.49a).

The special integral corresponds to the first factor in (5.49c), namely (5.56a):

$$p = \frac{x^2}{2}: \qquad\qquad 3y = 2x\left(\frac{x^2}{2}\right) - \frac{2}{x}\left(\frac{x^2}{2}\right)^2 = \frac{x^3}{2}, \qquad\qquad \text{(5.56a, b)}$$

that on substitution in the differential equation (5.49a) leads to (5.56b) ≡ (5.54b) ≡ (5.55b). From the general integral (5.51a) ≡ (5.51b) ≡ (5.52a) [differential equation (5.49a) ≡ (5.52c)] follow the C-discriminant (5.57a) [*p*-discriminant (5.57b)]:

$$0 = \frac{\partial f}{\partial C} = 8C + 4(3y - x^3), \qquad\qquad 0 = \frac{\partial F}{\partial p} = 2(2p - x^2); \qquad \text{(5.57a, b)}$$

eliminating C(*p*) between (5.52a; 5.57a) [(5.52c; 5.57b)] leads to (5.57c) [(5.57d)]:

$$0 = 9y^2 - 4C^2 = 9y^2 - (3y - x^3)^2 = x^3(6y - x^3), \qquad\qquad \text{(5.57c)}$$

$$0 = 2\left(\frac{x^2}{2}\right)^2 - 2x^2\left(\frac{x^2}{2}\right) + 3xy = 3xy - \frac{x^4}{2} = x\left(3y - \frac{x^3}{2}\right), \qquad \text{(5.57d)}$$

that coincides with (5.54a) ≡ (5.57c) [(5.55a) ≡ (5.57d)] and specifies the special integral (5.54b) ≡ (5.55b) [special curve (5.54c) ≡ (5.55c)] that is an envelope (cusp-locus).

5.4.3 Equation Solvable for the Dependent Variable
and Its Special Integral

As an example of equation of the type (5.47a, b) solvable for the independent
variable consider (5.58a):

$$\frac{8}{27x} = p^3 \equiv \left(\frac{dy}{dx}\right)^3, \qquad dy = \frac{2}{3}x^{-\frac{1}{3}}\,dx = d\left(x^{\frac{2}{3}}\right), \qquad (5.58\text{a, b})$$

that is separable (5.58b); it has general integral (5.59a) that is a cubic in the
arbitrary constant of integration C in (5.59b).

$$y = C + x^{2/3}: \quad x^2 = (y - C)^3, \quad \frac{dy}{dx} = \frac{2x}{3(y-C)^2} = \frac{2x}{3x^{4/3}} = \frac{2}{3}x^{-1/3};$$

$$y(0) = C, \quad y'(0) = \infty,$$

$$(5.59\text{a–e})$$

and slope (5.59c). The integral curves (5.59b) are a family of semi-cubical
parabolas (Figure 5.15), with cusps at (5.59d) along the y-axis, to which they
are tangent (5.59e). Thus the y-axis is a line of special points that is not an
envelope; yet, exceptionally, it is a solution $\infty = \infty$ of the differential equation (5.58a), because the integral curves happen to be tangent to the special
line at the special points. The differential equation (5.58a) [general integral
(5.59b)] is a cubic of the slope (arbitrary constant) and thus the particular quadratic case in the subsection 5.2.1 does not apply, and the $p(C)$-discriminant

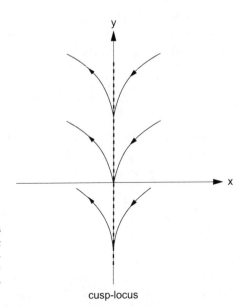

FIGURE 5.15
The family of cubics (5.59b) that has cusps
along the y-axis with vertical tangent
$-\infty(+\infty)$ on the right (left) side of the positive (negative) real axis, has the y-axis $x = 0$
as envelope that is a special integral of the
differential equation (5.58a).

[subsection 5.1.3 (5.1.2)] must be used. The C-discriminant is obtained by eliminating C between (5.59b) ≡ (5.60a) and (5.60b):

$$0 = f(x,y;C) = (y-C)^3 - x^2: \qquad 0 = \frac{\partial f}{\partial C} = 3(y-C)^2, \qquad y = C, \qquad x^2 = 0,$$

$$(5.60a\text{–}d)$$

leading (5.60c) to (5.60d) that shows that the y-axis is a double root. The p-discriminant is obtained by eliminating p between (5.58a) ≡ (5.61a) and (5.61b):

$$0 = f(x,y,p) = p^3 x - \frac{8}{27}: \qquad 0 = \frac{\partial F}{\partial p} = 3p^2 x, \qquad \frac{8}{9\,p} = 0, \qquad p = \infty, \qquad x = 0,$$

$$(5.61a\text{–}e)$$

leading to (5.61c), showing that the slope is infinite (5.61d) on the y-axis (5.61e). Thus the special line (5.60d) ≡ (5.61e) is the vertical axis to which all integral curves are tangent because they have infinite slope there (5.59d) ≡ (5.61d). The special line is a cusp-locus (Figure 5.15) to which the integral curves are tangent (Figure 5.8). It is not an envelope (Figures 5.1 and 5.4) because there are integral curves on both sides (Figure 5.15). Considering the sub-set of integral curves on the first and fourth $x > 0$ (second and third $x < 0$) quadrants the special line becomes an envelope.

5.4.4 Equation of Degree *N* Solvable for the Slope

Having considered the first-order differential equation (5.1a, b), in the cases when it is solvable for the dependent y in (5.45a, b) and dependent x in (5.47a, b) variables, the third case is solvable for the slope $y' = p$; thus is considered next (5.62a) the (standard CIII) first-order differential equation of degree M in the slope:

$$0 = \sum_{m=0}^{M} p^m A_m(x,y) = A_0(x,y) + y' A_1(x,y) + y'^2 A_2(x,y) + \ldots + y'^M A_M(x,y),$$

$$(5.62a, b)$$

that is a polynomial of degree M in $p = y'$ that can be factorized.

$$0 = A_M(x,y) \prod_{m=1}^{M} \left[p - a_m(x,y) \right]$$

$$(5.62c, d)$$

$$= A_M(x,y) \left[\frac{dy}{dx} - a_1(x,y) \right] \left[\frac{dy}{dx} - a_2(x,y) \right] \ldots \left[\frac{dy}{dx} - a_m(x,y) \right].$$

The differential equation (5.62a) ≡ (5.62b) is satisfied when any of the factors in (5.62c) ≡ (5.62d) vanishes, leading to M first-order differential equations of the first degree (5.63a) with general integrals (5.63b).

$$\frac{dy}{dx} = a_m(x,y) \quad \Leftrightarrow \quad f_m(x,y) = C; \qquad 0 = \prod_{n=0}^{N} \{f_m(x,y) - C\}, \qquad \text{(5.63a–c)}$$

any of the equalities (5.63b) is a solution of both the first-order differential equations of degree one (5.63a) and degree M in (5.62a–d). Thus the general integral of (5.62a–d) is their product (5.63c); that is, *the differential equation (standard CIII) of first-order and degree* M *in the slope (5.62a, b) has general integral (5.63c) formed by the product of the factors (5.63b) that are solutions of (5.62c, d)* ≡ *(5.63a), all with the same arbitrary constant of integration* C. It would appear that a different constant of integration C_m could be used in each factor in (5.63c); however, (5.63c) is satisfied if one of the factors vanishes, and since the constant C_m is arbitrary, it can be designated by C in all factors. This agrees with the known property (subsection 1.1.3) that the general integral (5.1c) of a first order differential equation (5.1b) involves one constant of integration.

As an example, consider the first-order differential equation of degree two (5.64a):

$$0 = p^2 + \left(y - \frac{1}{x}\right)p - \frac{y}{x} = (p+y)\left(p - \frac{1}{x}\right); \qquad \text{(5.64a, b)}$$

the two factors in (5.64b) correspond to the differential equations of first degree (5.65a) [(5.65b)]:

$$y' = -y, \frac{1}{x}: \qquad\qquad y(x;C) = Ce^{-x}, \quad C + \log x, \qquad \text{(5.65a–d)}$$

whose general integrals respectively (5.65c) [(5.65d)]. Thus:

$$\left(y - Ce^{-x}\right)\left(y - \log x - C\right) = 0, \qquad \text{(5.66)}$$

is the general integral of the differential equation (5.64a).

5.5 Dual Differentials and Thermodynamics

A variety of methods of solving a number of types of first-order differential equations has been presented as concerns the general (special) integrals [chapter 3 (sections 5.1–5.4)]. As a final method it is shown that to each equation is associated a dual form (subsection 5.5.2), and that if the latter can be solved, the former is solvable too (subsection 5.5.3). The dual and original differential equations are related by the Legendre transformation that interchanges the variable and the corresponding coefficients in an inexact differential (subsection 5.5.1).

The most important application of dual differentials is in thermodynamics (subsections 5.5.4–5.5.15). It can be illustrated for a simple thermodynamic system performing work (subsection 5.5.4) and exchanging heat (subsection 5.5.5). The simple thermodynamic system is specified by two extensive variables, namely the specific volume (entropy) that can be replaced by (subsection 5.5.6) the dual intensive variables, namely pressure (temperature); the latter specify mechanical (thermal) equilibrium (subsection 5.5.7). The four possible pairs of thermodynamic variables chosen between specific volume and pressure (entropy and temperature) lead (subsection 5.5.9) to four alternative and equivalent functions of state (subsection 5.5.8), namely the internal energy, enthalpy, free energy, and free enthalpy.

The function of state can be chosen so as to provide the simplest description of a particular thermodynamic process, for example: equivoluminar, adiabatic, isobaric, and isothermal (subsections 5.5.10–5.5.11) respectively for constant volume, entropy, pressure, or temperature. The heat exchanges are specified by the specific heats at constant volume and pressure (subsection 5.5.12); their ratio describes an adiabatic process (subsection 5.5.13); that is, without heat exchanges. The derivatives of the functions of state specify the thermodynamic coefficients (subsection 5.5.14) like the adiabatic sound speed and non-adiabatic coefficient (subsection 5.5.15).

The thermodynamic functions of state imply the existence of an equation of state relating any three thermodynamic variables, for example (subsection 5.5.14) the pressure as a function of the specific volume (or its inverse the mass density), plus another variable like entropy or temperature. The equation of state depends on the substance, and is particularly simple for a perfect (ideal) gas [subsection(s) 5.5.16–5.5.19 (5.5.18–5.5.25)] corresponding to non-interacting molecules (subsection 5.5.16) [without internal degrees-of-freedom (subsection 5.5.12)]. The perfect gas is specified by [subsection 5.5.17 (5.5.18)] the internal energy (equation if state), that lead to specific heats and adiabatic exponent dependent on temperature (subsection 5.5.19). These are constant for an ideal gas (subsection 5.5.18) simplifying: (i) the adiabatic relations (subsection 5.5.19); (ii) the entropy (subsection 5.5.20); (iii) the adiabatic exponent (subsections 5.5.21–5.5.23); and (iv) the non-adiabatic exponent and adiabatic and isothermal sound speeds (subsections 5.5.24–5.5.25). The ideal gas is a reasonable approximation to the atmosphere of the earth at low altitudes (subsection 5.5.26).

5.5.1 Legendre Transformation of an Exact Differential

A continuously differentiable function (5.61a) has exact differential (5.67b) with continuous coefficients (5.67a) specified by the partial derivatives with regard to the independent variables x_n:

$$\Phi(x_n)\in C^1\left(|R^N\right): \qquad d\Phi = \sum_{n=1}^{N} X_n\, dx_n, \qquad X_n \equiv \frac{\partial\Phi}{\partial x_n} \in C\left(|R^N\right). \qquad (5.67a\text{–}c)$$

*A variable can be (standard CIV) interchanged with the corresponding coefficient, for example (x_1, X_1) via the **Legendre transformation** (5.68):*

$$\Psi(X_1, x_2, ..., x_N) = \Phi(x_1, x_2, ..., x_N) - x_1, X_1, \qquad (5.68)$$

leading to:

$$d\Psi = d\Phi - X_1 dx_1 - x_1\, dX_1 = -x_1\, dX_1 + \sum_{m=2}^{N} x_m\, dX_m, \qquad (5.69)$$

showing that: (i) the independent variable x_1 changes to X_1 in (5.69) and coefficient X_1 changes to minus the independent variable $-x_1$ in (5.70a):

$$x_1 = -\frac{\partial\Psi}{\partial X_1}; \qquad m = 2, ..., N: \qquad \frac{\partial\Psi}{\partial x_m} = X_m = \frac{\partial\Phi}{\partial x_m}, \qquad (5.70a\text{–}c)$$

and (ii) the remaining $(N - 1)$ variables and coefficients (5.70b) are unaffected (5.70c). The Legendre transformation (5.68) can be applied to several variables. The Legendre transformation has multiple applications, for example dual differential equations (simple thermodynamic systems) [subsections 5.5.2–5.5.3 (5.5.4–5.5.25)].

5.5.2 Original and Dual Differential Equations

The idea of duality is to associate with a first-order differential equation (5.1b) with general integral (5.1c) a dual differential equation (5.71b) with general integral (5.71c):

$$P \equiv \frac{dY}{dX}: \qquad G(X, Y, P) = 0, \qquad g(X, Y; C) = 0, \qquad (5.71a\text{–}c)$$

such that the dependent variables are related by a Legendre transformation (5.68) with reversed sign (5.72a):

$$Y = xX - y: \qquad P\,dX = dY = x\,dX + X\,dx - dy = x\,dX + (X - p)\,dx, \qquad (5.72a, b)$$

from (5.72a; 5.1a; 5.71a) follows (5.72a), implying that: (i) the slopes inter-change with the independent variable (5.73a, b):

$$X = p, \qquad P = x; \qquad y = xX - Y = PX - Y, \qquad Y = px - y, \qquad \text{(5.73a–d)}$$

and (ii) the dependent variables are related by (5.73c, d).

Thus *the first-order differential equation (5.1a, b) has (standard CV) dual equation (5.74):*

$$0 = F(x,y,p) = F(P, PX - Y, X) \equiv G(X,Y,P); \qquad \text{(5.74)}$$

if the general integral (5.71c) of the dual equation (5.74) is known:

$$0 = \frac{\partial g}{\partial X} + \frac{\partial g}{\partial Y}\frac{dY}{dX} = \frac{\partial g}{\partial X} + P\frac{\partial g}{\partial X}: \qquad 0 = g(X,Y;C) = f(x,y;C), \qquad \text{(5.75a–c)}$$

the use of (5.73b, d; 5.75b) expresses (X,Y) *the general integral from the dual (5.71c) to the primal (5.1c) differential equation. For example, (standard CVI) for a primal first-order differential equation of the form (5.76a):*

$$\Phi(px-y) = x\Psi(p): \qquad \Phi(Y) = P\,\Psi(X) = \frac{dY}{dX}\Psi(X), \qquad \int \frac{dY}{\Phi(Y)} = \int \frac{dX}{\Psi(X)},$$
$$\text{(5.76a–c)}$$

the dual differential equation (5.76b) is separable and can be integrated (5.76c). An example of integration of a first-order differential equation of the form (5.76a) through its dual (5.74) is given next (subsection 5.5.3).

5.5.3 Solution of a Differential Equation from Its Dual

As an example, consider the primal first-order differential equation of degree two (5.77a) that is of the form (5.76a):

$$(y-px)^2 = px; \qquad Y^2 = XP = X\frac{dY}{dX}, \qquad \text{(5.77a, b)}$$

the dual differential equation (5.77b) is of degree one and separable (5.78a):

$$\frac{dX}{X} = \frac{dY}{Y^2}; \qquad \log C = \frac{1}{Y} + \log X, \qquad C = Xe^{1/Y}, \qquad \text{(5.78a–c)}$$

it has general integral (5.78b) where C is an arbitrary constant (5.78c). Differentiating (5.78b) with regard to X leads to (5.79a) ≡ (5.79b):

$$\frac{1}{X} = -\frac{\partial}{\partial X}\left(\frac{1}{Y}\right) = \frac{1}{Y^2}\frac{dY}{dX} = \frac{P}{Y^2}, \qquad\qquad 0 = Y^2 - P\,X = Y^2 - Y - y, \qquad (5.79a-c)$$

that can be re-written (5.79c), where (5.73c) was used. Solving the quadratic expression (5.79c) for Y yields (5.80a):

$$2\,Y = 1 \pm \sqrt{1+4\,y}; \qquad\qquad X = \frac{Y^2}{P} = \frac{Y^2}{x}, \qquad (5.80a-c)$$

substituting (5.73b) into (5.79b) ≡ (5.80b) leads to (5.80c). The expressions (5.80a, c) of dual X, Y in terms of primal x, y variables, substituted into (5.78c), give two solutions:

$$4C x = \frac{4CY^2}{X} = 4Y^2\,e^{1/Y} = \left(1 \pm \sqrt{1+4y}\right)^2 \exp\left(\frac{2}{1 \pm \sqrt{1+4y}}\right) \equiv f_\pm(y), \qquad (5.81)$$

of the primal differential equation (5.77a); since the latter is of degree two (5.62a, b), the general integral (5.63a–c) is:

$$0 = \left\{4\,C\,x - f_+(y)\right\}\left\{4\,C\,x - f_-(y)\right\}, \qquad (5.82)$$

is a product (5.82), with one constant of integration C involving the functions (5.81). Besides the dual differential equations (subsections 5.5.2–5.5.3), the Legendre transformation (subsection 5.5.1) has other applications, including simple thermodynamic systems that perform work and exchange heat (subsections 5.5.4–5.5.25).

5.5.4 Work of the Pressure in a Volume Change

A **simple thermodynamic system** is defined as one that: (i) can exchange heat (Notes 3.22–3.23); (ii) is subject only to one kind of force, associated with an isotropic pressure p, that is, (Figure 5.16) the force $d\vec{F}$ per unit area dA in the inward direction (5.83a), that is, opposite to the unit outward normal $\vec{N}$:

$$\vec{F} = -p\,\vec{N}\,dA; \qquad dW = \vec{F}.d\vec{x} = -p\,dA\left(\vec{N}.d\vec{x}\right) = -p\,dV, \qquad (5.83a-d)$$

the work (5.83b) of the pressure (5.83a) equals (5.83c) minus the pressure times the volume change (5.83d):

$$d\ell = \vec{N}.d\vec{x}, \qquad\qquad dV = dA\,d\ell = \left(\vec{N}.d\vec{x}\right)dA, \qquad (5.84a, b)$$

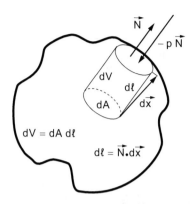

FIGURE 5.16
The pressure on a surface lies along the inward normal and its work is equal to minus the product by the displaced volume.

because: (i) the displacement along the outward normal is (5.84a); (ii) its product by the area is the volume (5.84b). A distinct *notation* $d(\vec{\pi})$ *could be used for exact (inexact) differentials,* for example the volume (5.84b) [work (5.83b)].

5.5.5 Simple and General Thermodynamic Systems

A general thermodynamic system can be subject to: (i) stresses (strains) more general (chapter II 4) that the pressure (volume changes); (iii) volume forces (notes III.8.3–III.8.15) such as gravity (chapter I.18), electric (chapter I.24); or (iii) chemical or other reactions between different substances. The general and simple thermodynamic systems can be treated similarly as regards dual differentials, and the latter is considered in the sequel (subsections 5.5.5–5.5.21). Thus a *simple thermodynamic system includes: (i) the work (5.83d)* ≡ *(5.85a) of the pressure* $p > 0$ *forces (5.83a), that is an inexact differential and is positive* $dW > 0$ *(negative* $dW < 0$*) in a compression* $dV < 0$ *(expansion* $dV > 0$*), that is a reduction (increase) in volume; (ii) adding (subsection 3.9.11) the heat (3.269a)* ≡ *(5.85b), that is also an inexact differential, involving the temperature T and entropy S leads to the internal energy (3.268)* ≡ *(5.85c), that is an exact differential (5.85d):*

$$dW = -p\,dV, \qquad dQ = T\,dS: \qquad dU = dW + dQ = -p\,dV + T\,dS. \quad (5.85\text{a–d})$$

The meaning of the thermodynamic variables in (5.85d) is discussed next (subsection 5.5.6).

5.5.6 Extensive and Intensive Thermodynamic Variables

Consider an isolated thermodynamic system consisting of two (Figure 5.17) or more interacting sub-systems. The **thermodynamic variables** *can be divided in two sets: (i) the* **extensive** *thermodynamic variables that are additive, namely internal energy (5.86a), specific volume (5.86b) and entropy (5.86c):*

$$U = U_1 + U_2, \quad V = V_1 + V_2, \quad S = S_1 + S_2; \quad p_1 = p_2, \quad T_1 = T_2, \qquad (5.86\text{a–e})$$

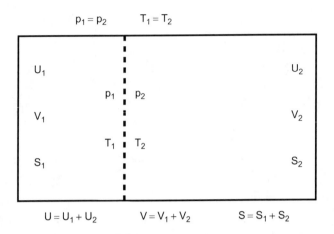

FIGURE 5.17
An isolated thermodynamic system conserves the total internal energy specific volume and entropy. If it consists of two or more interacting sub-systems, mechanical (thermal) equilibrium requires the equality of pressures (temperatures).

*and (ii) the **intensive** thermodynamic variables that are equal in equilibrium, namely the pressure (5.86d) and temperature (5.86e).* The statement (ii) is a consequence of (i) as is proved in the sequel: (a) consider an adiabatic process in which both subsystems do not exchange heat and hence the entropy is constant (5.87a, b), so that internal energy (5.85d) reduces to the work (5.87c):

$$dS_1 = 0 = dS_2: \qquad 0 = dU = -p_1\,dV_1 - p_2\,dV_2; \quad 0 = dV = dV_1 + dV_2, \qquad \text{(5.87a–d)}$$

$$0 = dU = (p_2 - p_1)dV_1: \qquad\qquad\qquad dV_1 \neq 0 \quad \Rightarrow \quad p_1 = p_2. \qquad \text{(5.87e, g)}$$

Both the total volume (5.87d) and internal energy (5.87c) ≡ (5.87e) are constant because the system is isolated; (c) a change of volume of one system (5.78f) requires that the pressures be equal (5.87g) ≡ (5.86d) for mechanical equilibrium. A similar proof leads to (5.86e) for an equivoluminar process that exchanges only heat instead of work (subsection 5.5.7).

5.5.7 Mechanical and Thermal Equilibrium of a System

In the case of (a) an equivoluminar process in which both subsystems have constant volume (5.88a, b), the internal energy (5.85d) reduces to the heat exchanges (5.88c):

$$dV_1 = 0 = dV_2: \qquad 0 = dU = T_1\,dS_1 + T_2\,dS_2; \qquad 0 = dS = dS_1 + dS_2, \qquad \text{(5.88a–d)}$$

$$0 = dU = (T_1 - T_2)\,dS_1: \qquad\qquad\qquad dS_1 \neq 0 \quad \Rightarrow \quad T_1 = T_2, \qquad \text{(5.88e–g)}$$

(b) since the total system is isolated, both the total entropy (5.88d) and internal energy (5.88c) ≡ (5.88e) are constant (5.88f); (c) the heat exchange (5.88f) between the two sub-systems leads to thermal equilibrium if they are at the same temperature (5.88g) ≡ (5.86e). It has been shown that *the* **mechanical (thermal) equilibrium** *of an isolated simple thermodynamic system consisting of several interacting subsystems requires the equality of pressures (temperatures).* So far the simple thermodynamic system has been described in terms of the internal energy (5.86d) for which the independent variables are both extensive, namely the specific volume and entropy; the Legendre transformation (subsection 5.5.1) allows the interchange of any extensive thermodynamic variable by the corresponding intensive thermodynamic variable, leading to three more equivalent and alternative thermodynamic functions of state (subsection 5.5.8).

5.5.8 Internal Energy, Enthalpy, Free Energy, and Free Enthalpy

The Legendre transformation (5.68) may be used to define the **enthalpy** (5.89a) exchanging as independent variable (5.89b) the specific volume for the pressure:

$$H(p,S) = U(V,S) + pV: \qquad dH = dU + p\,dV + V\,dp = T\,dS + V\,dp, \qquad \text{(5.89a, b)}$$

$$F(V,T) = U(V,S) - TS: \qquad dF = dU - T\,dS - S\,dT = -p\,dV - S\,dT. \qquad \text{(5.90a, b)}$$

The **free energy** (5.90a) or **Helmholtz function** is the Legendre transform (5.68) of the internal energy (5.86d), exchanging the entropy for the temperature (5.90b). The combination of (5.89a, b; 5.90a, b) specifies the **free enthalpy** (5.91a) or **Gibbs function** that is the Legendre transform (5.68) of the internal energy (5.86d), exchanging (5.91b) both specific volume (entropy) for pressure (temperature):

$$G(p,T) = U(V,S) + pV - TS: \qquad dG = V\,dp - S\,dT. \qquad \text{(5.91a, b)}$$

The four equivalent and alternative **thermodynamic functions of state** are related by (5.89a; 5.91a) ≡ (5.92a, b):

$$G(p,T) = H(p,S) - TS = F(V,T) + pV: \qquad V \leftrightarrow p, \qquad T \leftrightarrow S, \qquad \text{(5.92a–d)}$$

and correspond to the four distinct combinations of (5.92c, d) the two pairs of dual extensive–intensive variables. The intensive variables, pressure and temperature, are easier to measure than the extensive variables, specific volume and entropy (subsection 5.5.9).

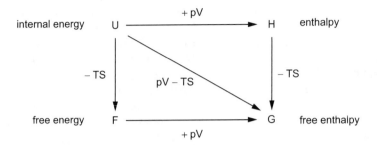

DIAGRAM 5.1
Starting with the internal energy and exchanging the specific volume for pressure (entropy for temperature) leads to the enthalpy (free energy). Both changes together specify the free enthalpy as the fourth function of state of a simple thermodynamic system.

5.5.9 Specific Volume, Pressure, Temperature, and Entropy

It has been shown that *a simple system is described equivalently and alternatively by four thermodynamic functions of state: (i) the internal energy (5.85d) as a function of the specific volume and entropy; (ii) the enthalpy (5.89a) as a function of the pressure and entropy (5.89b); (iii) the free energy (5.90a) as a function of the specific volume and temperature (5.90b); and (iv) the free enthalpy (5.91a) as a function of the pressure and temperature (5.91b). The four thermodynamic functions of state (Diagram 5.1) are related by (5.89a; 5.90a; 5.91a)* ≡ *(5.92a, b); they use as independent variables (Diagram 5.2) all distinct pairs of dual thermodynamic variable (5.92c, d).* The thermodynamic variables can be interpreted as follows: (i) the pressure (5.86d) specifies mechanical equilibrium (5.87a–g); (ii) its product by minus the change in specific volume or volume per unit mass determines the work (5.85a) that is an inexact differential; (iii) the temperature (5.86e) specifies thermal equilibrium (5.88a–g); (iv) to obtain a function of state, namely the internal energy (5.85c), it is necessary to add the heat (5.85b) to the work (5.85a); (v) hence the heat is an inexact differential (5.85b), but its ratio by the temperature specifies an exact differential, namely the entropy; and (vi–viii) the remaining functions of state, namely the enthalpy and free enthalpy, are convenient representations for specific thermodynamic processes (subsection 5.5.10).

DIAGRAM 5.2
The two pairs of extensive (intensive) thermodynamic variables are the specific volume (pressure) and entropy (temperature). The choice of one thermodynamic variable from each pair leads to the four functions of state (Diagram 5.1).

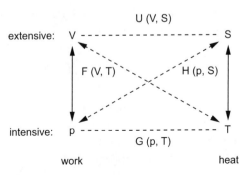

5.5.10 Equivoluminar, Isobaric, Isothemal, and Adiabatic Processes

The simplest thermodynamic processes are those for which one of the four thermodynamic variables is constant, namely two extensive and two intensive. Concerning the two extensive thermodynamic variables, namely the specific volume (entropy): (i) they are constant in an **equivoluminar (adiabatic) process** (5.93a) [(5.94a)] for which the work is zero (5.93b) [there are no heat exchanges (5.94b)]; (ii) conversely the heat (5.93d) [work (5.94d)] is an exact differential in this particular case because it coincides with a function of state, namely the internal energy (5.93c) [(5.94c)]; and (iii) besides the internal energy, the other simplest function of state depending only on one variable is the free energy (enthalpy) that is a function of the temperature (5.93e) [pressure (5.94e)]:

$$dV = 0: \qquad dW = 0, \qquad dU = T\,dS = dQ, \qquad dF = -S\,dT, \qquad (5.93\text{a--e})$$

$$dS = 0: \qquad dQ = 0, \qquad dU = -p\,dV = dW, \qquad dH = V\,dp; \qquad (5.94\text{a--e})$$

$$dp = 0: \qquad dH = T\,dS = dQ, \qquad dG = -S\,dT, \qquad (5.95\text{a--d})$$

$$dT = 0: \qquad dF = -p\,dV = dW, \qquad dG = V\,dp. \qquad (5.96\text{a--d})$$

Concerning the intensive thermodynamic variables, namely the pressure (temperature): (i) they are constant in an **isobaric (isothermal) process** (5.95a) [(5.96a)]; (ii) the heat exchanged (5.95c) [work performed (5.96c)] is an exact differential in this particular case, because it coincides with a function of state, namely the enthalpy (5.95b) [free energy (5.96b)]; and (iii) the other simplest function of state depending only on one variable is the free enthalpy, that depends only on the temperature (5.95d) [pressure (5.96d)]. Thus, although the work and heat are generally inexact differentials (subsections 5.5.4–5.5.5) they may become exact differentials for specific thermodynamic processes (subsection 5.5.11).

5.5.11 Heat and Work in a Thermodynamic Process

It has been shown that the *four simplest thermodynamic process are (i) equivoluminar (5.93a–c), (ii) isobaric (5.95a–d); (iii) isothermal (5.96a–d), and (iv) adiabatic (5.95a–e); that is, respectively at constant (i) specific volume, (ii) pressure, (iii) temperature, and (iv) entropy or without heat exchanges. The work (5.85a) [heat (5.85b)] are: (i) generally inexact differentials, and depend on the path between two thermodynamic equilibrium states; (ii) may coincide with a function of state for a particular thermodynamic process (5.94c, d; 5.96b, c) [(5.93b, c; 5.95b, c)], thus becoming an exact differential, and independent of the path between the same initial and final equilibrium states. The heat may or may not be an exact differential depending* on the thermodynamic process, but the entropy is always an exact differential given in any thermodynamic process by (5.85d) ≡ (5.97a) or (5.89b) ≡ (5.97b) that involve only functions of state:

$$dS = \frac{dU}{T} + \frac{p}{T}dV = \frac{dH}{T} - \frac{V}{T}dp; \qquad (5.97a, b)$$

$$\rho V = 1: \qquad dS = \frac{dU}{T} - \frac{P}{\rho^2 T}d\rho, \qquad dF = \frac{p}{\rho^2}d\rho - SdT. \qquad (5.98a-c)$$

Introducing the **mass density** or mass per unit volume; that is, (5.98a) the inverse of the specific volume or volume per unit mass leads to (5.98b) ≡ (5.97a) for the entropy or internal energy (5.85d) and to (5.98c) ≡ (5.90b) for the free energy. The non-adiabatic (adiabatic) thermodynamic process (subsection 5.5.12 (5.5.13)] that is with (without) heat exchanges are described preferably in terms of the entropy, that is a function of state, unlike the heat.

5.5.12 Specific Heats at Constant Volume and Pressure

Any of the four functions of state, namely the internal energy, enthalpy, free energy, or free enthalpy, can be used to calculate **thermodynamic derivatives** with regard to the four thermodynamic variables (pressure, temperature, entropy, and specific volume). The entropy is the function of state specifying the heat (5.85a) ≡ (5.99a) and is used to define the **specific heat at constant volume (pressure)** as the derivative of the internal energy (5.99b) [enthalpy (5.99c)] with regard to the temperature:

$$dS = \frac{dQ}{T}: \qquad C_v \equiv T\left(\frac{\partial S}{\partial T}\right)_v = \left(\frac{\partial U}{\partial T}\right)_v, \qquad C_p \equiv T\left(\frac{\partial S}{\partial T}\right)_P = \left(\frac{\partial H}{\partial T}\right)_p. \qquad (5.99a-c)$$

An adiabatic process (5.94a) ≡ (5.100a) that is without heat exchanges holds the equalities (5.94c) ≡ (5.100b) [(5.94e) ≡ (5.100d)] leading (5.99b) [(5.99c)] to (5.100c) [(5.100e)]:

$$dS = 0: \qquad -pdV = dU = C_v dT, \qquad V dp = dH = C_p dT. \qquad (5.100a-e)$$

It follows that the **adiabatic exponent** defined as the ratio of the specific heats at constant pressure and volume (5.101a) satisfies (5.101b) [(5.101c)]:

$$\gamma \equiv \frac{C_p}{C_v} = -\frac{V dp}{pdV}: \qquad \frac{dp}{p} = -\gamma\frac{dV}{V} = \gamma\frac{d\rho}{\rho}, \qquad (5.101a-c)$$

in terms of the pressure and specific volume (mass density) in (5.98a). The adiabatic exponent is the only thermodynamic coefficient appearing in an adiabatic process (subsection 5.5.13).

5.5.13 Adiabatic Exponent and Thermodynamic Relations

It has been shown that *the adiabatic exponent defined (5.101a) as the ratio of the specific heats at constant pressure (5.101c) and volume (5.101b): (i) appears in the adiabatic relation (5.101b) [(5.101c)] between the pressure and the specific volume (mass density); (ii) if it is constant (5.102a) it leads to (5.102b, c):*

$$\gamma = const: \qquad \log p + \gamma \log V = const = \log p - \gamma \log \rho, \qquad (5.102\text{a–c})$$

*to the **adiabatic relations** between pressure and specific volume (5.103b) [mass density (5.103c)]:*

$$\gamma = const: \qquad pV^{\gamma} = p_0 V_0^{\gamma}, \qquad \frac{p}{p_0} = \left(\frac{\rho}{\rho_0}\right)^{\gamma}, \qquad (5.103\text{a–c})$$

where the subscript "0" indicates any reference equilibrium state. Thus, pressure or mass density (or specific volume) may be replaced by the temperature in the adiabatic relations (subsection 5.5.17), provided that an equation of state is specified relating them (subsection 5.5.14).

5.5.14 Thermodynamic Derivatives and Equation of State

If the internal energy (5.71c) has continuous first-order derivatives (5.104a) they specify the pressure (5.104b) and temperature (5.104c):

$$U(V,S) \in C^1\left(|R^2\right): \qquad -\left(\frac{\partial U}{\partial V}\right)_S = p(V,S), \qquad \left(\frac{\partial U}{\partial S}\right)_v = T(V,S),$$
$$(5.104\text{a–c})$$

showing that they also depend on the entropy and specific volume. If the internal energy has continuous second-order derivatives (5.104d), the equality of cross-derivatives (5.104e) leads to the **thermodynamic equality** (5.104f):

$$U(V,S) \in C^2\left(|R^2\right): \qquad \frac{\partial^2 U}{\partial V \partial S} = \frac{\partial^2 U}{\partial S \partial V} \quad \Rightarrow \quad \left(\frac{\partial T}{\partial V}\right)_S = -\left(\frac{\partial P}{\partial S}\right)_V. \qquad (5.104\text{d–f})$$

*The **equation of state** is a relation between any three of the four thermodynamic variables, pressure, temperature, entropy, and mass density (or specific volume), and depends on the substance, for example, gas, liquid, solid, or a mixture. Choosing the* *equation of state in the form (5.105a) of the pressure as a function of the mass density and entropy:*

$$p = p(\rho, S): \qquad\qquad dp = c_s^2\, d\rho + \beta\, dS; \qquad\qquad (5.105a, b)$$

it leads by differentiation to (5.105b):

$$c_s^2 \equiv \left(\frac{\partial p}{\partial \rho}\right)_s = \left[\frac{\partial p}{\partial(1/V)}\right]_S = -V^2\left(\frac{\partial p}{\partial V}\right)_S, \qquad \beta \equiv \left(\frac{\partial p}{\partial S}\right)_\rho = \left(\frac{\partial p}{\partial S}\right)_V, \qquad (5.106a\text{–}e)$$

involving: (i) the **adiabatic sound speed** *(5.106a) ≡ (5.106b) ≡ (III.7.303e), that is a measure of the compressibility of the medium (Notes III.7.14) and larger for denser media, for example water versus air; and (ii) the* **non-adiabatic coefficient** *(5.106d) ≡ (5.106e) that measures the deviation from adiabatic conditions.*

5.5.15 Adiabatic Sound Speed and Non-Adiabatic Coefficient

The adiabatic sound speed (5.106a) ≡ (5.107a) follows from the adiabatic relation (5.101b) [≡(5.101c)] leading to (5.107b) [≡(5.107c)]:

$$c_s^2 \equiv \left(\frac{\partial p}{\partial \rho}\right)_s = \gamma\frac{p}{\rho} = \gamma p V; \qquad \beta \equiv \left(\frac{\partial p}{\partial S}\right)_v = \left(\frac{\partial p}{\partial S}\right)_\rho = -\left(\frac{\partial T}{\partial V}\right)_s, \qquad (5.107a\text{–}f)$$

the non-adiabatic coefficient (5.106d) ≡ (5.107d) is given by (5.104c) ≡ (5.107f) and also (5.107e) because constant specific volume is equivalent to constant mass density (5.98a). The preceding *thermodynamic relations valid for any substance, for example gas, liquid, or solid, include: (i) the functions of state, namely the internal energy (5.85a–d), enthalpy (5.89a, b), free energy (5.90a, b), and free enthalpy (5.91a, b); (ii) the adiabatic relation (5.101b) ≡ (5.101c) involving the adiabatic exponent (5.101a), defined by the ratio of the specific heats at constant pressure (5.99c) and volume (5.99b); (iii) the adiabatic relation simplifies to (5.103b) ≡ (5.103c) in the case of constant adiabatic exponent (5.103a); and (iv) the adiabatic exponent need not be constant in the equation of state (5.105a) ≡ (5.105b) involving the adiabatic sound speed (5.106a–c) ≡ (5.107a–c) and non-adiabatic coefficient (5.106d, e) ≡ (5.107d, e).* In order to obtain explicit expressions for these thermodynamic quantities, the equation of state relating three thermodynamic quantities out of four (p, ρ, T, S) must be specified; it depends on the substance, the simplest being a perfect (ideal) gas [subsections 5.5.16–5.5.19 (5.5.20–5.5.25)].

5.5.16 Perfect Gas Consisting of Non-Interacting Molecules

The perfect gas consists of molecules with low density so that all interactions, such as mechanical collisions or electric, magnetic, or gravity attractions or repulsions, can be neglected, implying that: (i) the internal energy is due only to the kinetic energy of the molecules; (ii) the **temperature** is defined as twice the average kinetic energy of the microscopic molecular motion (5.108a) with the **Boltzmann constant** (5.108c) as coefficient with the dimensions of energy (Joule) per degree of absolute temperature (Kelvin):

$$\left\langle m v^2 \right\rangle = kT \geq 0, \qquad\qquad k = 1.381 \times 10^{-23}\, J\,K^{-1}; \qquad (5.108a\text{--}c)$$

(iii) thus the **absolute temperature** (5.108a) is always non-negative (5.108b), and increases from zero for molecules at rest to larger values for stronger thermal agitation; and (iv) the internal energy (5.86d) ≡ (5.109a):

perfect gas: $\qquad\qquad -p\,dV + T\,dS = dU = C_v\,dT\,, \qquad\qquad$ (5.109a, b)

can depend only on the temperature (5.109b) ≡ (5.99b) through the specific heat at constant volume. The perfect gas is specified [subsection 5.5.17 (5.5.18)] by the internal energy (equation of state) together.

5.5.17 Internal Energy and Equation of State

The macroscopic temperature corresponds (5.108a) to the microscopic kinetic energy, and the macroscopic **pressure** is the microscopic linear momentum imparted per unit time and unit area by molecules colliding with a wall. In the case of a **perfect gas**: (i) the pressure (5.110a) is the product of twice the average kinetic energy of molecules (5.108a) by the number of particles per unit volume (5.108b):

$$p = kT\nu, \qquad\qquad \nu \equiv \frac{dN}{dV} = \frac{dN}{dm}\frac{dm}{dV} = \rho\frac{dN}{dm}; \qquad (5.110a\text{--}c)$$

(ii) the number of particles per unit volume (5.110b) is the mass density times the number of particles per unit mass (5.110c):

$$\frac{dN}{dm} = \frac{A}{M}: \qquad\qquad A = 6.022 \times 10^{23}\ mole^{-1}, \qquad\qquad (5.110d, e)$$

(iii) the number of particles per unit mass (5.110d) is the **Avogadro number** (5.110e) or number of particles per **mole**, divided by the **molecular mass** or mass of one mole. Substituting (5.110d) in (5.110c) and (5.110a) leads to the *equation of state of perfect gas (5.111a):*

$$p = kT\rho\frac{A}{M} = \rho RT = \frac{RT}{V}, \qquad\qquad RM = kA = 8.316\, J\,K^{-1}\,mole^{-1}, \qquad (5.111a\text{--}d)$$

*where (5.111b) ≡ (5.111c) the **gas constant** (5.111d) multiplied by the molecular mass (5.111c) equals the product of the Boltzmann constant (5.108c) by the Avogadro number (5.110d) and has the dimensions of energy per mole per unit temperature.*

5.5.18 Properties of Perfect and Ideal Gases

A perfect gas: (i) satisfies the equation of state (5.111a–d); (ii) has internal energy that depends only on the temperature and the derivative is the specific heat at constant volume (5.109b) ≡ (5.112a) ≡ (5.112c):

$$\{dU, dH\} = \{C_v(T), C_p(T)\}dT: \qquad C_v(T) = \frac{dU}{dT}, \quad C_p(T) = \frac{dH}{dT}. \qquad (5.112a\text{–}d)$$

It follows that: (i) the enthalpy is also a function of temperature only (5.112b) ≡ (5.113b) and the derivative is the specific heat at constant pressure:

$$U(T) + p\,V = U(T) + R\,T = H(T), \qquad \frac{dH}{dT} = \frac{dU}{dT} + R = C_v + R = C_p; \qquad (5.113a, b)$$

(ii) the difference of the specific heats at constant pressure and volume is the gas constant (5.113b) ≡ (5.114a), whereas the ratio or adiabatic exponent may depend on temperature (5.114b) ≡ (5.114c):

$$R = C_p(T) - C_v(T) = C_v(T)\left[\gamma(T) - 1\right] = C_p(T)\left[1 - \frac{1}{\gamma(T)}\right]. \qquad (5.114a\text{–}c)$$

*An **ideal gas** is a particular case of a perfect gas for which the adiabatic exponent is constant (5.115a), implying that: (i) the specific heats at constant pressure (5.115c) and volume (5.115c) are also constant:*

$$\text{ideal gas:} \quad \gamma = const, \quad C_v = \frac{R}{\gamma - 1} = const, \quad C_p = \frac{\gamma R}{\gamma - 1} = const. \qquad (5.115a\text{–}c)$$

$$U(T) = U(T_0) + C_v(T - T_0), \qquad H(T) = H(T_0) + C_p(T - T_0); \qquad (5.115d, e)$$

and (ii) the internal energy (5.115d) [enthalpy (5.115e)] is a linear function of the temperature with the constant specific heat at constant volume (pressure) as coefficient. Next are considered in more detail some properties of ideal gases, namely; (i) adiabatic relations involving the temperature (subsection 5.5.19); (ii) entropy as a function of temperature and mass density or specific volume (subsection 5.5.20); (iii) internal energy (enthalpy) and (subsection 5.5.21) specific heats at constant volume (pressure); (iv) adiabatic exponent for polyatomic molecules (subsection 5.5.22), (v) evaluation of thermodynamic derivatives including non-adiabatic coefficient (subsection 5.5.23) and adiabatic and isothermal sound speed (subsection 5.5.25); and (v) application to the atmosphere of the earth at sea level (subsection 5.5.26).

5.5.19 Adiabatic Perfect and Ideal Gases

The equation of state of a perfect gas (5.111a) ≡ (5.116a) [(5.111b) ≡ (5.116b)] leads by logarithmic differentiation to (5.116c) [(5.116d)]:

$$\log p - \log T - \log R = -\log V = \log \rho: \qquad \frac{dp}{p} - \frac{dT}{T} = -\frac{dV}{V} = \frac{d\rho}{\rho}; \qquad (5.116a\text{–}d)$$

substitution of (5.116c, d) in (5.101c, d) leads to the **adiabatic relations** *between temperature and specific volume (5.117a), mass density (5.117b), or pressure (5.118a) for a perfect gas:*

$$\frac{dT}{T} = (1-\gamma)\frac{dV}{V} = (\gamma-1)\frac{d\rho}{\rho}; \quad \gamma = const: \quad TV^{\gamma-1} = T_0 V_0^{\gamma-1}, \quad \frac{T}{T_0} = \left(\frac{\rho}{\rho_0}\right)^{\gamma-1},$$

$$(5.117a\text{–}e)$$

$$\frac{dT}{T} = \left(1-\frac{1}{\gamma}\right)\frac{dp}{p}; \qquad \gamma = const: \qquad \left(\frac{T}{T_0}\right)^{\gamma} = \left(\frac{p}{p_0}\right)^{\gamma-1}, \qquad (5.118a\text{–}c)$$

in the case of constant adiabatic exponent (5.115a) ≡ (5.117b) [≡(5.118b)] the adiabatic relation simplifies to (5.117c) ≡ (5.117d) [(5.118c)] for an ideal gas. The adiabatic relations for an ideal gas can be checked from the conservation of entropy, which is calculated next (subsection 5.5.20).

5.5.20 Entropy of an Ideal Gas

The entropy is given in general (5.97a) [(5.97b)] by: (i) for any substance (5.99b) [(5.99c)] by (5.119a) [(5.119b):

$$dS = C_v \frac{dT}{T} + \frac{p}{T}dV = C_p \frac{dT}{T} - \frac{V}{T}dp, \qquad (5.119a, b)$$

(ii) for a perfect gas (5.111c) ≡ (5.119c) by (5.119d)[(5.119e)]:

$$pV = RT: \qquad dS = C_v \frac{dT}{T} + R\frac{dV}{V} = C_p \frac{dT}{T} - R\frac{dp}{p} = C_v \frac{dp}{p} + C_p \frac{dV}{V}, \qquad (5.119c\text{–}f)$$

and (5.119f) follows from (5.116c; 5.114a); (iii) for an ideal gas (5.115a–c) the coefficients in (5.119a, b) are all constant, leading by integration to:

$$S - S_0 = C_v \log\left(\frac{T}{T_0}\right) + R\log\left(\frac{V}{V_0}\right) = R\left[\frac{1}{\gamma-1}\log\left(\frac{T}{T_0}\right) - \log\left(\frac{\rho}{\rho_0}\right)\right]$$

$$= C_p \log\left(\frac{T}{T_0}\right) - R\log\left(\frac{p}{p_0}\right) = R\left[\frac{\gamma}{\gamma-1}\log\left(\frac{T}{T_0}\right) - \log\left(\frac{p}{p_0}\right)\right] \qquad (5.120a\text{–}f)$$

$$= C_v \log\left(\frac{p}{p_0}\right) + C_p \log\left(\frac{V}{V_0}\right) = \frac{R}{\gamma-1}\left[\log\left(\frac{p}{p_0}\right) - \gamma\log\left(\frac{\rho}{\rho_0}\right)\right].$$

In an adiabatic process $S = S_0$ of an ideal gas (5.120a–f) lead respectively to (5.117d, e; 5.118c; 5.103b, c). Besides the entropy, the internal energy and enthalpy and specific heats at constant pressure and volume (an adiabatic exponent) take simple forms for an ideal gas [subsection 5.5.21 (5.5.22)].

5.5.21 Microscopic Statistics of Perfect/Ideal Gases

In the thermodynamic classification of substances (Table 5.2), a perfect gas consists of non-interacting molecules so that only the kinetic energy contributes to the internal energy through the temperature, implying a low density. If, in addition, the temperature is not too high the molecular vibrations and other internal degrees-of-freedom can be neglected for an ideal gas. The ideas gas has only translational and rotational degrees of freedom, and the average kinetic energy is equal for all degrees of freedom. Since the kinetic

TABLE 5.2

Thermodynamic Classification of Substance

Case	I	II	III
Physical processes	Molecular collisions and interactions through force field	Internal degrees of freedom: vibrations and deformations	External degrees of freedom: rotations and translations
Notions	Constrained	Elastic	Rigid body
Arbitrary substance and real gas	yes	yes	yes
Perfect gas	no	yes	yes
Ideal gas	no	no	yes

Note: An ideal gas consists of molecules having only external translational and rotational degrees of freedom like rigid bodies. A perfect gas adds internal degrees of freedom like vibrations and deformations. A real gas or generic solid or liquid substance adds collisions of molecules and/or interactions through force fields.

energy per degree of freedom specifies the temperature (5.108a), the total internal energy with n degrees of freedom is given by (5.121a):

$$U = n\frac{A}{M} < \frac{1}{2}mv^2 >= \frac{n}{2}\frac{kA}{M}T = \frac{n}{2}RT = \frac{n}{2}pV, \qquad (5.121a\text{–}d)$$

where were used (5.111b) in (5.121c) and the equation of state (5.119c) in (5.121d). It has been shown that *an ideal gas has internal energy (5.121d)* ≡ *(5.122a) [enthalpy (5.113a)* ≡ *(5.122c)] proportional to the temperature:*

$$U = \frac{1}{2}nRT = C_vT, \qquad H = \left(1+\frac{n}{2}\right)R\,T = C_pT; \qquad (5.122a\text{–}d)$$

(ii) the coefficient is the specific heat at constant volume (5.112c) ≡ *(5.122e) [constant pressure (5.112d)* ≡ *(5.122f)] that is constant in agreement with (5.115b) [(5.115c)]:*

$$C_v = \frac{dU}{dT} = \frac{n}{2}R, \qquad C_p = \frac{dH}{dT} = \left(1+\frac{n}{2}\right)R; \qquad \gamma \equiv \frac{C_p}{C_v} = 1+\frac{2}{n}, \quad (5.122e\text{–}g)$$

(iii) the adiabatic exponent (5.101a) ≡ *(5.122g) is also constant (5.115a) and depends only on the number of degrees of freedom of a molecule; (iv) the specific heats at constant volume (5.122e) and pressure (5.122f) involve also the gas constant (5.111d); and (v) the internal energy (5.122b) [enthalpy (5.122d)] multiplies by the temperature.* The adiabatic exponent is considered next for monatomic, diatomic, and polyatomic molecules (subsection 5.5.22).

5.5.22 Monatomic, Diatomic, and Polyatomic Molecules

It has been shown that an ideal gas has specific heat at constant pressure (5.122f) [volume (5.122e)] that depends only on the gas constant (5.111d) and number of degrees of freedom of a molecule. The gas constant is a common factor that disappears from the ratio for the adiabatic exponent (5.122g) that depends only on the number of degrees of freedom of a molecule. Thus, the adiabatic exponent of an ideal gas is given by:

$$\gamma = 1+\frac{2}{n} = \begin{cases} \dfrac{5}{3} & \text{if} \quad n=3: \quad \text{monatomic,} \\[2mm] \dfrac{7}{5} & \text{if} \quad n=5: \quad \text{diatomic,} \\[2mm] \dfrac{4}{3} & \text{if} \quad n=6: \quad \text{polyatomic,} \end{cases} \qquad (5.123a\text{–}d)$$

where n is the number of degrees of freedom of a molecule, leading to three cases: (i) a monatomic molecule (5.123b) has only $n=3$ translational degrees

TABLE 5.3

Thermodynamic Parameters of an Ideal Gas

Degrees of Freedom		$n = 3$	$n = 5$	$n = 6$
Molecule		Monatomic	Diatomic or Linear Polyatomic	Three Dimensional Polyatomic
Specific heat at constant	volume $\dfrac{n}{2}R$	$\dfrac{3}{2}R$	$\dfrac{5}{2}R$	$3\,R$
	pressure $\left(1+\dfrac{n}{2}\right)R$	$\dfrac{5}{2}R$	$\dfrac{7}{2}R$	$4\,R$
Adiabatic exponent	$\gamma = 1+\dfrac{2}{N}$	$\dfrac{5}{3}$	$\dfrac{7}{5}$	$\dfrac{4}{3}$

R – gas constant (5.111d).

Note: An ideal gas has constant adiabatic exponent and specific heats at constant volume and pressure proportional to the gas constant (5.122a–c). The coefficient depends on the number of translation and rotational degrees of freedom of a molecule.

of freedom; (ii) two rotational degrees of freedom are added $n = 5$ for a (5.123c) diatomic molecule or a polyatomic molecule with all atoms aligned in a row; or (iii) a three-dimensional polyatomic molecule, with atoms not all in a row, adds another rotational degree of freedom for a total $n = 6$ as (5.123d) for a rigid body. Thus *the adiabatic exponent equals (5/3, 7/5, 4/3) respectively (5.123b, c, d) for a monatomic, diatomic, and polyatomic ideal gas (5.115a–c) and the corresponding specific heats at constant volume (5.122e) [pressure (5.122f)] are indicated in Table 5.3.*

5.5.23 Evaluation of Thermodynamic Derivatives Using Jacobians

The Jacobian is defined by the determinant of partial derivatives:

$$\frac{\partial(A,B)}{\partial(C,D)} \equiv \begin{vmatrix} \dfrac{\partial A}{\partial C} & \dfrac{\partial A}{\partial D} \\[2mm] \dfrac{\partial B}{\partial C} & \dfrac{\partial B}{\partial D} \end{vmatrix} = \frac{\partial A}{\partial C}\frac{\partial B}{\partial D} - \frac{\partial A}{\partial D}\frac{\partial B}{\partial C}. \tag{5.124}$$

The properties:

$$-\frac{\partial(B,A)}{\partial(C,D)} = \frac{\partial(A,B)}{\partial(C,D)} = -\frac{\partial(B,A)}{\partial(D,C)}, \qquad \frac{\partial(A,B)}{\partial(C,D)} = \frac{\partial(A,B)}{\partial(E,F)}\frac{\partial(E,F)}{\partial(C,D)}, \tag{5.125a, b}$$

provide a general method of evaluation of thermodynamic derivatives:

$$\frac{\partial(A,B)}{\partial(C,B)} = \frac{\partial A}{\partial C}\frac{\partial B}{\partial B} - \frac{\partial A}{\partial B}\frac{\partial B}{\partial C} = \left(\frac{\partial A}{\partial C}\right)_B. \tag{5.126}$$

Two examples of the use of the *general method of Jacobians (5.124, 5.125a, b) to calculate thermodynamic derivatives are the non-adiabatic coefficient (5.106e) [adiabatic sound speed (5.106a)]:*

$$\beta = \frac{\partial(p,V)}{\partial(S,V)} = \frac{\partial(p,V)}{\partial(T,V)}\frac{\partial(T,V)}{\partial(S,V)} = \left(\frac{\partial p}{\partial T}\right)_V\left(\frac{\partial T}{\partial S}\right)_V = \frac{T}{C_v}\left(\frac{\partial p}{\partial T}\right)_\rho, \tag{5.127a}$$

$$c_s^2 = \frac{\partial(P,S)}{\partial(\rho,S)} = \frac{\partial(P,S)}{\partial(P,T)}\frac{\partial(P,T)}{\partial(\rho,T)}\frac{\partial(\rho,T)}{\partial(\rho,S)}$$

$$= \left[\left(\frac{\partial S}{\partial T}\right)_p\bigg/\left(\frac{\partial S}{\partial T}\right)_V\right]\left(\frac{\partial P}{\partial \rho}\right)_T = \frac{C_p}{C_v}\left(\frac{\partial P}{\partial \rho}\right)_T = \gamma\left(\frac{\partial P}{\partial \rho}\right)_T, \tag{5.127b}$$

where (5.99b, c) and (5.101a) were used; the expressions (5.127a) [(5.127b)] are alternatives to (5.107a–c) [(5.107d–f)].

5.5.24 Arbitrary Substances versus Perfect/Ideal Gases

Thus *the equation of state (5.105a) in a differential form (5.105b) involves as coefficients the adiabatic sound speed (5.106a–c) ≡ (5.107a–c) ≡ (5.128a) [non-adiabatic coefficient (5.106d–f) ≡ (5.128b)]:*

$$c_s^2 = \gamma\left(\frac{\partial p}{\partial \rho}\right)_T, \qquad \beta = \frac{T}{C_v}\left(\frac{\partial p}{\partial T}\right)_\rho. \tag{5.128a, b}$$

In the case of a perfect gas, using (5.128a; 5.111b) or (5.107c; 5.111d) [(5.107f; 5.117a) or (5.128b; 5.111c)] simplifies the adiabatic sound speed (non-adiabatic coefficient) to (5.129a) [(5.129b–d)]:

$$c_s^2 = \gamma RT, \qquad \beta = -(1-\gamma)\frac{T}{V} = \frac{\gamma-1}{R}p = \frac{p}{C_v}. \tag{5.129a–d}$$

In the case of an ideal gas (5.115a–c), the coefficients in (5.129a–d) are all constant and the square of the adiabatic sound speed (non-adiabatic coefficient) is proportional to the temperature (pressure). The adiabatic and isothermal sound speeds are compared next (subsection 5.5.25).

5.5.25 Adiabatic and Isothermal Sound Speeds

The adiabatic (isothermal) sound speed is the square root of the derivative of the pressure with regard to the mass density at constant entropy (5.106a) [temperature (5.130a)]:

$$c_t^2 = \left(\frac{\partial p}{\partial \rho}\right)_T = RT = \frac{p}{\rho} = \frac{c_s^2}{\gamma}, \qquad (5.130a\text{--}d)$$

and: (i) for a perfect gas (5.111b) simplifies to (5.129a) [5.130b) ≡ (5.130c)] so that their ratio (5.130d) is the adiabatic exponent. *The **isothermal sound speed** (5.130b) is analogous to the natural frequency of the harmonic oscillator (2.54a) ≡ (5.131a):*

$$\omega_0^2 = \frac{k}{m}: \qquad \omega_0 \leftrightarrow c_t, \qquad m \leftrightarrow \rho, \qquad k \leftrightarrow p, \qquad (5.131a\text{--}d)$$

replacing (5.131b): (i) the mass by the mass density (5.131c); and (ii) the resilience of the spring by the pressure (5.131d). The adiabatic sound speed (5.130d) multiplies the isothermal sound speed (5.130a) ≡ (5.130b) ≡ (5.130c) by the adiabatic exponent. Sound consists of compressions and rarefactions and thus: (i) if there is little or no dissipation the adiabatic sound speed (5.107a–c; 5.129a) is appropriate and there are associated temperature changes (5.117a–e; 5.118a–c); and (ii) if dissipation is strong enough to smooth out the temperature fluctuations in a time scale shorter than a period, then the isothermal sound speed (5.130a–c) is more appropriate. The isothermal sound speed was obtained **(Newton 1687)** using the analogy with the harmonic oscillator (5.131a–d) that does not require thermodynamics. The adiabatic sound speed **(Poisson 1807)** involves the thermodynamic properties of the medium of propagation. The atmosphere of the earth up to and excluding the ionosphere is reasonably approximated by an ideal diatomic gas (subsection 5.5.26); since dissipation is weak the adiabatic sound speed is relevant.

5.5.26 Atmosphere of the Earth at Sea Level

The atmosphere of the earth at sea level can be reasonably approximated by an ideal gas, whose gas constant (5.111d) is calculated next, starting with the mole: (i) the mole of nitrogen (oxygen), that is, the mass of the Avogadro number of atoms is (5.132a) [(5.132b)]:

$$\{M_N, M_O\} = \{14, 16\}\, g\, mole^{-1}; \qquad (5.132a, b)$$

(ii) air consists of about 80% (20%) of diatomic nitrogen (oxygen) leading to (5.132c) for a mole of air:

$$M_{air} = 0.8\,M_{N_2} + 0.2\,M_{O_2} = (0.8 \times 2 \times 14 + 0.2 \times 2 \times 16)\,g\,mole^{-1} = 28.8\,g\,mole^{-1};$$
(5.132c)

(iii) substituting (5.132c) in (5.111d) determines the gas constant of air:

$$R_{Air} = \frac{8316\,g\,m^2 s^{-2}\,K^{-1}\,mole^{-1}}{28.8\,g\,mole^{-1}} = 289\,m^2\,s^{-2}\,K^{-1};$$
(5.132d)

and (iv) since air is diatomic, the adiabatic exponent is (5.123c) ≡ (5.133a) and for a sea level temperature (5.133b):

$$\gamma = 1.4, \qquad T_0 = 15C = 288\,K: \qquad c_s = \sqrt{\gamma R T_0} = 341\,m\,s^{-1},$$
(5.133a–c)

leads (5.129a) to the adiabatic sound speed (5.133c).

Concerning the non-adiabatic coefficient, the starting point is the pressure at sea level (5.134d) that corresponds to the weight of a column of mercury of density (5.134a) and height (5.134b) in the gravity field (5.134c):

$$\rho_{Hg} = 13.6\,g\,cm^{-3}, \qquad h = 76\,cm, \qquad g = 981\,cm\,s^{-2}:$$
$$p_0 = \rho_{Hg} h g = 1.01 \times 10^6\,g\,cm^{-1} s^{-2} = 1.01 \times 10^5\,kg\,m^{-1} s^{-2}.$$
(5.134a–d)

The non-isentropic coefficient (5.129c) is given by:

$$\beta = 0.4\frac{p_0}{R} = 1,4 \times 10^3\,kg\,m^{-1}\,K.$$
(5.135)

Thus *the adiabatic sound speed (5.106a–c; 5.107a–c; 5.128a; 5.129a) [non-isentropic coefficient (5.106d, e; 5.107d, e; 5.128b; 5.129b–d)] is given by (5.133c) [(5.135)] in the atmosphere of the earth at sea level.* A similar calculation could be applied at other altitudes to obtain a profile of the variation of thermodynamic properties.

5.6 Equation of the Second-Order Missing Slope or One Variable

Besides first-order differential equations (chapter 3 and sections 5.1–5.5), higher order differential equations have been considered in the linear case with constant (homogeneous power) coefficients for any order [sections 1.3–1.5 (1.6–1.8)]. The first-order equations solved did include linear with variable coefficients and non-linear equations. Next are considered second-order equations (section 5.6). A second-order differential equation can always be reduced to a first-order differential equation (subsection 5.6.1) that may or may not be easier to solve. The cases when the reduction of a second-order differential equation to first-order leads to an easier integration, for example by quadratures, includes missing: (i) independent variable (subsection 5.6.2); (ii) also the slope (subsection 5.6.3); (iii) instead the dependent variable (subsection 5.6.4).

5.6.1 Reduction of Second-Order to First-Order Differential Equation

Proceeding from first-order to second-order differential equations (5.136a):

$$F(x,y,y',y'') = 0, \qquad f(x,y;C_1 C_2) = 0. \qquad (5.136\text{a, b})$$

the general integral involves (5.136b) two arbitrary constants of integration. For example, the equation of one-dimensional motion of a particle of mass m with acceleration (5.137b) due (5.137c) to a force that may depend on time t, position x, and velocity (5.137a):

$$\dot{x} \equiv \frac{dx}{dt}, \qquad \ddot{x} = \frac{d^2 x}{dt^2}: \qquad m\,\ddot{x} = G(t,x,\dot{x}); \qquad x = x(t;x,\dot{x}_0), \qquad (5.137\text{a–d})$$

the solution specifies the position as a function of time (5.137d) for a given initial position x_0 and velocity $\dot{x}_0$. The curvature y'' must be present in (5.136a); for this to be a second-order differential equation; this term can be written in the form (5.138a):

$$y'' \equiv \frac{dy'}{dx} = \frac{dy'}{dy}\frac{dy}{dx} = y'\frac{dy'}{dy}; \qquad F\left(x,y,y',y'\frac{dy'}{dy}\right) = 0, \qquad (5.138\text{a, b})$$

showing that *the solution of a second-order differential equation (5.136a) can always (standard CVII) be reduced to the solution (5.139a) of a first-order differential equation followed (5.138b) by a quadrature (5.139b):*

$$y' = f(x;C_1): \qquad y(x;C_1,C_2) = C_2 + \int^x f(\xi;C_1)\,d\xi. \qquad (5.139\text{a, b})$$

The latter may be more complicated than the former; any linear second-order differential equation with variable coefficients (3.98a) can be transformed to a non-linear first-order differential equation of Ricatti type (3.100). It may happen that one is simpler to solve than the other, but it is not obvious *a priori*: (i) that this is the case; (ii) which of the two is simpler.

For example, the linear second-order differential equation (5.140a):

$$y'' = xy' + y, \qquad \frac{dy'}{dy} = x + \frac{y}{y'}, \qquad (5.140a, b)$$

is equivalent to the non-linear first-order equation (5.140b); the latter can be written in the form (5.141a):

$$dy' = x\,dy + \frac{y}{y'}\,dy = x\,dy + y\,dx = d(\dot{x}y), \qquad y' = C_1 + xy, \qquad (5.141a, b)$$

that has a first integral (5.141b). This is a linear first-order equation (5.77b) ≡ (3.27) whose solution is (3.31a, b; 3.20b) is (5.142):

$$y = \exp\!\left(\frac{x^2}{2}\right)\!\left\{ C_2 + C_1 \int^x e^{-\xi^2/2}\, d\xi \right\}; \qquad (5.142)$$

this specifies the general integral (5.142) of the second-order differential equation (5.140a).

5.6.2 Second-Order Differential Equation with Independent Variable Missing

If the second-order differential equation (5.136a) omits (standard CVIII) the independent variable (5.143a), the corresponding (5.138a) first-order differential equation is (5.143b):

$$0 = F(y', y, y'') = F\!\left(y', y, y'\frac{dy'}{dx} \right), \qquad m\ddot{x} = G(x, \dot{x}), \qquad (5.143a\text{--}c)$$

corresponding to the one-dimensional motion of a particle of mass m under forces that do not depend on time, but may depend on position and velocity (5.143c). The differential equation (5.143b) has general integral of the form (5.144a):

$$y' = f(y; C_1): \qquad x + C_2 = \int dx = \int \frac{dy}{y'} = \int^y \frac{d\xi}{f(\xi; C_1)}; \qquad (5.144a, b)$$

thus a single quadrature (5.144b) yields the general integral of the second-order differential equation (5.143a). Thus, *if the second-order differential equation (5.136a) ≡ (5.137b) omits (standard CVIII) the independent variable (5.143a), the general integral is given by (5.144b), in terms of a solution (5.144a) of the first-order equation (5.143b).*

As an example of second-order differential equation omitting the indepen-dent variable (5.143a) consider (5.145a):

$$\frac{y''}{y'}=2\,y, \qquad \frac{dy'}{dy}=2\,y, \qquad y'+C_1^2=y^2, \qquad \text{(5.145a–c)}$$

whose associated first-order equation is (5.145b), leads to a first integral (5.145c), a single quadrature (5.155a):

$$x+\frac{C_2}{C_1}=\int\frac{dy}{y'}=\int\frac{dy}{y^2-C_1^2}=\frac{1}{C_1}\,arc\,tanh\left(\frac{y}{C_1}\right), \qquad \text{(5.146a)}$$

specifies the general integral:

$$y=C_1\tanh\left\{C_1\left(x+\frac{C_2}{C_1}\right)\right\}=C_1\tanh\left(C_1\,x+C_2\right), \qquad \text{(5.146b)}$$

of the second-order differential equation (5.145a).

5.6.3 Both Independent Variable and Slope Missing

If the second-order differential equation (5.136a) ≡ (5.136b) omits not only the slope (5.143a) ≡ (5.143b) but also (standard CIX) the independent variable (5.147a) ≡ (5.147a) ≡ (5.147b):

$$h(y)=y''=y'\frac{dy'}{y}, \qquad m\ddot{x}=G(x), \qquad \text{(5.147a–c)}$$

it corresponds to one-dimensional motion (5.147c) under a force that depends only on position. The first integral of (5.147b) is (5.148a) that may be solved (5.148b) for y':

$$y'^2-C_1=2\int^y h(\xi)d\xi: \qquad y'=\left|C_1+2\int^y h(\xi)d\xi\right|^{1/2}=\frac{dy}{dx}; \qquad \text{(5.148a–c)}$$

a further integration of (5.148c) leads to:

$$x+C_2=\int dx=\int\frac{dy}{y'}=\int^y\left|C_1+2\int^\eta h(\xi)d\xi\right|^{-1/2}d\eta, \qquad \text{(5.149)}$$

that is, the general integral (5.149) of (5.147a). Thus, *a second-order differential equation (5.147a) expressing curvature as a function of the dependent variable alone (standard CIX) is solved by two quadratures (5.149).*

As an example, consider the second-order equation with constant coefficients (5.150a):

$$y'' + y = 0, \qquad x + C_2 = \int^y \left| C_1^2 - \xi^2 \right|^{-1/2} d\xi = \arcsin\left(\frac{y}{C_1}\right), \qquad \text{(5.150a, b)}$$

whose solution (5.149) is (5.150b); the solution can be put into the form (5.151a):

$$y = C_1 \sin(x + C_2) = C \cos(x - \delta), \qquad \{C_1, C_2\} = \left\{ C, \frac{\pi}{2} - \delta \right\}, \qquad \text{(5.151a–d)}$$

that is equivalent to (5.151b) using the alternative constants of integration (5.151c, d). The general integral (5.151b) of (5.150a) corresponds: (i) to (1.74a; 1.81) with $\alpha = 0, \beta = 1, \delta = \beta$; (ii) to the harmonic oscillator (2.54c; 2.56b) with $\omega_0 = 1, y = x, x = t, \delta = \alpha$. Two instances (5.143a; 5.147a) of a second-order equation omitting the independent variable x (case I) have been considered so far; if the slope (case II) is omitted in (5.136a) there is in general no simplification; that is, the equation (5.152a) ≡ (5.152b) is generally as difficult to solve as (5.136a) ≡ (5.136b):

$$0 = F(x, y, y'') = F\left(x, y, y' \frac{dy'}{dy}\right); \qquad m\ddot{x} = G(t, x), \qquad \text{(5.152a–c)}$$

an equivalent statement is that is if the force (5.137c) does not depend on the velocity (5.152e), the integration of the equation of motion is not significantly simplified. The remaining case (III) is that of dependent variable missing and is considered next (subsection 5.6.4).

5.6.4 Second-Order Differential Equation with Dependent Variable Missing

In the case (III) for *the second-order differential equation (5.153a) without dependent variable (standard CX), the solution reduces to that of a first-order equation (5.153b) plus a quadrature (5.153c)*

$$0 = F(x, y', y'') = F(x, w, w'), \qquad w \equiv y'; \qquad \text{(5.153a–c)}$$

this corresponds to a one-dimensional motion of a particle under a force that does not depend on position (5.154a):

$$m\ddot{x} = G(\dot{x}, t), \qquad m\dot{v} = G(v, t), \qquad v = \dot{x}, \qquad \text{(5.154a–c)}$$

leading to a first-order differential equation (5.154b) for the velocity (5.154c). *If in the second-order differential equation (5.136a) both the dependent variable and the slope are absent (5.155a) and the curvature is explicit (standard CXI), the solution follows by two quadratures (5.155b):*

$$y'' = h(x), \qquad y(x) = C_1 + C_2 x + \int^x d\xi \int^\xi h(\eta)\, d\eta. \qquad \text{(5.155a, b)}$$

This corresponds to (5.156a) the one-dimensional motion of a particle:

$$m\ddot{x} = G(t), \qquad x = x_0 + v_0 t + \int^t d\xi \int^\xi G(\eta)\, d\eta, \qquad \text{(5.156a, b)}$$

in the simplest case (5.156b) when the force depends only on time.

An example of second-order differential equation of type (5.153a) that is without dependent variable is (5.157a) $\equiv$ (5.157b):

$$x = y'' = y'\frac{dy'}{dx}: \qquad y'^2 = C_1 + x^2: \qquad y - \frac{C_2}{2} = \int^x \sqrt{C_1 + \xi^2}\, d\xi, \qquad \text{(5.157a–d)}$$

that has first integral (5.157c) leading to (5.157d). The integral (5.157d) is evaluated (5.158c, d) via the change of variable (5.158c):

$$\xi = \sqrt{C_1}\, \sinh\alpha, d\xi = \sqrt{C_1}\, \cosh\alpha\, d\alpha:$$

$$\int^x \sqrt{C_1 + \xi^2}\, d\xi = C_1 \int \cosh^2\alpha\, d\alpha = C_1 \int \frac{1 + \cosh(2\alpha)}{2}\, d\alpha \qquad \text{(5.158a–c)}$$

$$= C_1 \left[\frac{\alpha}{2} + \frac{\sinh(2\alpha)}{4} \right] = C_1 \left[\frac{\alpha}{2} + \frac{\cosh\alpha \sinh\alpha}{2} \right].$$

Substituting (5.158c) in (5.157d) and using (5.158a) $\equiv$ (5.159a–c):

$$\alpha = \arg\sinh\left(\frac{x}{\sqrt{C_1}} \right), \qquad \sinh\alpha = \frac{x}{\sqrt{C_1}}, \qquad \cosh\alpha = \left| 1 + \frac{\xi^2}{C_1} \right|^{1/2},$$

$$\text{(5.159a–c)}$$

leads to:

$$2y = C_2 + x\sqrt{x^2 + C_1} + C_1 \operatorname{arg\,sinh}\left(\frac{x}{\sqrt{C_1}}\right), \qquad (5.160)$$

as the general integral of (5.157a). A second-order differential equation of the type (5.155a) involving neither the dependent variable nor the slope is (5.161a):

$$y'' = \frac{1}{x^2}, \qquad y' = -\frac{1}{x} + C_1, \qquad y = -\log x + C_1 x + C_2, \qquad (5.161a\text{--}c)$$

whose general integral is obtained by two quadratures (5.161b, c).

5.7 Equation of Order N Depressed to Lower Order

The methods of solution of a second-order differential equation by quadratures and/or reduction to a differential equation of first-order (section 5.6) can also be applied to differential equations of order N if some derivatives of lower order are not present (section 5.7). The simplest extensions are a differential equation of order $2(N)$ not involving lower order derivatives, which can be solved by $2(N)$ quadratures [subsection 5.6.4 (5.7.1)]. If in the differential equation of order N the only lower order derivatives are of order $N-1$ $(N-2)$ it can be reduced to a first (second) order differential equation followed by $N-1$ $(N-2)$ quadratures [subsection 5.7.2 (5.7.4)]. Further simplification arises if the independent variable is not present (subsection 5.7.3). In a similar way, if the lowest order derivative that appears is of order $N-P$, the differential equation of order N can be reduced to a differential equation of order P plus $N-P$ quadratures (subsection 5.7.5).

5.7.1 Differential Equation of Order N Involving Only the Independent Variable

A first instance of the extension of the methods used to solve differential equations of order two (section 5.6), to equations of order N is the case when, besides the N-th derivative, only the independent variable is present. The generalization of (5.155a) is the *(standard CXII) differential equation of order N involving only the independent variable (5.162a)*:

$$y^{(N)}(x) = f(x): \qquad y(x) = \sum_{n=0}^{N-1} C_{n+1} x^n + \int^x dx_1 \int^{x_1} dx_2 ... \int^{x_{n-1}} dx_N\, f(x_N), \qquad (5.162a, b)$$

that is solvable by N quadratures and involves N constants of integration (5.162b).
An example is the differential equation (5.163a) of order N:

$$y^{(N)}(x) = a x^b: \qquad y(x) = \frac{a x^{b+N}}{(b+1)(b+2)...(b+N-1)(b+N)} + \sum_{n=0}^{N-1} C_{n+1} x^n,$$

$$(5.163a, b)$$

whose general integral is (5.163b).

5.7.2 Differential Equation Not Involving Derivatives up to Order $N - 2$

A generalization of (5.153a) is *an N-th order differential equation (5.164b) involving (standard CXIII) only the independent variable x and N-th and (N − 1)-th derivatives (5.164a):*

$$w \equiv y^{(N-1)}(x): \qquad 0 = F\left(x, \; y^{(N-1)}(x), y^{(N)}(x)\right) = F(w', w, x); \qquad (5.164a–c)$$

*the solution reduces to that (5.165a) of a first-order equation (5.164c) and (N − 1)
quadratures (5.165b):*

$$w = f(x; C_1): \qquad y(x) = \sum_{n=0}^{N-2} C_{n+2} x^n + \int^x dx_1 ... \int^{x_{N-2}} dx_{N-1} \, f(x_{N-1}; C_1). \qquad (5.165a, b)$$

For example, the differential equation of third order (5.166a) involving only
the second-order derivative and independent variable (5.166b) has integral
(5.166c):

$$y'' = x y''' = x \frac{d y''}{dx}: \qquad \frac{d y''}{y''} = \frac{dx}{x}, \qquad \log y'' = \log x + \log C_1 ; \qquad (5.166a–c)$$

the first integral (5.166c) $\equiv$ (5.167a) leads by two quadratures:

$$y'' = C_1 x: \qquad y = C_1 \frac{x^3}{6} + C_2 x + C_3 , \qquad (5.167a, b)$$

to the general integral (5.167b) of (5.166a). The differential equation (5.166a) is
also satisfied by $y'' = 0$ that is a particular case $C_1 = 0$ of (5.167a); thus it is not
a special integral but rather a particular integral of the general integral that
corresponds to (5.167b) with $C_1 = 0$.

5.7.3 Differential Equation not Involving the Independent Variable

The case of the independent variable x is missing from (5.164b), leads *to an N-th order equation (5.168a) involving (standard CXIV) only N-th and $(N-1)$-th derivatives:*

$$0 = y^{(N)}(x) - h\left(y^{(N-1)}(x)\right) = w' - h(w): \qquad x + C_1 = \int^{w} \frac{d\xi}{h(\xi)}, \qquad (5.168a\text{–}c)$$

that reduces to a first-order differential equation (5.168b); the first integral (5.168c) solved for x in (5.165a) specifies the general integral (5.165b) of (5.168a) involving a further $(N-1)$ quadratures. As an example, we consider the equation (5.169a):

$$y''^2 = y''' = \frac{dy''}{dx}, \qquad dx = \frac{dy''}{y''^2}, \qquad C_1 - x = \frac{1}{y''}, \qquad (5.169a\text{–}c)$$

that is separable (5.169b), leading to a first integral (5.169c); a further two quadratures of (5.169c) $\equiv$ (5.170a):

$$y'' = -\frac{1}{x - C_1}, \qquad y' = C_2 - \log(x - C_1), \qquad (5.170a, b)$$

$$y = C_3 + C_2 x - (x - C_1)\left[\log(x - C_1) - 1\right], \qquad (5.170c)$$

yield (5.170b) the general integral (5.170c) of (5.169a).

5.7.4 Differential Equation Involving Only Derivatives of Orders N and $N-2$

In (5.168a), replacing the $(N-1)$-th derivative by the $(N-2)$-th derivative leads to an N-th order differential equation relating (Standard XCV) the N-th to the $(N-2)$-th derivative (5.171b):

$$w \equiv y^{(N-2)}(x): \qquad 0 = y^{(N)}(x) - h\left(y^{(N-2)}(x)\right) = w'' - f(w), \qquad (5.171a\text{–}c)$$

that reduces to a second-order equation (5.171c) for (5.171a). The solution of the latter is given by (5.149) $\equiv$ (5.172a):

$$x + C_2 = \int^{w}\left|C_1^2 + 2\int^{u} h(\xi)\,d\xi\right|^{-\frac{1}{2}} d\xi, \qquad w = w(x; C_1, C_2), \qquad (5.172a, b)$$

that may be solved (5.172b) for w; a further $N-2$ quadratures (5.173) specify the general integral of (5.171b):

$$y(x) = \sum_{n=0}^{N-3} C_{n+3} x^n + \int^x dx_1 \int^{x_1} dx_2 \dots \int^{x_{N-3}} dx_{N-2}\, w(x_{N-2}; C_1, C_2).$$

$$(5.173)$$

It has been shown that *the N-th order differential equation relating (standard CXV) the N-th to the (N − 2)-th derivative (5.171b), can be solved by N quadratures as follows: (i) the two quadratures (5.172a) specify the independent variable x as a function of the (N − 2)-th derivative (5.171a); (ii) solving for (5.172b) and performing N − 2 quadratures yields the general integral (5.173) of (5.171b).*
As an example, consider the third-order differential equation (5.174a):

$$y''' = y', \qquad x + C_2 = \int^{y'} \left| C_1^2 + w^2 \right|^{-\frac{1}{2}} dw = \operatorname{arc\,sinh}\left(\frac{y'}{C_1}\right), \qquad (5.174a, b)$$

with first integral (5.172a) given by (5.174b); solving (5.174b) for y' gives (5.175a):

$$y' = C_1 \sinh(x + C_2), \qquad y = C_3 + C_1 \cosh(x + C_2), \qquad (5.175a, b)$$

a further quadrature yields the general integral (5.175b) of the third-order differential equation (5.174a). The general integral can also be obtained, noting that (5.174a) ≡ (5.176a) ≡ (1.54) in a linear third-order differential equation with constant coefficients with characteristic polynomial (5.176b):

$$0 = y''' - y' = \left\{ P_3\left(\frac{d}{dx}\right) \right\} y(x), \qquad P_3(D) = D^3 - D = D(D-1)(D+1);$$

$$(5.176a{-}c)$$

the roots (5.176c) of the characteristic polynomial lead to the particular integrals (5.177a–c) and general integral (5.177d):

$$y_{1-3}(x) = 1, e^x, e^{-x}: \qquad y(x) = C_3 + C_+ e^x + C_- e^{-x}. \qquad (5.177a{-}d)$$

The general integral (5.177d) can be rewritten (5.177d) ≡ (5.178a):

$$y(x) - C_3 = (C_+ + C_-)\cosh x + (C_+ - C_-)\sinh x$$

$$= C_1(\cosh x \cosh C_2 + \sinh x \sinh C_2), \qquad (5.178a, b)$$

that coincides with (5.175b) ≡ (5.178b), provided that the arbitrary constants of integration are related by (5.179a, b):

$$C_+ + C_- = C_1 \cosh C_2, \qquad C_+ - C_- = C_1 \sinh C_2, \qquad \text{(5.179a, b)}$$

$$C_1 = \left| (C_+ + C_-)^2 - (C_+ - C_-)^2 \right|^{1/2} = 2\sqrt{C_+ C_-}, \qquad \tanh C_2 = \frac{C_+ - C_-}{C_+ + C_-}, \qquad \text{(5.179c, d)}$$

that are equivalent to (5.179a, b) ≡ (5.179c, d).

5.7.5 Lowest-Order Derivative Appearing is *N – P*

The differential equations involving [subsection 5.7.3 (5.7.4)] besides the derivative of order *N* only *N* – 1 (*N* – 2), can be extended (standard XXVII) to the case when only derivatives of order *N* – *P* or higher are present with *P* ≥ 2; for example, derivatives of orders *N*, *N* – 1 and *N* – 2. *The solution a differential equation of order N where (5.180b) only (standard CXVI) derivatives (5.180a) of order N* – *P or higher appear:*

$$w \equiv y^{(N-P)}(x): \qquad 0 = F\left(x; y^{(N-P)}, ..., y^{(N-1)}, y^{(N)}\right), \quad F\left(x, w, ..., w^{(P-1)}, w^{(P)}\right),$$
$$\text{(5.180a–c)}$$

reduces to the solution of differential equation (5.106c) of order P. The solution (5.181a) of (5.180c) involves P arbitrary constants of integration:

$$w = w(x; C_1, ..., C_p): \quad y(x) = \sum_{n=0}^{N-P-1} C_{P+n+1}\, x^n$$

$$+ \int^x dx_1 \int^{x_1} dx_2 ... \int^{x_{N-P-1}} dx_{N-P}\, w\left(x_{N-P}; C_1, ..., C_p\right),$$
$$\text{(5.181a, b)}$$

and a further (N – *P) quadratures (5.181b) specify the general integral of (5.180b).*

An example is the third-order non-linear differential equation (5.182a) involving derivatives of the first and second order, but neither the dependent nor the independent variable:

$$\left(1 + y'^2\right) y''' = 2 y' y''^2; \qquad w \equiv y', \qquad \frac{2 w w'^2}{1 + w^2} = w'' = w' \frac{dw'}{dw}; \qquad \text{(5.182a–d)}$$

it is equivalent to a second-order differential equation (5.182c) and a quadrature (5.182b). The second-order differential equation (5.182c) ≡ (5.182d) has a special solution (5.183a) ≡ (5.183b) involving only two constants of integration (5.183c):

$$0 = w' = y'': \qquad\qquad y = C_1 + C_2 x; \qquad (5.183a\text{--}c)$$

it is clear that (5.183b) satisfies (5.182a).

The general integral involving three arbitrary constants of integration arises from (5.182d) omitting the common factor (5.183a), leading to (5.184a):

$$\frac{dw'}{w'} = \frac{2w\,dw}{1+w^2}, \quad \log w' = \log C_1 + \log\left(1+w^2\right), \quad w' = C_1\left(1+w^2\right) = \frac{dw}{dx},$$
$$(5.184a\text{--}d)$$

whose first integral is (5.184b) ≡ (5.184c). From (5.184c) ≡ (5.184d) follows a second integration (5.185a) ≡ (5.185b) ≡ (5.185c):

$$C_1\,dx = \frac{dw}{1+w^2}, \quad C_1 x + C_2 = \arg\tan w, \quad w = \tan\left(C_1 x + C_2\right) = \frac{dy}{dx}.$$
$$(5.185a\text{--}d)$$

From (5.185c) ≡ (5.185d) follows a third integration (5.186a):

$$y = C_3 + \int^x \tan\left(C_1\,\xi + C_2\right)d\xi = C_3 - \frac{1}{C_1}\log\left[\cos\left(C_1 x + C_2\right)\right], \qquad (5.186a,\,b)$$

that specifies the general integral of (5.182a). The solution (5.183c) is not included in (5.186b) and is a special integral.

5.8 Factorizable and Exact Differential Equations

The depression of the order of a differential equation of order two (any order) has been based [section 5.6 (5.7)] on the omission of the independent or dependent variable and/or of lower order derivatives. Two additional methods of reduction of the solution of a differential equation to lower order apply to the cases of: (i) linear factorizable equations, when the differential operator can be split into factors (subsection 5.8.1); (ii) exact equations, when the differential equation of order N arises by P derivations of a differential equation of order $N - P$, either linear or non-linear (subsection 5.8.2).

5.8.1 Differential Equation with Factorizable Operator

If an *N*-th order differential equation cannot be reduced to first or second or some lower order, it may still be possible to decompose its solution into equations of lower order. *The* **factorizable linear differential equation** *of order N + M, involving (standard CXVII) the successive application of two differential operators or orders N, M:*

$$\left\{ P_N\left(\frac{d}{dx}\right)\left\{Q_M\left(\frac{d}{dx}\right)\right\}\right\} y(x) = B(x),$$
(5.187)

may be decomposed into the solution of an N-th order equation (5.188a):

$$\left\{ P_N\left(\frac{d}{dx}\right)\right\} w(x) = B(x), \qquad \left\{Q_M\left(\frac{d}{dx}\right)\right\} y(x) = w(x),$$
(5.188a, b)

followed by the solution of an M-th order equation (5.188b). As an example, we consider the linear second-order differential equation (5.189a):

$$1 = \left\{ \left(x\frac{d}{dx}-1\right)\left(\frac{d}{dx}-1\right)\right\} y(x) = x y'' - (1+x)y' + y,$$
(5.189a, b)

that can be decomposed in two linear first-order differential equations with homogeneous (5.190a) [constant (5.190b)] coefficients:

$$xw' = w + 1, \qquad y' - y = w.$$
(5.190a, b)

The linear second-order differential equation (5.189b) obtained (5.189a) by composition of (5.190a, b) has neither constant nor homogeneous coefficients. The former is a linear equation with homogeneous coefficients (5.190a), whose solution (3.20, 3.31a, b) is (5.191):

$$w = x\left\{ C_1 + \int \frac{dx}{x^2}\right\} = C_1 x - 1;$$
(5.191)

substituting (5.191) into (5.190b) leads to another linear equation, with constant coefficients (5.192a):

$$y' = y + C_1 x - 1, \qquad y = C_2 e^x - C_1 x + 1 - C_1,$$
(5.192a, b)

whose solution (5.192b) is the general integral of (5.189).

5.8.2 Exact Differential Equation of Any Order

If it is not possible to solve an N-th order differential equation, it may be possible to depress its order. For example, the solution of *an exact differential equation of order N*:

$$0 = F\left(x; y, y', ..., y^{(N)}\right) = \frac{d}{dx}\left\{G\left(x; y, y', ..., y^{(N-1)}\right)\right\}, \tag{5.193}$$

that is the derivative of a function is specified by setting the function equal to a constant (5.194), leading to a differential equation of order N − 1:

$$G\left(x, y, y', ..., y^{(N-1)}\right) = C_1. \tag{5.194}$$

If the latter is also an exact differential, the order of the equation can be depressed by one unit more, and so on, until an inexact equation is obtained and the process ceases to apply. Thus *an **exact differential equation** (5.195):*

$$0 = F\left(x, y, y', ..., y^{(N)}\right) = \frac{d^p}{dx^p}\left\{G\left(x, y, y', ..., y^{(N-P)}\right)\right\}, \tag{5.195}$$

that is (standard CXVIII) the derivative of order P < N of a function, is specified by setting the function equal to a polynomial of degree P − 1:

$$G\left(x, y, y', ..., y^{(N-P)}\right) = \sum_{n=0}^{P-1} C_{n+1} x^n, \tag{5.196}$$

that is a differential equation (5.196) of order N − P. As an example of (5.193, 5.194) consider the second-order differential equation (5.197):

$$0 = x y'' + (2 + x)y' + y = \left\{x y' + y(1 + x)\right\}', \tag{5.197}$$

that is an exact differential and leads to a first-order differential equation (5.198):

$$C_1 = x y' + y(1 + x) = (x y)' + x y; \tag{5.198}$$

the latter (5.198) is a linear first-order differential equation with constant coefficients for xy, whose solution is (5.199a):

$$x y = C_2 e^{-x} + C_1, \qquad y = \frac{C_1}{x} + C_2 \frac{e^{-x}}{x}, \tag{5.199a, b}$$

so that (5.199b) is the general integral of (5.197). The method of solution of exact differential equations (subsection 5.8.2) applies both to non-linear and linear equations, whereas the decomposition of the operator into factors (subsection 5.8.1) was presented only for linear equations (5.187); it could also be extended to non-linear operators, like the method for non-linear homogeneous equations that follows next (section 5.9).

5.9 Two Kinds of Non-Linear Homogeneous Differential Equations

Besides the preceding (sections 5.6–5.8), two more cases (section 5.9) when the order of a differential equation of order N can be depressed by unity are the homogeneous differential equation of the first (second) kind [subsection 5.9.1 (5.9.2)]; these may be non-linear as in the examples chosen [subsection 5.9.1 (5.9.3)].

5.9.1 Homogeneous Differential Equation of the First Kind

A case in which the order of a differential equation can be depressed by unity is the homogeneous equation, in which all terms have the same dimensions. If the independent variable x is dimensionless, the dependent variable y, the slope (5.200a), and all higher derivatives (5.200b) have the same dimension; this leads (standard CXIX) to (5.200c) an **homogeneous differential equation of the first kind and order** N:

$$y' \equiv \frac{dy}{dx}, y^{(N)} = \frac{d^N y}{dx^N}: \qquad 0 = F\left(\frac{y}{x}, y', y'', \ldots, y^{(N)}\right) = G\left(x, \frac{y'}{y}, \frac{y''}{y}, \ldots, \frac{y^{(N)}}{y}\right),$$

$$(5.200\text{a–d})$$

that generalizes the first-order homogeneous equation (3.127) that was solved using the change of variable $v = y/x$. In the form (5.200d), it is preferable to make the change of variable (5.201a):

$$u = \frac{y'}{y}, \qquad \frac{y''}{y} = \left(\frac{y'}{y}\right)' + \left(\frac{y'}{y}\right)^2 = u' + u^2, \qquad (5.201\text{a, b})$$

which, together with (5.201b) and successive expressions, leads to (5.200d) $\equiv$ (5.202a):

$$0 = G\left(x, u, u' + u^2, \ldots, u^{(N-1)} + \ldots\right) = H\left(x, u, u', \ldots, u^{(N-1)}\right), \qquad (5.202\text{a, b})$$

a differential equation (5.202b) of order $(N - 1)$.

For example, the second-order homogeneous differential equation of first kind (5.203a) corresponding to (5.200d) with $N = 2$ becomes a first-order equation (5.203b) in the variable (5.201a):

$$0 = F\left(x, \frac{y'}{y}, \frac{y''}{y}\right) = F\left(x, u, u' + u^2\right) = G(x, u, u'): \quad y(x) = C_2 \exp\left\{\int^x u(\xi; C_1) d\xi\right\},$$

$$(5.203\text{a–c})$$

whose solution $u(x; C_1)$ specifies (5.203c) the general integral of (5.203a). Thus, *a homogeneous differential equation of the first kind and order N has (standard CXIX) a dimensionless independent variable x, and hence is of the form (5.200c) ≡ (5.200d); it leads (5.200d) ≡ (5.201a) to a differential equation (5.202a) ≡ (5.202b) of order N − 1 by the change of dependent variable (5.201a). For example, the solution of the second-order homogeneous differential equation of the first kind (5.203a) reduces to the solution of a first-order differential equation (5.203b) plus a quadrature (5.203c).*

For example, the second-order homogeneous differential equation of first kind (5.204a):

$$0 = x\frac{y''}{y} - x\left(\frac{y'}{y}\right)^2 + \frac{y'}{y} = x\left(u' + u^2\right) - xu^2 + u = xu' + u = (xu)',\quad (5.204\text{a, b})$$

leads to a first-order equation (5.204b); its solution (5.205a):

$$xu = C_1,\quad y = C_2 \exp\left(\int^x \frac{C_1}{\xi} d\xi\right) = C_2 x^{C_1},\quad (5.205\text{a, b})$$

leads through (5.203c), to the general integral (5.205b) of (5.204a).

5.9.2 Homogeneous Differential Equation of the Second Kind

If the independent variable x has dimensions, the slope has dimensions (5.206a):

$$[y'] = \left[\frac{dy}{dx}\right] = \frac{[y]}{[x]},\qquad [y''] = \left[\frac{dy'}{dx}\right] = \frac{[y']}{[x]} = \frac{[y]}{[x]^2},\quad (5.206\text{a, b})$$

and the curvature has dimensions (5.206b); it follows by induction that the n-th derivative has dimensions (5.207a):

$$[y^{(n)}] = \frac{[y]}{[x]^n}:\qquad \left[x^n \frac{d^n y}{dx^n}\right] = [y],\quad (5.207\text{a, b})$$

and that the factors (5.207b) have the same dimension for all $n = 0, 1,, \ldots$. This leads (standard CXX) to an **homogeneous differential equation of second kind and order N:**

$$0 = F\left(y, y'x, y''x^2, \ldots, y^{(N)}x^N\right),\qquad(5.208)$$

that reduces, in the linear case (5.209a), to the Euler type (5.209b) $\equiv$ (1.291a) with homogeneous coefficients:

$$0 = F\left(y, y'x, y''x^2, \ldots y^{(N)}x^N\right) = \sum_{n=0}^{N} A_n\, x^n\, y^{(n)}(x),\qquad(5.209a, b)$$

involving homogeneous derivatives (1.292a–c). The latter was solved using the change of independent variable (1.288a) $\equiv$ (5.132a) that implies (5.210b–d), and:

$$x = e^t: \qquad \frac{dx}{dt} = e^t = x, \qquad \frac{dy}{dx} = \frac{dy}{dt}\frac{dt}{dx} = \frac{1}{x}\frac{dy}{dt}, \qquad \frac{d^2y}{dx^2} = -\frac{1}{x^2}\frac{dy}{dt} + \frac{1}{x^2}\frac{d^2y}{dt^2};$$
$$(5.210a\text{–}d)$$

the formulas (5.210c, d) suggest the change of dependent variable:

$$w = \frac{dy}{dt}, \qquad \frac{d^2y}{dt^2} = \frac{dw}{dt} = \frac{dw}{dy}\frac{dy}{dt} = w\frac{dw}{dy};\qquad(5.211a, b)$$

these (5.211a, b), together with (5.210c, d) yield:

$$x\frac{dy}{dx} = w, \qquad x^2\frac{d^2y}{dx^2} = -w + w\frac{dw}{dy},\qquad(5.212a, b)$$

that may be substituted into (5.208).

It has been shown that (standard CXX) *the N-th order homogeneous differential equation of the second kind (5.208) can have its order depressed by unity (5.213) by means of the changes of dependent (5.211a) and independent (5.210a) variable:*

$$0 = F\left(y, w, w\frac{dw}{dy}, \ldots\right) = G\left(y, w, w', \ldots, w^{(N-1)}\right).\qquad(5.213)$$

For example, the second-order equation (5.214a) is transformed to first-order (5.214b):

$$0 = F\left(y, y'x, y''x^2\right) = F\left(y, w, w\frac{dw}{dy} - w\right): \qquad w = w(y; C_1).\qquad(5.214a, b)$$

The solution (5.214c) of (5.214b) specifies the solution y(x) of (5.208) by:

$$x = \exp\left\{\int dt\right\} = \exp\left\{\log C_2 + \int \frac{dy}{dy/dt}\right\} = C_2 \exp\left\{\int^y \frac{d\xi}{w(\xi;C_1)}\right\}, \qquad (5.215)$$

where (5.210a) and (5.211a) were used.

5.9.3 Depression of the Order of Homogeneous Differential Equations

The depression of the order by unity applies to the homogeneous differential equations both of the first (second) kind [subsection 5.9.1 (5.9.2)], including the non-linear cases chosen as examples [subsection 5.9.1 (5.9.3)]. Consider as example the second-order homogeneous differential equation of second kind (5.216a) that leads (5.212a, b) to (5.216b):

$$0 = x^2 y'' - 2xy'y = w\left(\frac{dw}{dy} - 1 - 2y\right); \qquad (5.216a, b)$$

the factor (5.217a) ≡ (5.217b) in (5.216b) represents a special integral (5.217c):

$$w = 0: \qquad\qquad y' = 0, \qquad\qquad y(x) = C_0, \qquad\qquad (5.217a\text{–}c)$$

involving only one constant of integration, instead of two for the general integral of a second-order equation. The general integral is obtained by solving the second factor in (5.216b), namely (5.218):

$$\frac{dw}{dy} = 1 + 2y: \qquad w = y^2 + y + \frac{1}{4} + (C_1)^2 = \left(y + \frac{1}{2}\right)^2 + (C_1)^2 = \frac{dy}{dt}, \qquad (5.218a\text{–}c)$$

whose integral is (5.218b); using (5.211a) leads to a differential equation (5.218c) for $y(t)$. The solution for $y(x)$ follows using (5.215):

$$x = \exp\left\{\int dt\right\} = \exp\left\{\int \frac{dy}{(y+1/2)^2 + (C_1)^2}\right\}$$

$$= \exp\left\{\frac{1}{C_1} arc\tan\left(\frac{y+1/2}{C_1}\right) + \log C_2\right\}, \qquad (5.219a)$$

leading to:

$$x = C_2 \exp\left\{\frac{1}{C_1} arc\tan\left(\frac{y+1/2}{C_1}\right)\right\}, \qquad (5.219b)$$

that specifies the general integral (5.219b) of (5.216a). The general integral (5.219b) does not contain the special integral (5.217c) for any finite value of the constants (C_1, C_2).

NOTE 5.1: Elementary Exact Solutions of Differential Equations

The consideration of ordinary differential equations has concentrated in cases for which exact analytical solutions may be obtained in finite terms using elementary functions, namely: (i) linear differential equations of any order with constant (homogeneous) coefficients [sections 1.3–1.5 (1.6–1.8)]; (ii) first-order differential equations including variable coefficients and non-linear and without (with) singular integrals [chapter 3 (section 5.1–5.5)]; and (iii) second and higher differential equations including non-linear and variable coefficients. The five methods of solution, namely variation of parameters and Green functions (Fourier series and integrals and Laplace transforms) apply to differential equations of any order but mostly [notes 1.1–1.8 (1.9–1.28)] linear with variable (constant) coefficients. The second-order differential equations have many important applications, including: (i) the second-order system with constant coefficients (chapter 2); and (ii) its extensions either with non-linear and/or with variable coefficients (chapter 4). Considering a linear second-order differential equation with variable coefficients, it has been shown that using different changes of dependent variable it can be transformed into: (i) a non-linear first-order differential equation of Ricatti type (subsections 3.6.1–3.6.4); (ii) a second-order linear self-adjoint differential equation (subsections III.7.7.1–III.7.7.6). Next are considered (notes 5.1–5.20) some additional properties of second-order linear differential equations with variable coefficients.

NOTE 5.2: Linear Second-Order Differential Equations with Variable Coefficients

If a particular integral is known for (note 5.3) a linear unforced second-order differential equation with variable coefficients: (i) another linearly independent particular integral can be obtained, leading to the general integral of the unforced differential equation (note 5.4); and (ii) a particular integral of the forced differential equation can also be obtained by the method of variation of parameters leading to the complete integral (notes 1.2–1.4) or otherwise (note 5.5). A linear second-order differential equation with variable coefficients can be transformed, via different changes of dependent variable, into three alternative equivalent forms: (i) a non-linear first-order integro-differential equation (note 5.6); (ii) a linear second-order differential equation with a self-adjoint operator (note 5.7); or (iii) a linear invariant second-order differential equation omitting the first-order derivative (note 5.8). Thus (iii) the second-order linear differential equation can be put into an invariant form with the independent variable appearing only in one coefficient, showing how two apparently distinct linear second-order differential equations that have the same invariant form can be transformed into each other (note 5.9).

A constant positive (negative) invariant leads (note 5.10) to an oscillation with constant amplitude (an exponential growth or decay). In the case
of a variable coefficient that is a function of the independent variable, its
zeros correspond to turning points (note 5.11) across which the nature of
solution of the differential equation changes: for a turning point of the
first (second) kind the oscillatory solution on one side changes the a decay
(instability) on the other side (note 5.11). An example of a turning point of
the second kind is the transition from propagating to evanescent electromagnetic waves (note 5.12) in a medium with variable propagation speed
(note 5.13). The waves are sinusoidal (non-sinusoidal) in a medium with
constant (variable) propagation speed (note 5.14). The case of propagation
speed varying slowly in the scale of a wavelength (note 5.16) leads to the
ray approximation (note 5.15) that can be extended from the first (note 5.17)
to the second (note 5.18) order approximation. The ray approximation
applies (note 5.20) to high-frequency waves in weakly inhomogeneous
media (note 5.19), that is to light (sound) rays in the case of electromagnetic
(acoustic) waves (note 5.16).

NOTE 5.3: Singularities of a Linear Second-Order Differential Equation

A linear forced second-order differential equation (5.220b) corresponds to
(1.33) with $N = 2$:

$$A_2(x) \neq 0: \qquad A_2(x)\, y''(x) + A_1(x) y'(x) + A_0(x)\, y(x) = B(x). \qquad \text{(5.220a, b)}$$

*The linear differential equation (5.110b) of the second-order is non-singular if the
coefficient of the highest-order derivative is non-zero (5.220a), allowing (problem 161)
division (5.221a) so that the coefficient of the highest order derivative becomes unity
in (5.221b):*

$$\{P, Q, F\} = \frac{1}{A_2}\{A_1, A_0, B\}: \quad y''(x) + P(x)\, y'(x) + Q(x)\, y(x) = F(x). \qquad \text{(5.221a, b)}$$

A point where the coefficient of the highest-order derivative (5.220a) vanishes $A(x_c) = 0$ is a **singularity** of the differential equation (5.220b), where
some or all the coefficients (5.221a) of the alternative form (5.221b) of the same
differential equation may become infinite. The second-order derivative cannot be calculated from the differential equation (5.220a, b) $\equiv$ (5.221a, b) at a
singular point $x = x_s$ because $A(x_s) = 0$; thus, a Taylor series expansion about
the singular point may fail at the second term, and the solution of the differential equation may not exist in an analytic or non-singular form. The
solution of the general second-order linear differential equation (5.220a, b) $\equiv$
(5.221a, b) is not known; however, if a particular integral is known (note 5.4)
both the general (complete) integrals of the unforced (forced) differential

equation (5.220a, b) ≡ (5.221a, b) can be obtained [note 5.5 (5.6)] starting with a transformed equation indicated next. Replacing the dependent variable by the product of two functions (5.222a), the differential equation (5.221b) leads to (5.222b):

$$y = uv: \qquad v(u'' + Pu' + Qu) + v'(2u' + Pu) + v''u = F, \qquad (5.222a, b)$$

that will be used: (i) to obtain the complete integral of the forced differential equation from a particular integral of the unforced equation (note 5.4); (ii) to reduce the differential equation to an invariant form omitting the first-order derivative (note 5.5).

NOTE 5.4: General Integral Derived from a Particular Integral

Assuming that a particular integral of the unforced differential equation (5.220b) is known (5.223a):

$$y_1'' + Py_1' + Qy_1 = 0: \qquad y = y_1 v, \qquad v'(2y_1' + Py_1) + v''y_1 = F, \qquad (5.223a–c)$$

choosing $y_1 \equiv u$ and $y_2 \equiv v$ in (5.222a) leads (5.233b) to (5.223c). The latter (5.223c) ≡ (5.224a) is a linear differential equation for v' with coefficients (5.224b, c):

$$v'' = P_1 v' + Q_1: \qquad P_1 = -P - 2\frac{y_1'}{y_1}, \qquad Q_1 = \frac{F}{y_1}. \qquad (5.224a–c)$$

The method of integration (3.20a; 3.31a, b) leads to (5.225a–c):

$$X(x) = \exp\left\{ -\int^x \left[P(\xi) + 2\frac{y_1'}{y_1(\xi)} \right] d\xi \right\} = \frac{1}{[y_1(x)]^2} \exp\left\{ -\int^x P(\xi)\, d\xi \right\}, \qquad (5.225a)$$

$$Y(x) = \int^x \frac{F(\xi)}{y_1(\xi)} \frac{d\xi}{X(\xi)} = \int^x f(\xi) y_1(\xi) \exp\left(\int^\xi P(\eta)\, d\eta \right) d\xi, \qquad (5.225b)$$

$$v(x) = C_1 + \int^\xi v'(\xi)\, d\xi = C_1 + \int^x X(\xi)[C_2 + Y(\xi)]\, d\xi = \frac{y(x)}{y_1(x)}; \qquad (5.225c)$$

from (5.225d) follows the general (compete) integral of the unforced (forced) differential equation (5.221b) with $f = 0 (f \neq 0)$.

NOTE 5.5: Passage from a Particular to the Complete Integral

It has been shown that *if a particular integral of a linear unforced second-order differential equation with variable coefficients (5.223a) is known then: (i) another integral (problem 162) is given by the second term of (5.225c) ≡ (5.226a–c):*

$$y_2(x) = y_1(x) \int^x X(\xi)\, d\xi \quad X(x) = \frac{\Phi(x)}{\left[y_1(x)\right]^2}, \quad \Phi(x) \equiv \exp\left\{ -\int^x P(\xi)\, d\xi \right\};$$

$$(5.226a–c)$$

(ii) the two particular integrals are linearly independent and thus the general integral (problem 163) of the unforced differential equation is given by the first two terms of (5.225c) ≡ (5.227) where (C_1, C_2) are arbitrary constants of integration:

$$y(x) = C_1\, y_1(x) + C_2\, y_2(x) + y_*(x); \qquad (5.227)$$

(iii) adding the third term in (5.227) ≡ (5.225c) specifies the complete integral (problem 164) of the forced differential equation (5.221b), where (5.228a) involves (5.225a) ≡ (5.226a) and (5.225b) ≡ (5.228b):

$$y_*(x) = y_1(x) \int^x X(\xi) Y(\xi)\, d\xi, \quad Y(x) = \int^x \frac{F(\xi)}{y_1(\xi)} \frac{d\xi}{X(\xi)} = \int^x F(\xi) \frac{y_1(\xi)}{\Phi(\xi)}\, d\xi,$$

$$(5.228a–c)$$

is a particular integral of the forced differential equation involving no constants of integration. For example, the linear forced second-order differential equation (5.229a) has variable coefficients (5.229b–d):

$$y'' - xy' + y = x^a: \qquad \{P, Q, F\} = \{-x, 1, x^a\}. \qquad (5.229a–d)$$

The unforced equation (5.229a) has particular integral (5.230a) leading (5.226a, b) to another linearly independent particular integral (5.230b, c):

$$y_1(x) = x, \quad X(x) = \frac{1}{x^2} \exp\left(\int^x \xi\, d\xi \right) = \frac{1}{x^2} \exp\left(\frac{x^2}{2} \right), \quad y_2(x) = x \int^x \exp\left(\frac{\xi^2}{2} \right) \frac{d\xi}{\xi^2};$$

$$(5.230a–c)$$

the general integral of the unforced differential equation corresponds to the first two terms of (5.227) with (5.230a, c). The complete integral (5.227) of the forced differential equation (5.229a) adds (5.228a, b), that is:

$$Y(x) = \int^x \xi^{a+1} \exp\left(-\frac{\xi^2}{2}\right) d\xi, \qquad y_*(x) = x \int^x X(\xi) Y(\xi) d\xi, \qquad (5.231a, b)$$

involving (5.230b). The linear second-order differential equation (5.221b) can be written in three alternative and equivalent forms: (i) as a non-linear first-order differential or integro–differential equation (note 5.6); (ii) a linear second-order differential equation involving a self-adjoint operator (note 5.7); or (iii) as an invariant linear second-order differential equation omitting the term with the first-order derivative (note 5.8).

NOTE 5.6: Transformation to a Non-linear First-Order Integro-Differential Equation

The linear second-order differential equation (5.221b) can be rewritten:

$$\frac{F}{y} = \frac{y''}{y} + P\frac{y'}{y} + Q = Q + P\frac{y'}{y} + \left(\frac{y'}{y}\right)' + \left(\frac{y'}{y}\right)^2, \qquad (5.232)$$

suggesting the change of dependent variable:

$$u = \frac{y'}{y} = (\log y)': \qquad y(x) = \exp\left\{\int^x u(\xi) d\xi\right\}. \qquad (5.233a\text{–}c)$$

Substituting (5.233a, c) in (5.232) leads to:

$$u' + u^2 + Pu + Q = F(x) \exp\left\{-\int^x u(\xi) d\xi\right\}. \qquad (5.234)$$

It has been shown that *a forced linear second-order differential equation with variable coefficients (5.321b) is transformed via the change of dependent variable (5.233a–c) into (problem 164) a non-linear first-order integro-differential equation (5.234). In the absence of forcing (5.235a):*

$$F = 0: \qquad y'' + Py' + Q = 0 \quad \leftrightarrow \quad u' = -Q - Pu - u^2, \qquad (5.235a\text{–}c)$$

the linear second-order differential equation with variable coefficients (5.235b) is transformed, via the change of dependent variable (5.233c), into a non-linear first-order differential equation (5.235c) of Riccati type (3.58), in agreement with subsection 3.6.1–3.6.4.

NOTE 5.7: Transformation to a Self-Adjoint Differential Operator

A linear second-order self-adjoint differential operator (subsections III.7.7.1–III.7.7.5) is (problem 165) specified by (III.7.97b) ≡ (5.236a, b):

$$0 = \left(Ry'\right)' + Sy - T = Ry'' + R'y' + Sy - T. \tag{5.236a, b}$$

The general linear second-order differential equation with variable coefficients (5.221b) can be transformed into a self-adjoint form (5.236a) if and only if (5.236b) equals P times (5.221b):

$$Ry'' + R'y' + Sy - T = R\left(y'' + Py' + Q - F\right). \tag{5.237}$$

In (5.237) the coefficients (P,Q,F) of the general linear second-order differential equation with variable coefficients (5.221b) are assumed to be known, and the coefficients (R,S,T) of the self-adjoint form (5.236a) ≡ (5.236b) are to be determined. They are related by three equations:

$$R' = RP, \qquad S = RQ, \qquad T = RF. \tag{5.238a–c}$$

The first equation (5.238a) leads to (5.239a):

$$P = \frac{R'}{R} = \left(\log R\right)' : \qquad R(x) = \exp\left\{\int^x P(\xi)d\xi\right\}, \tag{5.239a, b}$$

suggesting that (5.221b) be multiplied by (5.239b):

$$\exp\left(\int^x P(\xi)d\xi\right)(F - Qy) = \exp\left(\int^x P(\xi)d\xi\right)(y'' + Py')$$

$$= \frac{d}{dx}\left[y'\exp\left(\int^x P(\xi)d\xi\right)\right]. \tag{5.239c}$$

The latter (5.239c) ≡ (5.236a) is in self-adjoint form with coefficients (5.239b) and (5.240a):

$$\{T(x), S(x)\} = \exp\left(\int^x P(\xi)d\xi\right)\{F(x), Q(x)\} = R(x)\{F(x), Q(x)\}, \tag{5.240a, b}$$

in agreement with (5.240b) ≡ (5.238b, c). It has been shown that *multiplication of the linear second-order differential equation with variable coefficients (5.221b) by (5.239b) leads (problem 165) to the self-adjoint form (5.236a) ≡ (5.236b) with coefficients (5.240a, b).*

NOTE 5.8: Invariant Form of a Linear Second-Order Differential Equation

Another use of (5.222b) is to eliminate the coefficient of v' by choosing (5.241a):

$$2u' + P\,u = 0, \qquad \frac{du}{u} = -\frac{P}{2}dx, \qquad u(x) = \exp\left\{-\frac{1}{2}\int^x P(\xi)d\xi\right\},$$
$$(5.241a\text{--}c)$$

that implies (5.241b), leading to (5.241c) where the constant of integration was omitted. Using (5.241c) in (5.222a) it follows that *the change of dependent variable (5.242a) transforms the general linear forced second-order differential equation (5.221b) into (problem 166) the **invariant form** (5.242b):*

$$v(x) = y(x)\exp\left\{\frac{1}{2}\int^x P(\xi)\,d\xi\right\}: \qquad v''(x) + I(x)v(x) = G(x), \qquad (5.242a, b)$$

that: (i) omits the first-order derivative; (ii) hence has a single non-forcing invariant coefficient (5.243a) and changes the forcing term to (5.243b):

$$I(x) = Q(x) - \frac{P'(x)}{2} - \frac{1}{4}[P(x)]^2, \quad G(x) = F(x)\exp\left\{\frac{1}{2}\int^x P(\xi)d\xi\right\}. \quad (5.243a, b)$$

The proof follows substituting (5.241a) in (5.222b) that simplifies to (5.244a):

$$v'' + \left(Q + P\frac{u'}{u} + \frac{u''}{u}\right)v = \frac{F}{u}: \qquad G = \frac{F}{u}, \qquad (5.244a, b)$$

that coincides with (5.242b) with the: (i) forcing term (5.244b; 5.241c) ≡ (5.243b); (ii) coefficient (5.245a):

$$I = Q + P\frac{u'}{u} + \frac{u''}{u} = Q - \frac{P^2}{2} + \left(\frac{u'}{u}\right)' + \left(\frac{u'}{u}\right)^2 = Q - \frac{P^2}{4} - \frac{P'}{2}, \qquad (5.245a\text{--}c)$$

where (5.241a) was used to obtain (5.245b) ≡ (5.245c) ≡ (5.243a). For example, in the case of the linear second-order differential equation (5.229a) with coefficients (5.229b–d) ≡ (5.245a) ≡ (5.243a), the standard invariant form (5.242b) can be used (Note 5.9) to: (i) compare two linear second-order differential equations; (ii) find a transformation between the two differential equations and their solutions.

NOTE 5.9: Transformation or Equivalence of Differential Equations

As an example of reduction to the invariant form (5.242b), consider the linear second-order differential equation (5.229a) with coefficients (5.229b–d). The change (5.242a) of dependent variable (5.246a) suppresses the first-order derivative in (5.246b):

$$v(x) = y(x)\exp\left(-\frac{x^2}{4}\right): \qquad v'' + \left(\frac{1}{2} - \frac{x^2}{4}\right)v = x^a\exp\left(-\frac{x^2}{4}\right), \qquad (5.246a, b)$$

using the invariant (5.243a) and forcing term (5.234b). Next consider the linear second-order differential equation (5.247):

$$z'' + \frac{4}{x}z' + \left(\frac{1}{2} + \frac{2}{x^2} - \frac{x^2}{4}\right)z = x^{a-2}\exp\left(-\frac{x^2}{4}\right), \qquad (5.247)$$

that includes the first-order derivative:

$$\{P_2, Q_2, F_2\} = \left\{\frac{4}{x}, \frac{1}{2} + \frac{2}{x^2} - \frac{x^2}{4}, x^{a-2}\exp\left(-\frac{x^2}{4}\right)\right\}. \qquad (5.248a–c)$$

It is transformed to the invariant form (5.242b); (i) using (5.242a) the change of dependent variable (5.249a); (ii) leading (5.243a) to the invariant (5.249b); (iii) and (5.242b) to the forcing term (5.249c):

$$v(x) = z(x)\exp\left(-2\int^x \frac{d\xi}{\xi}\right) = \frac{z(x)}{x^2}; \qquad (5.249a)$$

$$I(x) = Q_2(x) - \frac{[P_2(x)]^2}{4} - \frac{P_2'(x)}{2} = \frac{1}{2} - \frac{x^2}{4}; \qquad (5.249b)$$

$$G_2(x) = F_2(x)\exp\left(-2\int^x \frac{d\xi}{\xi}\right) = x^2 F_2(x) = x^a\exp\left(-\frac{x^2}{4}\right). \qquad (5.249c)$$

The invariant (5.249b) and forcing term (5.249c) lead to the same invariant differential equation (5.246b). Thus *the distinct linear second-order differential equations (5.229a) ≠ (5.247) have the same invariant form (5.246b) and therefore (problem 167) their solutions are related by (5.246a) ≡ (5.249a) ≡ (5.250):*

$$y(x)\exp\left(-\frac{x^2}{4}\right) = v(x) = \frac{z(x)}{x^2}. \tag{5.250}$$

Since a linear differential equation of the second-order (5.220a, b) ≡ (5.221a, b) can always be reduced to the simpler invariant form (5.242b), the latter is used in the sequel to give a physical interpretation (notes 5.10–5.20) of the preceding mathematical results (notes 5.2–5.9) in terms of waves.

NOTE 5.10: Cases of Constant/Variable Positive/Negative Invariant

Considering the linear second-order ordinary differential equation (5.251b) with constant invariant (5.251a) there are (problem 168) three possibilities:

$$I(x)=const:\quad \Psi''(x)+I(x)\Psi(x)=0;\quad \begin{cases} I=k^2>0: & \Psi(x)=C_+\,e^{ikx}+C_-\,e^{-ikx}, \\ I=0: & \Psi(x)=C_1+C_2\,x, \\ I=-k^2<0: & \Psi(x)=C_+e^{Kx}+C_-\,e^{-Kx}, \end{cases}$$
$$\tag{5.251a–e}$$

namely (Figure 5.18): (i) if the invariant is positive the solution is oscillatory (5.251c); (ii) if the invariant is negative the solution is exponentially increasing or decreasing (5.251e); (iii) in the intermediate case of zero invariant the solution is linear (5.251d). Considering a non-constant (5.252a) invariant (Figure 5.19) of the differential equation (5.252b):

$$I(x)\ne const:\quad \Psi''+I(x)\Psi=0:\quad \begin{cases} I(x)>0 & \Psi \text{ is oscillatory,} \\ I(x_r)=0 & \Psi \text{ has a turning point,} \\ I(x)<0 & \Psi \text{ is monotonic,} \end{cases}$$
$$\tag{5.252a–e}$$

*three cases (problem 169) arise: (i) where it is positive (5.252c) there are oscillatory solutions like (5.251c); (iii) where it is negative (5.252e) there are monotonic solutions like (5.251e); (ii) where it vanishes (5.252d) there is a **turning point** separating oscillatory from exponentially (a) decaying or (b) growing solutions, that are considered next (note 5.11).*

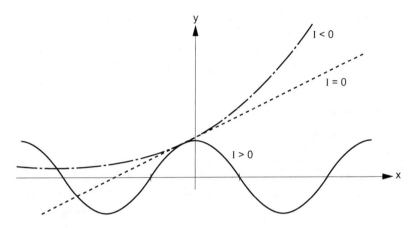

FIGURE 5.18
The linear unforced second-order differential equation in invariant form (5.251b) with constant invariant (5.251a) leads to: (i) oscillations with constant amplitude for positive invariant (5.251c); (iii) exponential growth or decay for negative invariant (5.251e) (ii) linear variation (5.251d) for zero invariant; that is, in the case separating (i) and (iii).

NOTE 5.11: **Turning Points of Two Kinds**

A turning point is (5.252d) a root of the invariant, and if it is a simple root the latter is of the form (5.253a):

$$I(x) \sim \alpha^2 (x - x_r): \qquad\qquad \Psi'' + \alpha^2 (x - x_r)\Psi = 0, \qquad\qquad (5.253a, b)$$

leading (problem 170) to an **Airy (1838) differential equation** (5.253b), whose exact solution will be considered subsequently (subsection 9.4.14). A first approximation, that will be improved in the sequel (notes 5.13–5.17),

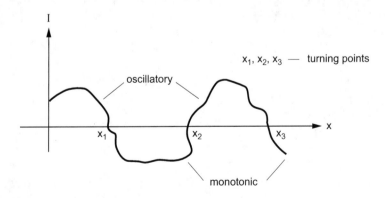

FIGURE 5.19
The vanishing (5.252d) of the invariant of the linear unforced second-order differential equation (5.252b) specifies turning points separating regions of oscillatory (5.252c) and monotonic (5.252e) solutions.

is to treat the invariant (5.253a) as a constant (5.251a, b) leading to (5.151c, e) ≡ (5.254a, b):

$$\Psi_\pm(x) \sim \begin{cases} A\exp\left[\pm i\alpha|x-x_r|^{1/2}\right] & \text{if} \quad x>x_r, \\ A\exp\left[\pm\alpha|x-x_r|^{1/2}\right] & \text{if} \quad x<x_r, \end{cases}$$

(5.254a, b)

solutions that are: (i) oscillatory after the turning point (5.255a) with constant amplitude (5.255b):

$$x>x_r: \qquad |\Psi_\pm(x)| = A; \qquad \lim_{x\to-\infty}\Psi_+(x)=\infty, \qquad \lim_{x\to-\infty}\Psi_-(x)=0,$$

(5.255a–d)

(ii) exponentially growing (a) [decaying (b)] for Ψ_+ (Ψ_-) before the turning point (5.255c) [(5.255d)]. The cases (a) [(b)] of (5.254b) lead to the turning point of the first (second) kind [Figure 5.20 (5.21)] that are considered (note 5.12) after discussion of the oscillatory regime (5.254a) that applies in both cases. In the oscillatory regime (5.156a) may be introduced (5.254a) ≡ (5.256b):

$$x>x_r: \qquad A\exp\left\{\pm i\alpha|x-x_r|^{1/2}\right\} = \Psi_\pm(x) = A\exp\left[\pm i(x-x_r)K(x)\right],$$

(5.256a, b)

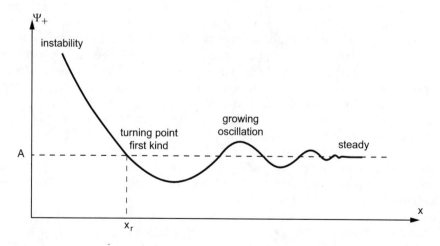

FIGURE 5.20
One example of turning point of the first kind is a steady state that develops growing oscillations as the turning point is approached, leading to a monotonic instability beyond, which is asymptotically exponentially growing.

a **local wavenumber** (5.157a) and a **local wavelength** (5.257b) ≡ (5.257c):

$$K(x) = \alpha |x - x_r|^{-1/2} = \frac{2\pi}{\lambda(x)}: \qquad \lambda(x) = \frac{2\pi}{\alpha} |x - x_r|^{1/2} ; \qquad (5.257a\text{–}c)$$

the designation local wavenumber (wavelength) emphasizes that the oscillation is not sinusoidal, so there is no global wavenumber (wavelength) and (5.257a) [(5.257c)] is just a local approximation. As the turning point is approached the wavelength tends to zero (5.257b), the wavenumber diverges (5.257c), and the wave field reduces to the amplitude (5.257c) with zero phase:

$$\lim_{x \to x_r + 0} \{ \Psi_\pm(x), \ \lambda(x), \ K(x) \} = \{ A, 0, \infty \}; \qquad (5.257a\text{–}c)$$

$$\lim_{x \to \infty} \{ |\Psi_\pm(x)|, \ \lambda(x), \ K(x) \} = \{ A, \infty, 0 \}, \qquad (5.258a\text{–}c)$$

far from the turning point on the propagation side the wavenumber tends to zero (5.258c) as the wavelength tends to infinity (5.258b) with constant amplitude (5.257a) and increasing phase.

NOTE 5.12: Transitions from Steadiness to Instability and Between Light and Darkness

The case (a) of a **turning point of first kind** is illustrated in Figure 5.20: (i) the system is in a steady state with constant amplitude far from the turning point $x \gg x_r$; (ii) as the turning point is approached $x \to x_r + 0$ there are oscillations with constant amplitude; (iii) beyond the turning point $x < x_r$ there is monotonic instability; (iv) at large distance $x \ll x_r$ there is growth like the exponential of a square root. The linear description remains valid as long as the amplitude is not too large. The opposite case (b) is a **turning point of the second kind** illustrated in Figure 5.21 as the transition from light to shadow behind an opaque obstacle (i) far from the turning point $\theta \gg \theta_r$ the light is steady with constant intensity; (ii) as the turning point is approached $\theta \to \theta_r + 0$ the interference with waves diffracted by the edge of the obstacle leads to oscillations of intensity; (iii) beyond the turning point into the shadow zone the intensity decays; (iv) far into the shadow zone the exponential decay leads to darkness. A similar transition occurs for the total reflection (zone of silence) for wave scattering by the interface between two media (chapter I.22), the turning point is the angle of incidence for total reflection (zone of silence). Another case of turning point concerns the vibrations of a membrane under variable tension (example 10.12). Next is given as an example of turning point of the second kind the propagation of electromagnetic waves in a refracting medium with non-uniform speed of light (note 5.13).

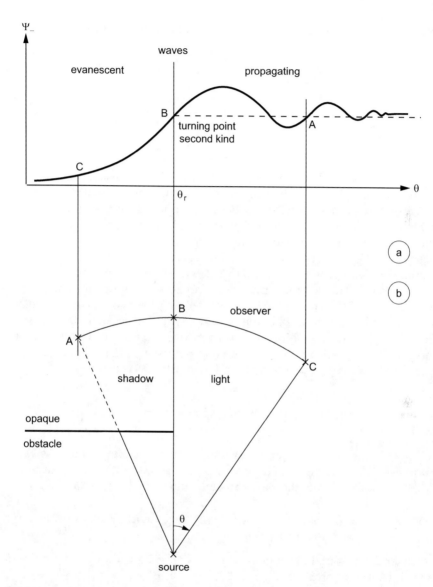

FIGURE 5.21
The examples of a turning point of the second kind (Figure 5.21) opposite to the first kind (Figure 5.20) include the transition from light to shadow due to the presence of an obstacle: (i) far from the obstacle at *C*, the observer receives light with constant intensity; (ii) as the observer approaches the position *B* corresponding to a turning point θ_r for the direction angle θ the waves diffracted from the edge of the obstacle interfere causing growing oscillations; (iii) beyond the boundary *B* between light and shadow the oscillations cease and the waves become evanescent; (iv) as the observer moves to the position *A*, into the shadow zone far from the line-of-sight *B* from the edge of the obstacle, the exponential decay leads to total darkness.

NOTE 5.13: **Electromagnetic Waves in a Medium with Non-Uniform Wave Speed**

The propagation of electromagnetic waves (2.39a, b) ≡ (5.258e) is described (problem 171) by the classical wave equation:

$$\Phi = \{\vec{E}, \vec{B}\}, q = 0 = \vec{J}, \alpha_e = 0, c_{em} = c(x): \quad \frac{1}{\left[c(x)\right]^2} \frac{\partial^2 \Phi}{\partial t^2} = \frac{\partial^2 \Phi}{\partial x^2} + \frac{\partial^2 \Phi}{\partial y^2} + \frac{\partial^2 \Phi}{\partial z^2},$$

$$(5.258a-e)$$

where: (i) the dependent or wave variable is any Cartesian component (5.258a) of the electric field or magnetic induction; (ii) there are no wave sources, that is, the medium is devoid (5.258b) of electric charges or currents; (iii) the electrical resistivity is neglected (5.258c), corresponding to infinite conductivity so that waves are not dissipated as they propagate; and (iv) in the classical wave equation (5.258e) the speed of propagation of electromagnetic waves (5.258d) is assumed to depend only on one coordinate x in the direction of non-uniformity of the medium. The electromagnetic wave equation in a steady inhomogeneous medium (note 7.14) is not of the form (5.258e); the latter will be considered next as the expression often used in the literature with the variation of wave speed interpreted as **index of refraction** of the medium. Since the properties of the medium do not depend on time t or on the transverse Cartesian coordinates (y, z) a Fourier integral representation (1.549c) ≡ (5.259) is used:

$$\Phi(x,y,z,t) = \int_{-\infty}^{+\infty} d\omega \int_{-\infty}^{+\infty} dk_y \int_{-\infty}^{+\infty} dk_z \, \Psi(x; k_x, k_y, \omega) \exp\left[i\left(k_y y + k_z z - \omega t\right)\right], \quad (5.259)$$

where Ψ is the **spectrum** for a wave of **frequency** ω and **transverse wave-numbers** (k_y, k_z) in the directions (y, z) at the position x. The implication of (5.259) is (Note 5.14) that the waves are non-sinusoidal (sinusoidal) in x (y, z, t).

NOTE 5.14: **Non-sinusoidal (Sinusoidal) Waves with Variable (Constant) Speed of Propagation**

Consider a sinusoidal oscillation with constant frequency ω and amplitude A at (5.260a) position $x = 0$:

$$\Phi(0,t) = A\cos(\omega t): \qquad \Phi(x;t) = A\cos\left\{\omega\left[t \mp \int_0^x \frac{d\xi}{c(\xi)}\right]\right\}, \qquad (5.260a, b)$$

and add a non-uniform speed of propagation $c(x)$ in (5.260b). In (5.260b) the upper- (lower +) sign corresponds to propagation to the right (left); that is, the positive (negative) x-direction. The effect of the speed of propagation can be simulated (Figure 5.22) assuming a harmonic oscillation (5.260a) with frequency ω and amplitude A and pulling the paper with propagation velocity

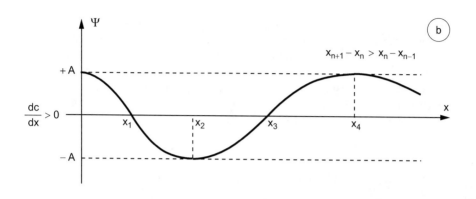

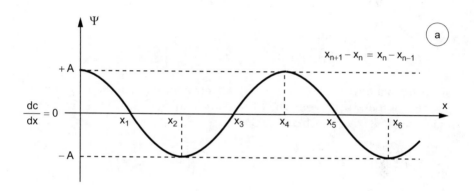

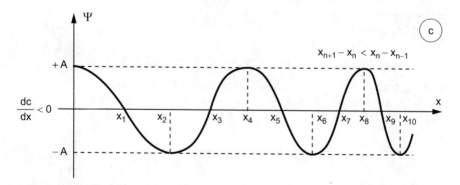

FIGURE 5.22
Consider a harmonic oscillation in time with frequency ω and amplitude A at $x = 0$: (i) pulling the paper with uniform velocity c leads to a sinusoidal wave with equally spaced zeros or nodes (Figure 5.22b); (ii/iii) pulling the paper with increasing (decreasing) velocity leads (Figure 5.22a (c)] to a non-sinusoidal wave with nodes increasingly (decreasingly) spaced.

$c(x)$ in the x-direction. If the speed of propagation is constant (Figure 5.22b) the waves are sinusoidal with equally spaced zeros or **nodes**; if the propagation speed increases (decreases) with distance [Figure 5.22a (c)] the nodes become progressively more (less) spaced and the waves are no longer sinusoidal.

Since the wave speed does not depend on time t [and on the transverse coordinates (y, z)] the waves are sinusoidal, and differentiation corresponds (5.261a–c) to multiplication by the frequency (transverse wavenumber) times $-i(+i)$:

$$\left\{\frac{\partial}{\partial t},\frac{\partial}{\partial y},\frac{\partial}{\partial z},\frac{\partial}{\partial x}\right\}\Phi(x,y,z,t) \;\leftrightarrow\; \left\{-i\omega,ik_y,ik_z,\frac{d}{dx}\right\}\Psi(x;k_y,k_z,\omega);$$

$$(5.261\text{a–c})$$

substitution of (5.261a–c) in (5.258e) leads to:

$$\frac{d^2\Psi}{dx^2}+\left[\frac{\omega^2}{\left[c(x)\right]^2}-\left(k_x\right)^2-\left(k_y\right)^2\right]\Psi=0, \qquad (5.262)$$

showing that (problem 172) the waves are not sinusoidal in the x-direction of variable of the wave speed. The differential equation (5.262) is of the invariant form (5.242b) ≡ (5.252b) ≡ (5.263a):

$$\frac{d^2\Psi}{dx^2}+\left[K(x)\right]^2\Psi=0:\quad I(x)=\left[K(x)\right]^2=\frac{\omega^2}{\left[c(x)\right]^2}-k^2,\quad k^2\equiv\left(k_y\right)^2+\left(k_y\right)^2,$$

$$(5.263\text{a–c})$$

where: (i) the **transverse wavenumber** (5.263c) is constant; (ii) the **longitudinal wavenumber** (5.263b) depends on position, and its square plays the role of invariant.

NOTE 5.15: Transition from Propagating to Evanescent Waves

The turning points correspond to zero longitudinal wavenumber. For example, if the wave speed is monotonic increasing (5.264a) there is a single turning point (5.264b):

$$\frac{dc}{dx}>0:\qquad K(x_r)=0 \quad\Leftrightarrow\quad c(x_r)=\pm\frac{\omega}{k}, \qquad (5.264\text{a–c})$$

where the propagation speed (5.264c) equals the wave frequency divided by the transverse wavenumber (Figure 5.23). Thus:

$$\Psi_\pm(x;k_y,k_x,\omega)\sim C_\pm\times\begin{cases}\exp\left(\pm i|K|x\right) & \text{if}\quad x\ll x_r & (5.265\text{a})\\[2mm]\exp\left(\mp|K|x\right) & \text{if}\quad x\gg x_r, & (5.265\text{b})\end{cases}$$

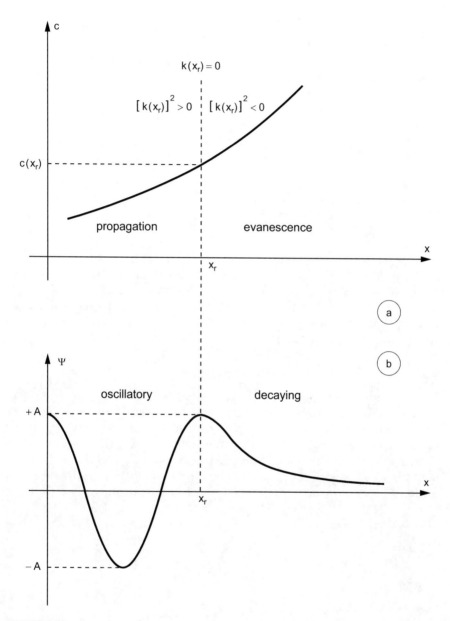

FIGURE 5.23
The transition between light (and darkness) occurs (Figure 5.21) for: (a) wave transmission (total reflection) at an interface between two media (Figure I.22.1), that is a discontinuity in wave speed; (b) for gradual variation of the wave speed in a non-uniform medium. An example of case (b) is a medium with wave speed increasing monotonically in a direction x, so that there is a single turning point (Figure 5.23a) where the longitudinal wavenumber vanishes. Far before (after) the turning point the wavenumber is real (imaginary) corresponding to propagating (evanescent) waves (Figure 5.23b).

(Figure 5.23b) the waves propagate (5.265a) [become evanescent (5.265b)] before (after) the turning (Figure 5.23a). The preceding conclusions are approximate and can be reviewed (Notes 7.1–7.55) in the context of the exact theory of waves in non-uniform media whose properties vary rapidly on the scale of a wavelength. The case of waves in a medium whose properties vary on a lengthscale L much larger the wavelength $K^2L^2 \gg 1$ leads to ray theory (Notes 5.16–5.20), that improves on the approximation (5.265a, b) of constant longitudinal wavenumber. Considering the relation (5.257b) ≡ (6.266a) between local wavelength and local wavenumber varying with position:

$$K(x) = \frac{2\pi}{\lambda(x)}: \qquad\qquad \lim_{\lambda \to \infty} K = 0, \qquad \lim_{\lambda \to 0} K = \infty, \qquad\qquad (5.266a\text{–}c)$$

there are two extremes: (i) oscillations cease at a turning point (Figures 5.18–5.23) that corresponds (Notes 5.10–5.15) to an infinite wavelength or zero longitudinal wavenumber (5.264b) ≡ (5.226b); (ii) the opposite case of infinite wavenumber or zero wavelength (5.266c) corresponds to high-frequency waves propagating along rays (Figures 5.24–5.27) in analogy with particles along paths (Notes 5.16–5.19).

NOTE 5.16: **Light and Sound in the Ray Limit**

The electromagnetic waves with very small wavelength propagating in a medium whose properties vary slowly in a wavelength can be interpreted as **light rays** (Figure 5.24) in an **optical system** or **sound rays** in **air** in analogy with particles travelling along a trajectory. The wave equation (5.258a–e) leads to an unforced linear second-order differential equation of the form (5.242b) with the invariant corresponding (5.267a) to the square of the longitudinal wavenumber (5.263b). Far from the turning points into the

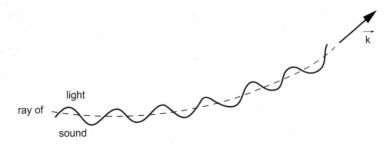

FIGURE 5.24
Far from the turning points into the propagation zone, high-frequency waves with wavelength (5.287c) small (5.287a) compared with the lengthscale (5.284b) variation of properties of the medium waves can be represented by rays, in analogy with particles along a trajectory.

propagation zone the solution of (5.263b) ≡ (5.267b) is sought in the form (5.267c) of "light rays," improving on (5.265a) that assumes constant longitudinal wavenumber:

$$I(x) = \left[K(x) \right]^2 : \quad \frac{d^2\Psi}{dx^2} + \left[K(x) \right]^2 \Psi(x) = 0, \quad \Psi_\pm(x) = C_\pm(x) \exp\left[\pm i \int^x K(\xi) d\xi \right].$$

$$(5.267\text{a–c})$$

The solution of the wave equation (5.267b) is sought in the form (5.267c) ≡ (5.268a) **first-order ray approximation** consisting (problem 173) of a phase (5.268b) and an amplitude:

$$\Psi_\pm(x) = C_\pm(x) \exp\{\pm i\Phi(x)\}, \quad \Phi(x) = \int^x K(\xi) d\xi. \qquad (5.268\text{a, b})$$

The phase (5.268a) has opposite signs for waves propagating in opposite directions +(−) for positive (negative) x; it equals the integral of the local longitudinal wavenumber along the ray path, that reduces to (5.265a) for constant wavenumber. In order to satisfy (5.267b), the constant amplitude in (5.265b) has to be replaced by an amplitude that is a function of position in (5.268a), as is the method of variation of parameters (notes 1.2–1.4; sections 2.9, 3.3; subsections 1.3.6, 4.3.12, 4.7.17). It may be expected that the amplitude varies slowly, in contrast with the phase (5.268a) that varies rapidly, because the longitudinal wavenumber is large:

$$\left\{ \Psi_\pm, \Psi'_\pm, \Psi''_\pm \right\} = \exp\left[\pm i\Phi(x) \right] \left\{ C_\pm, C'_\pm \pm i K C_\pm, C''_\pm \pm 2 i K C_\pm \pm i K' C_\pm - K^2 C_\pm \right\}.$$

$$(5.269\text{a–c})$$

The wave field (5.267c) ≡ (5.268a, b) ≡ (5.269a) and its first (second) order derivatives (5.269b) [(5.269c)] with regard to position, involve the longitudinal wavenumber (amplitudes) and their first (first and second) order derivatives. Substitution of (5.269a, b, c) in (5.267b) leads to:

$$0 = \Psi''_\pm + K^2 \Psi_\pm = \exp(\pm i\Phi)\left[C''_\pm \pm 2 i K C'_\pm \pm i K' C_\pm \right]. \qquad (5.270)$$

The term in square brackets in (5.270) must vanish. By slowly varying amplitudes it is meant that the second-order derivatives can be neglected (5.271a):

$$|C''_\pm| \ll 2K|C'_\pm|; \qquad A \equiv C_\pm: \qquad 2KA' + K'A = 0, \qquad (5.271\text{a–c})$$

it follows that the amplitudes (5.271b) of the waves propagating in the positive C_+ and negative C_- directions satisfy the same equation (5.271c). The latter equation (5.271a) ≡ (5.272a) may be integrated (5.272b):

$$\frac{dC_\pm}{C_\pm} = -\frac{dK}{2\,K}: \qquad \log C_\pm - \frac{1}{2}\log K = \log B_\pm, \qquad C_\pm(x) = \frac{B_\pm}{\sqrt{K(x)}}, \qquad (5.272\text{a--c})$$

implying that the amplitude varies the inverse square root of the longitudinal wavenumber (5.272c). Using (5.272c), the condition (5.271a) of slow amplitude variation may be re-stated:

$$1 \gg \left| \frac{C_\pm''}{2\,C_\pm'\,K} \right| = \left| \frac{\left(K^{-1/2}\right)''}{2K\left(K^{-1/2}\right)'} \right| = \left| \frac{1}{2}\frac{\left(K^{-3/2}\,K'\right)'}{K^{-1/2}\,K'} \right| = \left| \frac{K''}{2\,K'\,K} - \frac{3\,K'}{4\,K^2} \right|, \qquad (5.273)$$

in terms of the longitudinal wavenumber alone; it implies that the longitudinal wavenumber varies slowly and the wave is nearly sinusoidal locally. This completes the first-order ray approximation (5.267c; 5.272c; 5.273) that is interpreted next (note 5.17).

NOTE 5.17: Phase along Rays and Amplitude on Ray Tubes

The preceding (note 5.16) results (5.267c; 5.272c) ≡ (5.274b) and (5.273) ≡ (5.274a) may be interpreted as follows: *the linear second-order ordinary differential equation in invariant form (5.267b) has (problem 173) two linearly independent solutions (5.274b):*

$$1 \gg \frac{K''}{2\,K'\,K} - \frac{3\,K'}{4\,K^2}: \qquad \Psi_\pm(x) = B_\pm \left| K(x) \right|^{-1/2} \exp\left[\pm i \int^x K(\xi)\,d\xi \right], \qquad (5.274\text{a, b})$$

where $B_\pm$ are arbitrary constants; the solutions are valid if the condition (5.274a) is met, implying that K is a slowly varying function of x. Since K is the longitudinal wavenumber in (5.263b, c), its slow variation applies to a wave of short wavelength changing slowly in direction, like a ray of light or sound in Figure 5.24, hence the name **ray approximation**. *The physical interpretation of (5.274b) is that: (i) the phase of the oscillation (problem 174) is the integral of the wavenumber along the* **ray path** *(Figure 5.24) and varies rapidly for large wavenumber in the ray approximation; (ii) the waves propagating in the positive (negative) x-directions have arbitrary amplitudes B_+ (B_-) and opposite phases (5.268a, b); (iii) the amplitude varies (5.272c) like (problem 175) the inverse square root of the longitudinal wavenumber, that is, slowly along a* **ray tube** *(Figure 5.25) bounded by ray paths; (iv) since no energy crosses the rays at the sides of the ray tube, total energy must be constant in each*

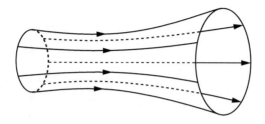

FIGURE 5.25
The phase of the waves varies along rays (Figure 5.24) that form ray tubes (Figure 5.25). The conservation of energy along ray tubes requires that the constancy of the product of the cross-sectional area by the square of the amplitude.

cross-section (5.275a); (v) the constant energy (5.275a) scales (5.275b) on the cross-sectional area times the square of the amplitude of the waves:

$$const = E = \left| \Psi_\pm(x) \right|^2 A(x) = A(x) \left| C_\pm(x) \right|^2 = \frac{\left| B_\pm \right|^2 A(x)}{K(x)} = \frac{\left| B_\pm \right|^2}{2\pi} A(x) \lambda(x);$$

$$(5.275\text{a–d})$$

(vi) thus the cross-section is proportional to the wavenumber (5.275c) and hence (5.266a) inversely proportional to the wavelength (5.275d); (viii) if a ray tube converges (diverges) that is [Figure 5.26a) (5.27a)] has a decreasing (increasing) cross-sectional area (5.276a) [(5.277a)] the amplitude increases (5.276b) [decreases (5.277b)]:

$$A_1 > A_2: \qquad \left| \Psi_1^\pm \right| < \left| \Psi_2^\pm \right|, \qquad K_1 > K_2, \qquad \lambda_1 < \lambda_2, \qquad c_1 < c_2, \qquad (5.276\text{a–e})$$

$$A_1 < A_2: \qquad \left| \Psi_1^\pm \right| > \left| \Psi_2^\pm \right|, \qquad K_1 < K_2, \qquad \lambda_1 > \lambda_2, \qquad c_1 > c_2, \qquad (5.277\text{a–e})$$

(viii) the longitudinal wavenumber decreases (5.276c) [increases (5.277c)] corresponding to longer (5.276d) [shorter (5.277d)] wavelength and increased (decreased) spacing of nodes; (ix) the decrease (5.277c) [increase (5.277c)] in the longitudinal wavenumber (5.263b) corresponds to an increase (5.276e) [decrease (5.277e)] of wave speed; (x) the increase (5.276b) [decrease (5.277b)] in amplitude and increase (5.276d) [decrease (5.2773d)] in wavelength have opposite effects on the steepness of the waveforms, that is comparable in the cases, leading to similar magnitudes for dissipation effects. The preceding solution (5.274a, b) is known as the **JWKB-approximation** (Jeffreys 1924, Wentzel 1926, Kramers 1926, Brillouin 1926) in quantum mechanics, and was implicitly used in wave theory long before, since it corresponds to the high-frequency limit of electromagnetic (sound) waves represented by light (sound) rays. The preceding **first-order ray approximation** (notes 5.15–5.17) can be extended to higher orders (note 5.19).

Higher-Order Differential Equations and Elasticity

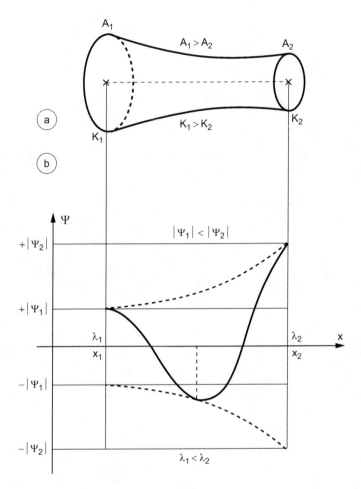

FIGURE 5.26
From Figures 5.24 and 5.25 it follows that in a converging ray tube (Figure 5.26a); that is, has decreasing cross-sectional area, the amplitude increases as the wavelength increases (Figure 5.26b), leading to small change in the slope of the waveform.

NOTE 5.18: Second-Order JWKB-Approximation (Jeffreys 1924, Wentzel 1926, Kramers 1926, Brilloun 1926)

The second-order ray approximation (5.278a, b) adds to the first-order (5.274b) a smaller perturbation:

$$\Psi_{\pm} = K^{-1/2}\psi_{\pm} + u, \qquad \psi_{\pm} \equiv B_{\pm}\exp\left(\pm i\Phi\right) = B_{\pm}\exp\left\{\pm i\int^{x} K(\xi)d\xi\right\};$$

$$(5.278a, b)$$

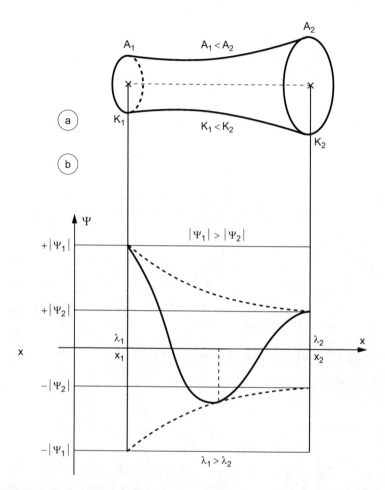

FIGURE 5.27
Conversely to the Figure 5.26, if the ray tube diverges; that is, has increasing cross-sectional area (Figure 5.27a), the amplitude decreases and the wavelength also decreases (Figure 5.26b), again tending to preserve the slope of the waveform.

the first-order ray approximation (5.274b) corresponds to the first term on the r.h.s. of (5.278a), consisting of a plane wave with constant amplitude (5.278b) and the amplitude factor $K^{-1/2}$, leading to (5.279a, b):

$$\psi'_\pm = \pm i K \psi_\pm, \qquad \psi''_\pm = \pm i K' \psi_\pm - K^2 \psi_\pm. \qquad (5.279\text{a, b})$$

Including the second-order correction u in (5.278a) and using (5.279a, b) follows:

$$\Psi'_\pm = u' + K^{-1/2}\psi'_\pm - \frac{1}{2}K^{-3/2} K' \psi_\pm = u' + \psi_\pm \left[\pm i K^{1/2} - \frac{1}{2} K^{-3/2} K' \right], \qquad (5.280\text{a})$$

$$\Psi''_\pm = u'' + K^{-1/2}\psi''_\pm - K^{-3/2}K'\psi'_\pm - \frac{1}{2}\left(K^{-3/2}K'\right)'\psi_\pm$$

$$= u'' - K^{3/2}\psi_\pm - \frac{1}{2}\left(K^{-3/2}K'\right)'\psi_\pm .$$

(5.280b)

Substituting (5.278a) and (5.280b) in (5.267b) leads to:

$$0 = \Psi''_\pm + K^2\Psi_\pm = u'' + K^2 u - \frac{1}{2}\left(K^{-3/2}K'\right)'\psi_\pm ,$$

(5.281)

as (problem 176) the second-order ray approximation. Assuming a slow variation of the second-order perturbation (5.282a) leads from (5.281) to (5.282b):

$$u'' \ll K^2 u: \qquad \frac{u}{\psi_\pm} = \frac{\left(K^{-3/2}K'\right)'}{2K^2} = \frac{1}{2}K^{-7/2}K'' - \frac{3}{4}K^{-9/2}K'^2 .$$

(5.282a, b)

Since (5.282b) is real, the second-order ray approximation changes the amplitude but not the phase.

NOTE 5.19: High-Frequency Waves in Weakly Non-Homogeneous Media

Substituting (5.282b) and (5.278b) in (5.278a) yields:

$$\Psi_\pm(x) = B_\pm \left[K^{-1/2} - \frac{1}{2}K^{-7/2}K'' + \frac{3}{4}K^{-9/2}K'^2 \right] \exp\left\{ \pm i \int^x K(\xi)d\xi \right\},$$

(5.283)

as (problem 176) *the **second-order ray approximation** to the solution (5.283) of the second-order linear ordinary differential equation in invariant form (5.267b) that consists of: (i) the first-order ray approximation (5.274a, b); and (ii) a second-order correction to the amplitude (5.282a, b) without phase change. The **lengthscale** of variation of the speed of propagation is defined by (5.284a) leading by integration to (5.270b):*

$$\frac{1}{L(x)} \equiv \frac{c'(x)}{c(x)} = \frac{d}{dx}\{ \log[c(x)] \}: \qquad c(x) = c(0)\exp\left[\int_0^x \frac{d\xi}{L(\xi)} \right].$$

(5.284a, b)

In the case of constant lengthscale (5.285a), the simplification of (5.284b) to (5.285b):

$$L = const: \qquad c(x) = c(0)\exp\left(\frac{x}{L}\right), \qquad \lim_{L\to\infty} c(x) = c(0),$$

(5.285a–c)

shows that: (i) a uniform wave speed corresponds to an infinite lengthscale (5.285c); and (ii) the variation of the wave speed is larger for shorter lengthscale.

NOTE 5.20: **Conditions of Validity of the Ray Approximation**

The longitudinal wavenumber (5.263b) depends on position through the wave speed leading to a comparable lengthscale (5.286a, b):

$$K' \sim \frac{K}{L}, |K''| \sim \frac{K}{L^2}: \qquad \frac{K''}{2K'K} \sim \frac{1}{KL} \sim \frac{3K'}{4K^2}, \qquad (5.286a\text{--}d)$$

so that the two terms in (5.274a) have comparable magnitudes (5.286c, d). Therefore, the condition of validity of the ray approximation (5.274a) that involves the difference of comparable terms (5.286c, d) is one order of magnitude smaller (5.287a):

$$1 \gg \frac{1}{K^2 L^2}: \qquad 1 \ll \left[K(x)L(x)\right]^2 = \left[\frac{2\pi L(x)}{\lambda(x)}\right]^2, \qquad (5.287a\text{--}c)$$

leading to (5.287b) [(5.287c)] in terms of (5.266a) the local longitudinal wavenumber (wavelength). Thus, *the ray approximation (5.287b) ≡ (5.287c) assumes (problem 177) that the local longitudinal wavelength (5.266a) is small compared with the lengthscale (5.284a) of variation of the wave speed; therefore it applies to high-frequency waves, that is, large wavenumber (5.263b) in weakly inhomogeneous media, that is, with large lengthscale (2.284a) of variation of properties.* Since the ray theory assumes a large wavenumber K varying slowly; that is, small K', the second-order ray approximation, corresponding to the second and third terms in square brackets in (5.283), is smaller than the first-order ray approximation corresponding to the first term; that is, (5.274b). The ray theory: (i) does not apply at a turning point $K = 0$ where the amplitude (5.272c) would be infinite; (ii) it also breaks down at foci (Figure 4.1c) where sound rays cross and at envelopes (Figure 5.1) that mark the transition from light to shadow. The consideration of these cases (i–iii) requires: (a) either further development of ray theory to include **caustics**; (b) or exact solutions of the wave equation (notes 7.1–7.15).

Conclusion 5

The solutions of a first-order differential equation form a family of integral curves with the arbitrary constant C as the parameter. The C-discriminant is the locus of points where two integral curves of the family coincide; that is, it may be an envelope (Figure 5.1 and 5.2), a node-locus (Figure 5.2), or a cusp-locus (Figure 5.6). The p-discriminant is the locus of points where the tangents to two curves coincide, and may be an envelope (Figure 5.4), a tac-locus

(Figure 5.5), or a cusp-locus (Figure 5.6). Generally, of these singular curves, only the envelope (Figure 5.1 and 5.4) is tangent to the integral curves and specifies a special integral; exceptionally, another special curve, such as a cusp-locus (Figure 5.8) or one branch of a node-locus (Figure 5.7) may be tangent to the integral curves and supply a special integral of the differential equation. Some examples of integral curves obtained as general integral of a differential equation are: (i) a set of parabolas with an envelope (Figure 5.9); (ii) a family of circles with two envelopes and a tac-locus (Figure 5.10); (iii) a family of lace-like curves with an envelope, a tac-locus, and a node-locus (Figure 5.11). These confirm that whereas the envelope will always supply a special integral, the other solutions of the *C*-discriminant or *p*-discriminant generally fail to satisfy the differential equation. Further examples of special integrals include a parabola (a straight line) that is the envelope of a family of straight (parabolic) integral curves [Figure 5.12 (5.13)]. Another two examples, both involving semi-cubical parabolas, are the cases of: (i) a cusp-locus distinct from the envelope, with the former (latter) not being (being) an integral (special integral) (Figure 5.14); and (ii) a cusp-locus tangent to the integral curves (Figure 5.15) that exceptionally is a special integral, since it is tangent to the integral curves, in this case on both sides.

The special integrals can occur not only for first-order differential equations (Table 5.1), but also for higher-order differential equations. A special integral of a differential equation of order N is a solution involving less than N arbitrary constants and not contained in the general integral. To the first-order differential equations without special integrals (chapter 3) may be added those have special integrals (sections 5.1 to 5.5). The solution on the last standard; that is, the dual differential equations, uses the Legendre transform, which has important applications in thermodynamics of simple systems, for which work is performed only by an isotropic inward pressure (Figure 5.16). A simple thermodynamic system is specified by the internal energy leading (Diagram 5.1) to three other functions of state, namely the enthalpy, free energy, and free enthalpy; these four functions of state depend on four distinct combinations of two pairs of extensive (intensive) thermodynamic variables: (i) the first pair is specific volume or mass density (pressure); (ii) the second pair is entropy (temperature). Although the four functions of state are interchangeable and equivalent, one may give a simpler representation of a particular thermodynamic process (Figure 5.17). The thermodynamic properties of a substance (Table 5.2) are specified by the equation of state; for example, for an ideal gas (Table 5.3).

To the first-order differential equations are added differential equations of order two (higher order). Of particular interest are the properties of linear differential equations of the second-order that include the invariant form. When the invariant is a constant the solutions (Figure 5.18) may be (i) oscillations with constant amplitude or (iii) exponential growth or decay, with the (ii) linear solution as the intermediate case. If the invariant is not constant (Figure 5.19) its zeros correspond to turning points where the solution changes between oscillatory and monotonic. A turning point may be: (i) of the first kind (Figure 5.20), if it leads from a steady state through growing oscillations to instability; or (ii) of the second kind (Figure 5.21a), if it leads from a constant to a decaying solution through intermediate oscillations, as in the transition from light to shadow (Figure 5.21b). The turning point of the second kind corresponding to the transition from light to shadow also occurs: (i) for total reflection of waves at the interface between two media (Figure I.22.2); (ii) for waves propagating in a medium with variable waves speed (Figure 5.23).

The waves propagating in a medium with constant (variable) wave speed are sinusoidal (non-sinusoidal) as can be seen [Figure 5.22b (a, c)] from the equal (unequal) spacing of the nodes; that is, the zeros of the waveform; an increasing (decreasing) wave speed leads to nodes that are more (less) spaced [Figure 5.21a(c)]. The limit when propagation ceases corresponds to the turning point (Figure 5.23a) where the waveform changes (Figure 5.23b) almost abruptly: the oscillations ceases corresponding to a limit of infinite wavelength and zero wavenumber. The limit opposite to the turning point is the ray approximation of large wavenumber or small wavelength; it corresponds to high-frequency waves propagating in a medium with slowly varying properties along rays (Figure 5.24) like particles along a path; for example, light and optics are the ray limit (Figures 5.24–5.27) of electromagnetic waves (Figures 5.21–5.23). The light or sound rays (Figure 5.24) form tubes (Figure 5.25); if a ray tube converges (diverges), that is, has decreasing (increasing) cross-sectional area [Figure 5.26a (5.27a)], the wave amplitude increases (decreases) and the wavelength also increases (decreases) that is [Figure 5.26b (5.27b)]. Thus, the waveforms have comparable slope leading to the same order of magnitude of dissipation.

6

Buckling of Beams and Plates

The uncoupled, one-dimensional mechanical oscillator or single electrical circuit satisfy ordinary differential equations of the second-order that are linear (non-linear) for small (large) perturbations [chapter 2 (4)]. The deformations of elastic bodies are specified by differential equations of the second (fourth) order in the absence (presence) of stiffness. The two main examples are one(two)-dimensional elastic bodies; that is, beams (plates) for which one (two) dimension(s) is (are) much larger, namely: (i) a slender string (beam) is long compared with the dimensions of the cross-section [chapter III.2 (III.4)]; (ii) a membrane (plate) has large dimensions compared with the thickness [sections II.6.1–II.6.3 (6.5–6.9)]. Starting with one-dimensional elastic bodies, the transverse deflection of a string (bar) that has no (has) bending stiffness is specified [chapter III.2 (III.4)] by a second (fourth) order differential equation; the axial, compression, or traction loads on a bar are specified (section 6.4) by a second-order differential equation, and together with the elastic string (chapter III.2) are the simplest problems in elasticity (chapter III.2); this relative simplicity facilitates the study of the non-linear deflection of strings (sections III.2.4–III.2.7) and axial loads in inhomogeneous bars with non-uniform material properties (notes III.4.4–III.4.7). A bar is a long thin elastic body (chapter III.4), which, unlike a string (chapter III.2), resists bending; for example, when acted upon by a transverse load. A longitudinal load may also be applied, either in traction or in compression. A beam is a bar under axial load either compression or traction. A beam under an axial compression load exhibits a new phenomenon, buckling, that is linear (non-linear) for small (large) slopes (section 6.1). In the absence of transverse loads, a beam under compression will remain straight until the axial load reaches a critical value, when it buckles. The critical load for buckling, or elastic instability, depends on the way the beam is supported: (i) it is lowest, that is, the beam buckles most easily, if it is clamped at one end and free at the other end; (ii/iii) the buckling load is increased relative to case (i) if both ends are pin-joined, or one is pin-joined and the other clamped; (iv) the greatest resistance to elastic instability applies to a beam clamped at both ends. The type [(i) to (iv)] of support of the beam affects its buckled shape; that is, the way in which it deforms from a straight line under a compression load exceeding the critical value for elastic stability. The buckling may be opposed (facilitated) by transverse loads toward (away) from the undeformed position (section 6.2). A beam under traction load does not buckle in the elastic case; that is, it remains straight unless transverse loads are applied. In order to bend a beam under traction, transverse loads have to be applied; for example, by a continuous distribution of repulsive springs. This leads to the consideration (section 6.3) of all possible combinations of axial traction or compression with transverse attractive or repulsive springs.

There are significant analogies between one(two)-dimensional elastic bodies; namely, strings (membranes) without stiffness and bars (plates) with stiffness, together with some important differences, such as ordinary (partial) differential equations apply in one (two) dimensions, leading to some different boundary conditions for finite bodies. The simplest case is axial (in plane) loads in a bar (plate), which are specified by second-order ordinary (partial) differential equations [section 6.4 (6.5)]. The in-plane loads; that is, tractions, compressions, and shears on a plate (section 6.5), are similar to plane elasticity (chapter II.4) with one difference: (i) in plane elasticity there is no transverse deformation, implying that a transverse stress may be needed; (ii) in the case of a plate the transverse stresses are small compared with longitudinal stresses and may be neglected altogether, by equating them to zero. The transverse instead of longitudinal deflection of a one(two)-dimensional elastic body without stiffness; that is, a string (membrane), is also specified by a second-order ordinary (partial) differential equation [chapter III.2 (sections II.6.1–II.6.3)]; a difference for a membrane is that the in-plane tension may be either isotropic (sections II.6.1–II.6.3) or anisotropic (section 6.6). The transverse deflection of a one(two)-dimensional elastic body with stiffness; that is, a bar (plate), is specified by a fourth-order ordinary (chapter III.4) [partial (sections 6.7–6.9)] differential equation. The bending of a bar with neither end free can give rise to longitudinal traction (sections III.4.5); the bending of a plate is weak (strong) if the in-plane deformation can (cannot) be neglected, that is the deflection is (is not) small compared with the thickness [sections 3.7–3.8 (3.9)]. The one(two)-dimensional buckling applies to a beam (thick plate) under axial (in-plane) compression [sections 6.1–6.3 (6.8)]. For the beam (plate), a linear deflection neglects the square of the slope (square of the modulus of the gradient the deflection with regard to the in-plane coordinates). The strong bending of a thick plate combines with in-plane deformation leading to a pair of fourth-order non-linear partial differential equations (section 6.9); a method of approximate solution is the use of two perturbation expansions, as for non-linear oscillations (section 4.5) and resonance (section 4.6).

6.1 Non-Linear Buckling of a Beam under Compression

The equation of equilibrium of a beam with bending stiffness under an axial load is derived (subsection 6.1.1) by combining earlier results for strings (chapter III.2) and bars (chapter III.4), including uniform and non-uniform cases (subsection 6.1.2). The case of axial compression is considered in the linear (non-linear) case of small (large) slope [subsection 6.1.3 (6.1.4)]; the linear case is considered first for the four classical support conditions (section III.4.2) as indicated by order of decreasing critical buckling load: (i) clamped-clamped (subsection 6.1.5); (ii) clamped-pinned (subsection 6.1.7); (iii) pinned-pinned (subsection 6.1.6); (iv) clamped-free (subsection 6.1.9) or cantilever beam. The linear (non-linear) boundary conditions at the free end (subsection 6.1.8) of a cantilever beam (subsection 6.1.10) are used for the comparison (subsection 6.1.12) of linear and non-linear buckling, including the lowest-order non-linear approximation and non-linear corrections of all orders (subsection 6.1.11). It is shown that both for the cantilever beam and other types of support the critical buckling load is not changed in the lowest order non-linear approximation because the onset of buckling occurs at a linear level (subsection 6.1.13). The non-linear effects do change the shape of the buckled elastic beam (subsection 6.1.14) by the addition of harmonics to the fundamental buckled mode (subsection 6.1.15).

6.1.1 Shape, Slope, and Curvature of the Elastica

Consider a beam that is straight in the absence of loads and subject to an **axial tension** T that may be either a **traction** $T > 0$ (**compression** $T < 0$) in Figure 6.1 a(b). The beam may be acted (Figure 6.1d) by a **transverse force** F causing bending (Figure 6.1c) associated with a bending moment M varying along the longitudinal coordinate x. The bending stretches (shortens) the longitudinal fibers on the outer (inner) side, so that one intermediate fiber, namely the **elastica** (dotted line on Figure 6.1c) has unchanged length; the equation of the elastica (6.1a) leads to the arc length (6.1c) where (6.1b) is the slope:

$$y = \zeta(x): \qquad \zeta' \equiv \frac{dy}{dx} = \tan\theta, \qquad ds = \left|(dx)^2 + (dy)^2\right|^{1/2} = \left|1 + \zeta'^2\right|^{1/2} dx.$$

$$(6.1a\text{–}c)$$

The tension is tangent to the elastica (Figure 6.1e) and thus has longitudinal (transversal) component (6.2a) [(6.2b)]:

$$T_x = T\cos\theta = T\frac{dx}{ds} = T\left|1 + \zeta'^2\right|^{-1/2}, \quad T_y = T\sin\theta = T\frac{dy}{ds} = T\zeta'\left|1 + \zeta'^2\right|^{-1/2},$$

$$(6.2a, b)$$

where θ in (6.1b; 6.2a, b) is the angle of the tangent to the elastica with the x-axis. The bending (Figure 6.1c) of the beam (Figure 6.1a, b) under transverse loads and/or axial tension (Figure 6.1d) causes the elastica to become curved.

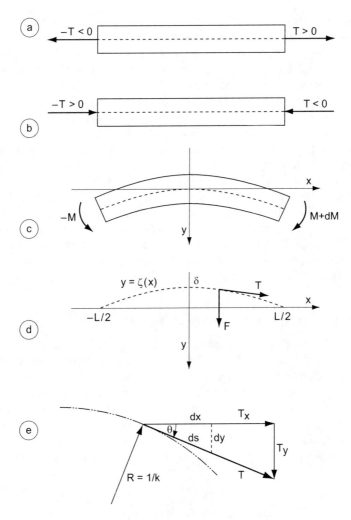

FIGURE 6.1
The bending moment on a beam can be due to transverse forces (c), and bending is opposed
(facilitated) by axial traction (a) [compression (b)]. The shape of the elastica is determined by
the balance (d) of the transverse force and tangential tension. The transverse component of
the tangential tension is negligible (not negligible) for linear (non-linear) bending with (large)
slope (e).

The simplest case of curvature is (Figure 6.2 a) a circle of radius R that multiplied by the angle θ specifies (6.3a) the arc length s, leading to (6.3b):

$$s = R\theta: \quad R = \frac{d\theta}{ds}; \quad k = \frac{1}{R} = \frac{d\theta}{ds} = \frac{dx}{ds}\frac{d\theta}{dx} = \left|1+\zeta'^2\right|^{-1/2}\frac{d}{dx}\left(arc\tan\zeta'\right) = \zeta''\left|1+\zeta'^2\right|^{-3/2},$$

$$(6.3a\text{--}c)$$

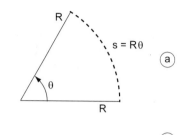

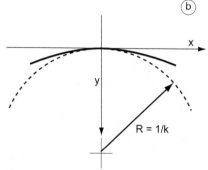

FIGURE 6.2
The bending moment equals (6.6a) minus the product of the Young modulus of the material by the moment of inertia of the cross-section by the curvature of the elastica. The curvature is the inverse of the radius of curvature (b), corresponding to the radius of the circle (a) tangent to the elastica at each point that best approximates the elastica in the neighborhood.

in the case of an arbitrary curve (Figure 6.2b), like the shape of the elastica (6.1a), the radius of curvature is not constant (6.3a) as for the circle (Figure 6.2a); the local radius of curvature for an arbitrary curve varies along its length and is determined at each point by the radius of the circle that most closely approximates the curve (subsection II.6.4.1). Substitution of (6.1b) in (6.3b) leads to (6.3c) that specifies (II.6.97a, b) ≡ (6.4a) ≡ (6.4b) the **radius of curvature** R, and its inverse; that is, the **curvature** k:

$$k = \frac{1}{R} = \zeta'' \left| 1 + \zeta'^2 \right|^{-3/2} = \left\{ \zeta' \left| 1 + \zeta'^2 \right|^{-1/2} \right\}'. \qquad (6.4a, b)$$

It has been shown that (problem 178) *the elastica (6.1a) has slope (6.1b) and arc length (6.1c) leading to: (i) the horizontal (6.2a) [vertical (6.2b)] components of a tangent vector such as the tension; and (ii) the curvature and radius of curvature (6.4a, b) ≡ (II.6.97a, b).*

6.1.2 Stiff Beam under Traction/Compression

The **transverse force** F and **tangential tension** T cause (Figure 6.1d) a **bending moment** M given (Figure 6.1c) by (6.5a):

$$0 = dM + \left(F + T_y \right) ds, \qquad F + T_y = -\frac{dM}{ds} = -\left| 1 + \zeta'^2 \right|^{-1/2} M', \qquad (6.5a\text{--}c)$$

that is equivalent to (6.5b) where (6.1c) prime denotes derivative (6.1b) ≡ (6.5c) with regard to x. The bending moment (chapter III.4) is equal (III.4.4b) ≡ (6.6a) to the product of the Young modulus E of the material, by the inertia moment I of the cross-section, by the curvature (6.4a) of the neutral line or elastica:

$$M(x) = -EIk, \qquad \frac{d}{ds}(EIk) - T_y = F, \qquad f = F' = \frac{d}{dx}\frac{d}{ds}(EIk) - T'_y, \qquad (6.6\text{a--d})$$

leading: (i) to (6.6b) for the transverse force; and (ii) to (6.6d) for the **shear stress** defined by (6.6c) as the transverse force per unit undeflected length. Substituting (6.2b) and (6.4a) in (6.6b) [(6.6d)] it follows that (problem 179) *the transverse force (shear stress) is related to the shape of the elastica by (6.7) [(6.8)]:*

$$F = \left|1 + \zeta'^2\right|^{-1/2}\left[EI\zeta''\left|1 + \zeta'^2\right|^{-3/2}\right]' - T\zeta'\left|1 + \zeta'^2\right|^{-1/2}, \qquad (6.7)$$

$$f = \left\{\left(1 + \zeta'^2\right)^{-1/2}\left[EI\zeta''\left|1 + \zeta'^2\right|^{-3/2}\right]'\right\}' - \left[T\zeta'\left|1 + \zeta'^2\right|^{-1/2}\right]', \qquad (6.8)$$

*where: (i) T is the tangential tension; (ii) the product of the **Young modulus** of the material by the **moment of inertia** of the cross-section (6.9b) defines the **bending stiffness** (6.9a):*

$$B(x) = E(x)I(x), \qquad\qquad I(x) = \int A y^2\, dS; \qquad (6.9\text{a, b})$$

(iii) the bending stiffness (6.9a) may vary along the length of the beam due to non-uniformity of the material or variations of cross-section.
   A **uniform beam** has: (i) uniform axial tension (6.10a); and (ii) constant bending stiffness (6.10b). A constant (6.10b) bending stiffness (6.9a) applies to: (ii-a) a homogeneous beam E = const with uniform cross-section I = const; (ii-b) an inhomogeneous beam whose Young modulus varies along the length inversely to the moment of inertia of the cross-section (6.9a). The **buckling parameter** p in (6.10c) has the dimensions of inverse length:

$$T = const, \quad EI = const: \qquad\qquad p^2 = -\frac{T}{EI}, \qquad (6.10\text{a--c})$$

is real $p^2 > 0$ (imaginary $p^2 < 0$) for compression $T < 0$ (traction $T > 0$) and is constant for a uniform beam (6.10a, b). *The buckling parameter (6.10c) for*

(problem 180) a uniform beam (6.10a, b) appears in the transverse force (6.11a–c)
[shear stress (6.12a–c)]:

$$\frac{F}{EI} = \left|1 + \zeta'^2\right|^{-1/2} \left[\zeta''\left|1 + \zeta'^2\right|^{-3/2}\right]' + p^2\,\zeta'\left|1 + \zeta'^2\right|^{-1/2}$$

$$= \left|1 + \zeta'^2\right|^{-1/2} k' + p^2 \eta = \left|1 + \zeta'^2\right|^{-1/2} \eta'' + p^2 \eta, \qquad (6.11a–c)$$

$$\frac{f}{EI} = \left\{\left|1 + \zeta'^2\right|^{-1/2} \left[\zeta''\left|1 + \zeta'^2\right|^{-3/2}\right]'\right\}' + p^2 \left[\zeta'\left|1 + \zeta'^2\right|^{-1/2}\right]'$$

$$= \left[\left|1 + \zeta'^2\right|^{-1/2} k'\right]' + p^2 \eta' = \left[\left|1 + \zeta'^2\right|^{-1/2} \eta''\right]' + p^2 \eta', \qquad (6.12a–c)$$

that have: (i) all terms non-linear in the slope (6.1b) of the elastica (6.1a); (ii) same terms linear using as variable the sine of the angle of inclination (6.2b) ≡ *(6.13a):*

$$\eta \equiv \zeta'\left|1 + \zeta'^2\right|^{-1/2} = \sin\theta = \frac{dy}{ds}; \qquad k = \eta' \qquad (6.13a, b)$$

(iii) the curvature (6.4a) is (6.4b) the derivative (6.13b) of (6.13a), that is, a non-linear function of the slope. Thus, the equation of the elastica for the transverse force (shear stress) is: (i) of the fourth (third) order in terms of the shape of the elastica (6.1a) and has all terms non-linear in (6.11a) [(6.12a)]; (ii) of the third (second) order (6.11c) [(6.12c)] involving some terms linear in an auxiliary variable, namely, the sine of the angle of inclination (6.13a), whose derivative (6.13b) is the curvature (6.4a) ≡ *(6.4b). Thus the non-linearity does not lie entirely in the auxiliary variable (6.13a). The linear (non-linear) cases of small (large) slope are considered next [subsection 6.1.3 (6.1.4)].*

6.1.3 Linear Bending for Small Slope

The linear bending corresponds to small slope (6.14a) in which case (problem 181): (i) the angle of inclination (6.1b; 6.13a) [curvature (6.4a)] of the elastica simplify to (6.14b) [(6.14c)] leading to the bending moment (6.14d); (ii) the transverse force (6.7) [shear stress (6.8)] simplify to (6.14e) [(6.14f)]:

$$\zeta'^2 \ll 1: \qquad \eta = \zeta' = \theta, \quad k = \zeta'', \quad M = -EI\zeta'',$$

$$F = \left(EI\zeta''\right)' - T\zeta', \quad f = \left(EI\zeta''\right)'' - \left(T\zeta'\right)'. \qquad (6.14a–f)$$

In the case of the linear deflection (6.14a) ≡ (6.15a) of a uniform beam (6.10a, b) ≡ (6.15b, c) the transverse force (shear stress) simplify further to (6.15d) [(6.15e)]:

$$\zeta'^2 \ll 1; \ EI \sim const, \ T \sim const: \quad F = EI\zeta''' - T\zeta', \quad f = EI\zeta'''' - T\zeta''. \quad (6.15a\text{--}e)$$

The beam is **elastically stable (unstable)** if there is no (there is) deflection in the absence of shear stress. For a uniform beam (6.10a, b) in the absence of shear stress $f = 0$ instability is possible only if the buckling parameter is positive $p^2 > 0$ in (6.12c), that is under compression $T < 0$, corresponding to (6.16a, b) and leading to (6.16c) for the shape of the elastica:

$$T = -|T|: \qquad p^2 = -\frac{|T|}{EI}, \qquad \zeta'''' + p^2\zeta'' = 0. \qquad (6.16a\text{--}c)$$

The linear homogeneous differential equation (6.16c) with constant coefficients (6.16b) ≡ (6.17a) is specified by the characteristic polynomial (6.17b):

$$p^2 = const: \quad 0 = \left(\frac{d^4}{dx^4} + p^2\frac{d^2}{dx^2}\right)\zeta(x) = \left\{\frac{d^2}{dx^2}\left(\frac{d}{dx} - ip\right)\left(\frac{d}{dx} + ip\right)\right\}\zeta(x),$$
$$(6.17a, b)$$

that has a double root zero and simple roots $\pm ip$, so that the general integral is:

$$\zeta(x) = A + Bx + C\cos(px) + D\sin(px), \qquad (6.18)$$

where A, B, C, D are arbitrary constants of integration. Thus *(problem 182) the **linear buckling** of a beam occurs for the lowest value of the buckling parameter (6.16b) for the solution (6.18) of the equation (6.16c) of the elastica is non-zero, corresponding to the **critical buckling load**.* An intermediate case between the exact non-linear (linear) theory of buckling [subsection 6.1.2 (6.1.3)] is the lowest-order non-linear approximation (subsection 6.1.4).

6.1.4 Non-Linear Buckling with Large Slope

In the linear (non-linear) case of small (large) slope without forcing, the elastica satisfies a linear (non-linear) differential equation with constant coefficients of order four (6.16c) for the transverse displacement [order three (6.12c) ≡ (6.19b) for the sine of the angle of inclination (6.13a) ≡ (6.19a) that is a non-linear variable]:

$$\zeta' = \eta\left|1 - \eta^2\right|^{-1/2}: \qquad \left\{\left|1 - \eta^2\right|^{1/2}\eta''\right\}' + p^2\eta' = 0. \qquad (6.19a, b)$$

The differential equation (6.19b) has (6.20a) a first integral (6.20b) where $\bar{A}$ is an arbitrary constant:

$$p^2 = const: \qquad \left(\frac{\bar{A}}{2} - p^2\,\eta\right)\left|1-\eta^2\right|^{-1/2} = \eta'' = \eta'\frac{d\eta'}{d\eta}. \qquad (6.20\text{a--c})$$

Re-arranging (6.20c) in the form (6.21a):

$$2\,\eta'\,d\eta' = \bar{A}\left|1-\eta^2\right|^{-1/2}d\eta - 2p^2\left|1-\eta^2\right|^{-1/2}\eta\,d\eta, \qquad (6.21)$$

it can be integrated (II.7.110a, b) as:

$$\eta'^2 = \bar{B} + \bar{A}\,arc\sin\eta + 2p^2\left|1-\eta^2\right|^{1/2}, \qquad (6.22)$$

where $\bar{B}$ is another arbitrary constant.

The linear approximation of small slope (6.14a) implies $\eta^2 < \zeta'^2 \ll 1$ in (6.13a) and the **lowest-order non-linear approximation** (6.23a) to (6.22) is (6.23b):

$$\zeta'^3 \sim \eta^3 \ll 1: \qquad \eta'^2 = \bar{B} + 2p^2 - p^2\,\eta^2 + \bar{A}\,\eta, \qquad (6.23\text{a, b})$$

using only the leading terms of the power series for the square root or binominal (I.25.38) [arc of circular sine (II.7.167a–c)]. The integration of (6.23b) introduces another arbitrary constant $\bar{C}$ in (6.24).

$$x + \bar{C} = \int\left|\bar{B} + 2p^2 + \bar{A}\,\eta - p^2\,\eta^2\right|^{-1/2}d\eta. \qquad (6.24)$$

The shape of the elastica is given by (6.19a) involving another constant of integration $\bar{D}$ in (6.25):

$$\zeta(x) = \bar{D} + \int^x \eta(\xi)\left|\,1-\left[\eta(\xi)\right]^2\right|^{-1/2}d\xi. \qquad (6.25)$$

Thus, *in the linear case of small slope (6.14a) [in the lowest-order non-linear approximation (6.23a)] the shape of the elastica is given [problem 182 (183)] by (6.18) [(6.24; 6.25)] involving four arbitrary constants. The four boundary conditions, two at each end the beam: (i) specify three constants in terms of one, that is, an arbitrary amplitude; (ii) determine the **eigenvalues** p, of which the smallest specifies (6.10c) the critical buckling load. It will be investigated in the sequel whether (i) the critical buckling load and (ii) the shape of the elastica are equal or different in the linear (non-linear) cases of small (6.14a) [moderate (6.23a)]* slope. This will be ascertained by considering both the linear (non-linear) cases for the four classical types of support (section II.4.2) of a beam: (i) clamped-clamped (subsection 6.1.5); (ii) clamped-pinned (subsection 6.1.7); (iii) pinned-pinned (subsection 6.1.6); (iv) clamped-free (subsection 6.1.9). These lead to decreasing critical buckling loads, as shown starting with the linear theory.

6.1.5 Critical Buckling Load for a Clamped Beam

In the case (Figure 6.3a) of a beam clamped at both ends at a distance L, the boundary conditions are zero displacement and slope at both ends $x = 0$ and $x = L$:

$$\zeta_1(0) = 0 = \zeta_1'(0), \qquad\qquad \zeta_1(L) = 0 = \zeta_1'(L). \qquad (6.26a-d)$$

In the linear case (6.18) the boundary conditions (6.26a, b) lead to (6.27a, b):

$$A + C = 0 = B + pD: \qquad \zeta_1(x) = C\big[\cos(px) - 1\big] + D\big[\sin(px) - px\big],$$
$$(6.27a-c)$$

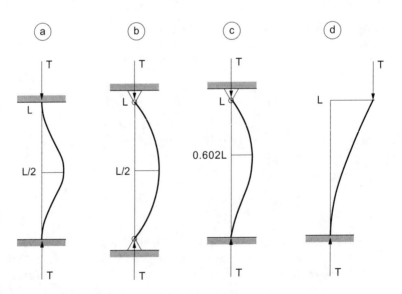

FIGURE 6.3
The critical buckling load for a beam under compression (Figure 6.1) depends on the type of support and is: (a) largest for clamping at both ends; (a) smaller if one end is pinned; (b) further reduced if both ends are pinned, (d) smallest for a cantilever beam clamped at one end and free at the other.

that simplify (6.18) to (6.27c). Substitution of (6.27c) in the boundary conditions (6.26c, d) leads to the linear homogeneous system of equations (6.28):

$$\begin{bmatrix} \cos(pL)-1 & \sin(pL)-pL \\ -\sin(pL) & \cos(pL)-1 \end{bmatrix}\begin{bmatrix} C \\ D \end{bmatrix}=0. \tag{6.28}$$

If $C=0=D$ then also $A=0=B$ by (6.27a, b) and a trivial solution (6.18) results $\zeta=0$. Thus $(C,D)\neq(0,0)$ cannot both vanish, and the determinant of the matrix (6.28) must vanish:

$$0=\left[\cos(pL)-1\right]^2+\sin(pL)\left[\sin(pL)-pL\right], \tag{6.29}$$

implying (6.29) ≡ (6.30a):

$$0=2\left[1-\cos(pL)\right]-pL\sin(pL): \qquad \cos(pL)-1=0=\sin(pL), \tag{6.30a–c}$$

and hence (6.30b, c); the roots of (6.30b) and (6.30c) coincide (6.31a):

$$p_{1,n}L=2\pi n: \qquad p_{1,1}=\frac{2\pi}{L}, \quad -T_1=EI\left(p_{1,1}\right)^2=\frac{4\pi^2 EI}{L^2}, \tag{6.31a–c}$$

and the smallest (6.31b) leads to the critical buckling load (6.31c) for a clamped beam in the linear case.

At the critical buckling condition (6.31b) ≡ (6.32a) the second equation of the system (6.28) is trivial and the first (6.32b) implies (6.32c), so that (6.27a, c) simplifies to (6.32d):

$$p_1L=2\pi;\ p_{1,1}LD=0: \qquad D=0, \qquad \zeta_1(x)=A\left[1-\cos(p_{1,1}x)\right]; \tag{6.32a–d}$$

from (6.32d) in the alternative forms (6.32e, f):

$$\zeta_1(x)=A\left\{1-\cos\left(\frac{2\pi x}{L}\right)\right\}=2A\sin^2\left(\frac{\pi x}{L}\right), \tag{6.32e, f}$$

it follows that the deflection (6.32e, f) vanishes at both ends (6.26a, c) and is maximum in the middle (6.33a), where the slope (6.33b) vanishes (6.33c):

$$\zeta_{1max}=\zeta\left(\frac{L}{2}\right)=2A: \qquad \zeta_1'(x)=\frac{2\pi A}{L}\sin\left(\frac{2\pi x}{L}\right), \qquad \zeta_1'\left(\frac{L}{2}\right)=0; \tag{6.33a–c}$$

the linear slope (6.33b) vanishes at both ends (6.26b, d) as well as in the middle (6.33c) and is maximum (minimum) at the one-quarter (three-quarter) points (6.33d–g):

$$\zeta'_{1\max} = \zeta'_1\left(\frac{L}{4}\right) = \frac{2\pi A}{L} = -\zeta'_1\left(\frac{3L}{4}\right) = -\zeta'_{1\min}. \qquad (6.33\text{d–g})$$

The extrema (6.33d–g) of the slope (6.33b, c) are points of inflexion, where the curvature and bending moment (6.14d) ≡ (6.34a–c):

$$M_1(x) = -EI\zeta''(x) = -\frac{4\pi^2 EI}{L^2}A\cos\left(\frac{2\pi x}{L}\right) = AT_1\cos\left(\frac{2\pi x}{L}\right), \qquad (6.34\text{a–c})$$

vanish (6.35a, b):

$$M_1\left(\frac{L}{4}\right) = 0 = M\left(\frac{3L}{4}\right): \quad M_{1\max} = M_1(0) = M_1(L) = AT_1 = -M_{1\min} = M_1\left(\frac{L}{2}\right),$$
$$(6.35\text{a–e})$$

and the maximum bending moment occurs at the supports (6.35c, d) and the minimum (6.35e) in the middle; the latter (6.35e) equals the reaction bending moment at the supports, since the extrema have the same modulus and opposite signs. Thus, *(problem 184) the critical buckling compression load for a uniform beam clamped at both ends (Figure 6.3a) is given by (6.31c) in the linear are case of small (6.14a) slope and: (i) the displacement is given by (6.32e, f; 6.3a); (ii) the slope is given by (6.33b–g); (iii) the bending moment by (6.34a–c; 6.35a–e). The critical buckling load decreases replacing two clamped by two pinned supports as shown next (subsection 6.1.6).*

6.1.6 Buckling of a Beam with Both Ends Pinned

In the case (Figure 6.3b) of a pinned beam, the boundary conditions are the vanishing of the displacement and bending moment or curvature at both ends:

$$\zeta_3(0) = 0 = \zeta''_3(0), \qquad\qquad \zeta_3(L) = 0 = \zeta''_3(L). \qquad (6.36\text{a–d})$$

In the linear case (6.18), the boundary conditions (6.36a, b) lead to (6.37a, b) and hence (6.18) to (6.37c):

$$C = 0 = A: \qquad\qquad \zeta(x) = Bx + D\sin(px). \qquad (6.37\text{a–c})$$

The boundary conditions (6.36c, d) applied to (6.37c) lead to (6.38a, b):

$$B = 0, \qquad D\sin(pL) = 0: \qquad D \neq 0, \qquad \sin(p_3 L) = 0, \qquad \text{(6.38a–d)}$$

so that a non-trivial solution (6.38c) leads to (6.38d). The roots of (6.38d) are (6.39a) and the smallest (6.39b):

$$p_{3,n} L = n\pi; \qquad p_{3,1} L = \pi, \qquad -T_3 = EI\left(p_{3,1}\right)^2 = \frac{\pi^2 EI}{L^2} = -\frac{T_1}{4}, \qquad \text{(6.39a–d)}$$

specifies the critical buckling load (6.39c) in the linear case for a pinned beam; that is, one-quarter (6.39d) of the value for the clamped case (6.31c).

The linear shape of the buckled beam (6.37c; 6.38a; 6.39b) is (6.40a):

$$\zeta_3(x) = D\sin(p_{3,1} x) = D\sin\left(\frac{\pi x}{L}\right), \qquad \zeta_{3\max} = \zeta\left(\frac{L}{2}\right) = D, \qquad \text{(6.40a, b)}$$

showing that the displacement is zero at both ends (6.36a, c) and maximum in the middle (6.40b). The converse applies to the slope (6.41a), that vanishes in the middle (6.41b) and has opposite extrema at the two ends (6.41c, d):

$$\zeta_3'(x) = \frac{\pi D}{L}\cos\left(\frac{\pi x}{L}\right): \qquad \zeta_3'\left(\frac{L}{2}\right) = 0, \qquad \zeta_{3\max}' = \zeta_3'(0) = \frac{\pi D}{L} = -\zeta_3'(L) = -\zeta_{3\min}'.$$

$$\text{(6.41a–d)}$$

The bending moment (6.42a) like the displacement is zero at the supports (6.36b, d) and minimum in the middle (6.42b):

$$M(x) = -EI\zeta_3''(x) = \frac{\pi^2 EI D}{L^2}\sin\left(\frac{\pi x}{L}\right) = -T_3 D\sin\left(\frac{\pi x}{L}\right), \qquad M_{3\min} = M\left(\frac{L}{2}\right) = T_3 D.$$

$$\text{(6.42a, b)}$$

Thus *(problem 185) the critical buckling compression load for a uniform beam (Figure 6.3b) pinned at both ends is (6.39c) one-quarter (6.39d) of the value (6.31c) with clamped supports. Also, in the linear case of small slope the displacement is given by (6.40a, b), the slope by (6.41a–d), and the curvature and bending moment by (6.42a, b).* The case intermediate between the clamped-clamped (pinned-pinned) beam [subsection 6.1.5 (6.1.6)] is the clamped-pinned beam (subsection 6.1.7).

6.1.7 Beam with One Clamped and One Pinned Support

In the case (Figure 6.3c) of one clamped (6.26a, b) ≡ (6.43a, b) and one pinned (6.36c, d) ≡ (6.43c, d) support the boundary conditions are:

$$\zeta_2(0) = 0 = \zeta_2'(0), \qquad\qquad \zeta_2(L) = 0 = \zeta_2''(L). \qquad (6.43a\text{--}d)$$

In the linear case (6.18) using (6.43a, b) leads to (6.44a, b) ≡ (6.27a, b) and hence to (6.27c). Substituting (6.27c) in the two remaining boundary conditions (6.43c, d) leads to (6.44c):

$$A + C = 0 = B + pD: \qquad \begin{bmatrix} \cos(pL) - 1 & \sin(pL) - pL \\ \cos(pL) & \sin(pL) \end{bmatrix} \begin{bmatrix} C \\ D \end{bmatrix} = 0. \qquad (6.44a\text{--}c)$$

If $C = 0 = D$ then $A = 0 = B$ and a trivial solution (6.18) results $\zeta = 0$. Thus a non-trivial solution requires that $(C, D) \neq (0,0)$ do not both vanish, and the determinant of the matrix in (6.44c) must vanish:

$$0 = \left[1 - \cos(pL)\right]\sin(pL) + \cos(pL)\left[\sin(pL) - pL\right] = \sin(pL) - pL\cos(pL),$$
$$(6.45a, b)$$

leading to (6.45a), which is a transcendental equation (6.45b) ≡ (6.46a):

$$\tan(p_{2,n} L) = p_{2,n} L: \qquad n\pi < p_{2,n}L < \left(n + \frac{1}{2}\right)\pi, \qquad \pi < p_{2,1}L < \frac{3\pi}{2}, \qquad (6.46a\text{--}c)$$

whose roots (Panel 6.1) lie in the range (6.46b), excluding the trivial root $pL = 0$.
   The smallest root of (6.46a) lies (6.46b) in the range (6.46c) corresponding to a critical buckling load:

$$-T_1 = \frac{4\pi^2 EI}{L^2} > \frac{9\pi^2 EI}{4L^2} > EI(p_{2,1})^2 = -T_2 > \pi^2 \frac{EI}{L^2} = -T_3, \qquad (6.47a, b)$$

that is larger (6.47b) than in the pinned case (6.39c) and smaller (6.47a) than in the clamped case (6.31c). The precise value (6.48a) of the smallest positive root of (6.46a) is 4.494 radians, corresponding to the angle 257.5° in the range $180° < p_n L < 270°$ in (6.46c) in agreement with θ_1 in the Panel 6.1, and leads to the critical buckling load (6.48b):

$$p_{2,1}L = 4.494\,\text{rad} = 257.5° \equiv a: \quad -T_2 = EI(p_{2,1})^2 = \frac{EIa^2}{L^2} = 20.196\frac{EI}{L^2} = 2.046\pi^2\frac{EI}{4L^2},$$
$$(6.48a\text{--}c)$$

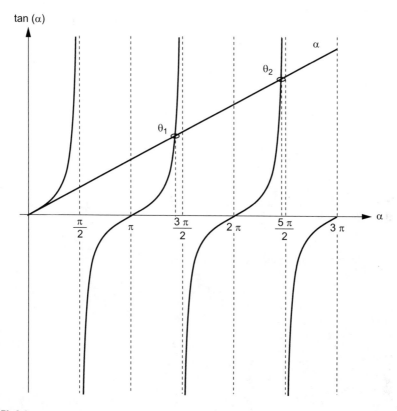

PANEL 6.1
The axial compressions corresponding to the buckling modes of a beam (Panel 6.3) are obtained as roots of a transcendental equation in this case for circular tangent equated to its variable.

that is close to the arithmetic mean (6.48c) of the pinned (6.39c) and clamped (6.31c) cases.

In the linear case, the shape of the elastica is given by (6.27c) where the constants are related by (6.44c) so only one is arbitrary. From the second line of (6.44c) follows (6.49a) where (6.46a) is used leading to (6.49b):

$$-C = D\frac{\sin(pL)}{\cos(pL)} = D\tan(pL) = pLD; \qquad -C = p_{2,1}LD = aD, \qquad (6.49\text{a–c})$$

the critical buckling load (6.48a) leads from (6.49b) to (6.49c) and hence (6.27c) to the linear displacement:

$$\zeta_2(x) = D\left[a - p_{2,1}x + \sin(p_{2,1}x) - a\cos(p_{2,1}x)\right]$$

$$= D\left[a\left(1 - \frac{x}{L}\right) + \sin\left(\frac{ax}{L}\right) - a\cos\left(\frac{ax}{L}\right)\right], \qquad (6.50\text{a, b})$$

that vanishes at $x = 0$ and $x = L$ because $\tan a = a$. The corresponding slope is:

$$\zeta_2'(x) = \frac{Da}{L}\left[\cos\left(\frac{ax}{L}\right) - 1 + a\sin\left(\frac{ax}{L}\right)\right], \tag{6.51}$$

and vanishes (6.52a) at the clamped end but not at the pinned end (6.68b):

$$\zeta_2'(0) = 0 \neq \zeta_2'(L) = \frac{Da}{L}(\cos a - 1 + a\,\sin a) = -16.195\frac{D}{L}. \tag{6.52a–c}$$

Using the value of the angle (6.48a) from Table II.5.1 follow (6.53b) ≡ (6.53c) [(6.54a) ≡ (6.54b)]:

$$\tan a = a: \quad \cos a = \cos\alpha\left|\cos^2\alpha + \sin^2\alpha\right|^{-1/2} = -\left|1 + \tan^2\alpha\right|^{-1/2}$$
$$= -\left|1 + a^2\right|^{-1/2} = -0.2172, \tag{6.53a–e}$$

$$\sin a = \sin\alpha\left|\cos^2\alpha + \sin^2\alpha\right|^{-1/2} = \tan\alpha\left|1 + \tan^2\alpha\right|^{-1/2}$$
$$= -a\left|1 + a^2\right|^{-1/2} = -0.9761 = a\cos a, \tag{6.54a–e}$$

leading to (6.53d) [(6.54c)] by (6.53a) in (6.46a) and to (6.53e) [(6.54d, e)] by (6.48a).

The slope (6.51) vanishes (6.55a) at the position (6.55b) corresponding (6.55c) to (6.55d) that lies (6.55e) in the upper half of the beam (Figure 6.3c) where the displacement (6.50b) is maximum (6.55f):

$$\zeta_2'(x_m) = 0: \qquad \frac{x_m\,a}{L} = b, \qquad \cos b + a\sin b = 1, \qquad b = 2.704, \tag{6.55a–d}$$

$$\frac{x_m}{L} = \frac{b}{a} = 0.602: \quad \zeta_{max} = \zeta(x_m) = \zeta\left(\frac{bL}{a}\right) = D(a - b + \sin b - a\cos b) = 6.284\,D. \tag{6.55e–f}$$

The bending moment:

$$M_2(x) = -EI\zeta_2''(x) = EI\frac{Da^2}{L^2}\left[a\cos\left(\frac{ax}{L}\right) - \sin\left(\frac{ax}{L}\right)\right]$$
$$= -T_2D\left[a\cos\left(\frac{ax}{L}\right) - \sin\left(\frac{ax}{L}\right)\right], \tag{6.56a, b}$$

vanishes (6.56c) at the pinned support $x = L$ because of (6.53a) and is non-zero (6.56d) at the clamped support:

$$M_2(L) = 0 \neq M_2(0) = -T_2 D \, a = -4.494 T_2 D. \qquad \text{(6.56c, d)}$$

Thus, *(problem 186) a uniform clamped free beam (Figure 6.3c) has a critical buckling load (6.48b, c) that is close to the arithmetic mean of those of the clamped (6.31c) and pinned (6.39c) beams. Also, in the linear case the displacement is given by (6.50b) and is maximum (6.55a–f) where the slope (6.51) vanishes. The slope (6.51) also vanishes at the clamped support but not at the pinned support (6.52a–c); the reverse applies (6.56a–d) to the curvature and to the bending moment.* The remaining of the four classical support conditions is the clamped-free or cantilever beam that has the lowest critical buckling load (subsection 6.1.9). The boundary conditions at the free end differ in the linear and non-linear cases (subsection 6.1.8).

6.1.8 Linear and Non-Linear Boundary Conditions at a Free End

A **cantilever beam** (Figure 6.3d) is clamped at one end and free at the other end where the bending moment (6.6a; 6.4a, b; 6.13b) $\equiv$ (6.57a–d):

$$M(x) = -EIk = -EI\zeta''\left|1+\zeta'^2\right|^{-3/2} = -EI\left[\zeta'\left|1+\zeta'^2\right|^{-1/2}\right]' = -EI\eta', \qquad \text{(6.57a–d)}$$

[the transverse force (6.11a–c)] must vanish (6.58a) [(6.58b)] leading to the non-linear boundary conditions (6.58c) [(6.58d)]:

$$M(L) = 0 = F(L): \qquad \eta'(L) = 0 = \left|1-\eta^2\right|^{1/2}\eta''(L) + p^2\,\eta(L). \qquad \text{(6.58a–d)}$$

In the linear case of small slope (6.59a) $\equiv$ (6.14a), the vanishing of the bending moment (6.59b) [transverse force (6.59c)] at a free end of a uniform beam (6.10a–c) lead to the boundary conditions (6.59d) [(6.59e)]:

$$\zeta'^2 \ll 1: \qquad M(L) = 0 = F(L): \qquad \zeta''(L) = 0 = \zeta'''(L) + p^2\,\zeta'(L). \qquad \text{(6.59a–e)}$$

In the non-linear case of unrestricted slope, the free end boundary condition of zero bending moment (6.60a) [transverse force (6.61a)] is (6.60b) [(6.61b)] in terms of (6.13a) the sine of the inclination of the elastica and (6.60c) [(6.61c)] in terms of the displacement of the elastica:

$$M(L) = 0: \qquad 0 = \eta'(L) = \zeta''(L)\left|1 + \left[\zeta'(L)\right]^2\right|^{-3/2}, \qquad \text{(6.60a–c)}$$

$$F(L) = 0: \quad 0 = \eta''(L) + p^2 \left|1 - \eta^2\right|^{-1/2} \eta(L)$$

$$= p^2 \zeta' + \left|1 + [\zeta'(L)]^2\right|^{-5/2} \left\{\zeta'''(L)\left(1 + [\zeta'(L)]^2\right) - 3\zeta'(L)[\zeta''(L)]^2\right\}.$$

$$\text{(6.61a–c)}$$

The passage from (6.60b) [(6.61b)] to (6.60c) [(6.61c)] uses (6.4a, b) [(6.62)]:

$$\eta'' = \left[\zeta''\left|1 + \zeta'^2\right|^{-3/2}\right]' = \left|1 + \zeta'^2\right|^{-5/2}\left[\zeta'''\left(1 + \zeta'^2\right) - 3\zeta'\zeta''^2\right]. \qquad \text{(6.62)}$$

The boundary conditions for the displacement at the free end in (problem 187) the linear (non-linear) cases of small (6.15a) [unrestricted] slope of a uniform (6.10a–c) beam: (i) coincide (6.59d) ≡ (6.60c) for the vanishing of the bending moment; (ii) do not coincide (6.59e) ≠ (6.61c) for the transverse force when the second term in (6.61c) differs from the first term in (6.59e).

6.1.9 Buckling of a Clamped-Free or Cantilever Beam

In the case of a cantilever beam (Figure 6.3d) that is clamped at one end and free at the other end, the linear boundary conditions are: (i) zero displacement and slope at the clamped end; and (ii) zero bending moment (6.6a; 6.4b) [transverse force (6.11a)] at the free end that in the linear case (6.15a) imply (6.59d) ≡ (6.63c) [(6.59e) ≡ (6.63d)]:

$$\zeta_4(0) = 0 = \zeta_4'(0), \qquad \zeta_4''(L) = 0 = \zeta_4'''(L) + p^2\zeta_4'(L). \qquad \text{(6.63a–d)}$$

In the linear case (6.18), the boundary conditions (6.63a–d) give:

$$B = 0 = B + pD, \qquad A + C = 0, \qquad C\cos(p_4 L) = 0. \qquad \text{(6.64a–d)}$$

If $C = 0$ then $A = 0$ and a trivial solution results. Thus, a non-trivial solution requires that $C \neq 0$ implying (6.64d).

$$p_{4,n}L = \frac{\pi}{2} + n\pi: \quad p_{4,1} = \frac{\pi}{2L}, \quad -T_4 = EI\left(p_{4,1}\right)^2 = \frac{\pi^2 EI}{4L^2} = -\frac{T_1}{4} = -\frac{T_2}{16}, \qquad \text{(6.65a–e)}$$

the smallest root (6.65b) specifies the critical buckling loading (6.65c); that is, one-quarter (6.65d) of that for pinned ends (6.39c) and one-sixteenth (6.65e) of that for clamped ends (6.31c).

The shape of the elastica (6.18) is given in the linear case (6.64a–c) by:

$$\zeta_4'(x) = A\left[1 - \cos(px)\right] = C\left[\cos(px) - 1\right]. \qquad \text{(6.66a, b)}$$

The linear displacement of the buckled beam is given by (6.66a) and (6.65b), leading to (6.67a):

$$\zeta_4(x) = A\left\{1 - \cos\left(\frac{\pi x}{2L}\right)\right\} = 2A\sin^2\left(\frac{\pi x}{4L}\right); \qquad \zeta_{4\max} = \zeta_4(L) = A; \qquad (6.67a, b)$$

the maximum deflection (6.67b) occurs at the free end and the value A is undetermined and appears as a factor in the slope (6.68a):

$$\zeta_4'(x) = \frac{\pi A}{2L}\sin\left(\frac{\pi x}{2L}\right), \qquad \zeta_{4\max}' = \zeta_4'(L) = \frac{\pi A}{2L}, \qquad (6.68a, b)$$

that is also maximum (6.68b) at the free end. The curvature specifies (6.6a) the bending moment (6.69a):

$$M_4(x) = -EI\zeta_4''(x) = -\frac{\pi^2 EIA}{4L^2}\cos\left(\frac{\pi x}{2L}\right) = T_4 A\cos\left(\frac{\pi x}{2L}\right),$$

$$M_{4\min} = M_4(0) = T_4 A,$$
(6.69a, b)

that decreases from zero at the free end to (6.69b) at the clamped end; that is, the reaction moment at the support is $T_4 A$, as can be confirmed from Figure 6.3d.

A clamped-free or cantilever uniform beam (Figure 6.3d) has (problem 188) linear buckled elastica with displacement (6.67a, b) and slope (6.68a, b) corresponding to the curvature and bending moment (6.69a, b). The critical buckling load (6.65c) is one-fourth (6.65d) [one-sixteenth (6.65e)] of a pinned (6.39c) [clamped (6.31c)] beam with the same length, with the clamped-pinned beam (6.48c) near the arithmetic mean:

$$-T_1 = \frac{4\pi^2 EI}{L^2} > -T_2 = 2.046\frac{\pi^2 EI}{L^2} > -T_3 = \frac{\pi^2 EI}{L^2} > -T_4 = \frac{\pi^2 EI}{4L^2}. \qquad (6.70a\text{–}d)$$

Comparing (problem 189) the critical buckling loads (6.70a–d) for beams of the same length made of the same material, it follows that the clamped-clamped (pinned-pinned) beam has a buckling load sixteen (four) times greater than the clamped-free beam and the clamped-pinned beam is in between (6.71b–d), assuming all have the same length (6.71a):

$$L_1 = L_2 = L_3 = L_4 \equiv L: \qquad \left\{\frac{T_1}{T_4}, \frac{T_1}{T_2}, \frac{T_1}{T_3}\right\} = \left\{16, \frac{4a^2}{\pi^2} = 8.185, 4\right\}; \qquad (6.71a\text{–}d)$$

$$T_1 = T_2 = T_3 = T_4 = T: \qquad \left\{\frac{L_1}{L_4}, \frac{L_1}{L_2}, \frac{L_1}{L_3}\right\} = \left\{4, \frac{2a}{\pi} = 2.860, 2\right\}, \qquad (6.72a\text{–}d)$$

bearing in mind that the critical buckling load varies like the inverse square of the length of the beam, the result (6.71a–d) can be re-stated (6.72a–d) as follows: for the same buckling load (6.72a), the clamped-clamped (pinned-pinned) beam can be four times (twice) as long as the clamped-free beam, and the length of the clamped-pinned beam lies in between these values (6.72b–d). Table 6.1 compares the clamped, pinned, clamped-pinned, and cantilever beams not only as concerns critical buckling loads (6.70a–d;·6.71a–d; 6.72a–d) but also for the boundary conditions, displacement, slope, and curvature of the elastica in the linear case of small slope. The critical buckling loads could be the same in the linear (non-linear) cases of small (large) slope since buckling must start with small slope and is thus a linear instability. The shape of the buckled elastica cannot be expected to be the same in the linear (non-linear) cases because in the curvature of the elastica (6.4a, b) the dependence on the square of the slope is not (is) important. These expectations are tested first (subsections 6.1.10–6.1.12) in the case of a cantilever beam, that has the least buckling load; for the same buckling load the cantilever beam has the largest deflection, making non-linear effects more relevant.

6.1.10 Non-Linear Elastica of a Cantilever Beam

The approximation (6.23a) ≡ (6.73a) in (6.12a) in the absence of shear stress (6.73b) leads to (6.73c):

$$\zeta'^3 \ll 1; \quad f(x) = 0: \quad 0 = \left\{ \left(1 - \frac{\zeta'^2}{2} \right) \left[\zeta'' \left(1 - \frac{3}{2} \zeta'^2 \right) \right] \right\}' + p^2 \left[\zeta' \left(1 - \frac{\zeta'^2}{2} \right) \right]',$$

$$(6.73a–c)$$

showing that *(problem 190) the lowest-order (6.73a) non-linear buckling (6.73b) of a uniform beam (6.10a, b) with buckling parameter (6.10c) is specified by the elastica as the solution of the fourth-order non-linear differential equation (6.73c).* The solution can be obtained from first integrals (subsection 6.1.4) as shown next, starting with a cantilever beam. The first integral of the differential equation for the elastica (6.20c) ≡ (6.74a) arising from the integration of (6.19c) for a uniform beam (6.20c) involves a constant $\bar{A}$:

$$\left| 1 - \eta^2 \right|^{1/2} \quad \eta'' + p^2 \, \eta = \frac{\bar{A}}{2} = 0 \qquad (6.74a, b)$$

that vanishes (6.74b) in the case of a cantilever beam (6.58d), since the transverse force must vanish at the free end. The condition (6.74b) simplifies the second integral (6.22) and in the lowest-order non-linear approximation (6.23a, b) simplifies (6.24) to (6.75b) involving the constant (6.75a):

$$q \equiv \frac{p}{\sqrt{B + 2p^2}}: \quad (x + \bar{C}) \sqrt{B + 2p^2} = \int \left| 1 - q^2 \, \eta^2 \right|^{-1/2} d\eta = \frac{1}{q} \arcsin(q\,\eta). \qquad (6.75a–c)$$

TABLE 6.1

Linear and Non-Linear Buckling of Beams

Case		General	I	II	III	IV
Support		–	clamped-clamped	clamped-pinned	pinned-pinned	clamped-free (cantilever)
Figure		6.3	6.3a	6.3b	6.3c	6.3d
Critical buckling load						
Linear: 6.1.3	subsection	6.1.5	6.1.7	6.1.6	6.1.8–6.1.9	
	boundary conditions		(6.26a–d)	(6.43a–d)	(6.36a–d)	(6.63a–d)
	displacement		(6.32e; 6.33a)	(6.50a, b; 6.55a–f)	(6.40a, b)	(6.66a, b; 6.67a, b)
	slope		(6.33b–g)	(6.51; 6.52a–c)	(6.41a–d)	(6.68a, b)
	bending moment		(6.34a–c; 6.35a–e)	(6.56a, b)	(6.42a, b)	(6.69a, b)
Non-linear: 6.1.1–6.1.2	subsection(s)	6.1.10–6.1.12	6.1.13	6.1.13–6.1.15	6.1.13–6.1.15	
(lowest order: 6.1.4)	boundary conditions		(6.26a–d)	(6.43a–d)	(6.36a–d)	(6.63a–c; 6.61c)
	harmonics		(6.112a–c)	(6.46a–c)	(6.113a–c)	(6.111a–c)
	displacement		(6.114a)	(6.107)	(6.114b)	(6.85a, b; 6.89a–e; 6.90) ≡ (6.115f)
	slope/curvature		(6.99a–d)	(6.99a–d)	(6.99a–d)	(6.99a–d)

Note: The linear (non-linear) buckling of beams with large (small) slope leads to (i) the same critical buckling load that depends on the type of support (Figure 6.2); (ii) the shape of the buckled elastica is modified in the non-linear case (Panel 6.1).

The primitive (6.75c) of (6.75b) leads to (6.76a, b):

$$\eta(x) = \frac{1}{q}\sin\left[q\left(x+\bar{C}\right)\sqrt{\bar{B}+2p^2}\right] = \sqrt{2+\frac{\bar{B}}{p^2}}\sin\left[p\left(x+\bar{C}\right)\right]. \qquad \text{(6.76a, b)}$$

The clamping boundary condition (6.77a) implies (6.77b) by (6.13a) and hence (6.77c):

$$\zeta'(0) = 0: \qquad 0 = \eta(0) = \sqrt{2+\frac{\bar{B}}{p^2}}\sin(p\bar{C}), \quad \bar{C} = 0. \qquad \text{(6.77a-c)}$$

Substituting (6.77c) in (6.76b) and introducing another arbitrary constant (6.78a) leads to (6.78b)

$$G \equiv \sqrt{2+\bar{B}/p^2}: \qquad \eta(x) = G\sin(px). \qquad \text{(6.78a, b)}$$

The boundary condition stating that the bending moment vanishes at the free end (6.60a) is (6.60b) ≡ (6.79a) in the non-linear case and applied to (6.78b) ≡ (6.79b).

$$\eta'(L) = 0: \qquad \eta'(x) = pG\cos(px), \quad \cos(pL) = 0, \qquad \text{(6.79a-c)}$$

leads to (6.79c) ≡ (6.64d). Thus the critical buckling load is the same (6.65a, b) in the linear and non-linear cases for a cantilever beam that is free to move the free end.

The non-linear slope (6.80) is obtained by substituting (6.78b) in (6.19a):

$$\zeta_4'(x) = G\sin(px)\left|1-G^2\sin^2(px)\right|^{-1/2}. \qquad \text{(6.80)}$$

In the linear case (6.15a) ≡ (6.80a), the factor with the square root can be omitted and (6.80) leads to (6.81b) ≡ (6.81c):

$$\left(\zeta_4'\right)^2 \ll 1: \qquad \zeta_4'(x) = G\sin(p_{4,1}x) = G\sin\left(\frac{\pi x}{2L}\right), \quad G = \frac{\pi A}{2L}, \qquad \text{(6.81a-d)}$$

proving the agreement of (6.68a) ≡ (6.81c) relating the arbitrary constants by (6.81d). In the non-linear case, the square root in (6.80) cannot be omitted. The assumption (6.82a) that the slope does not exceed unity leads (6.13a) to (6.82b):

$$\zeta_4' < 1: \qquad G = \left|\eta_4(x)\right|_{max} \leq \left|\zeta_4'\right|\left|1+\zeta_4'^2\right|^{-1/2} < \left|\zeta_4'\right| < 1, \qquad \text{(6.82a, b)}$$

and thus the inverse square root in (6.80) can be expanded in a binomial series (I.25.37a–c) ≡ (6.83a):

$$\left|1-G^2\sin^2(px)\right|^{-1/2}=\sum_{m=0}^{\infty}a_m G^{2m}\sin^{2m}(px),\tag{6.83a}$$

with coefficients (4.248a, b); the first coefficients are (II.6.57a–g) ≡ (6.83b):

$$a_{0-6}=\left\{1,\frac{1}{2},\frac{3}{8},\frac{5}{16},\frac{35}{128},\frac{63}{256},\frac{231}{1024}\right\},\tag{6.83b}$$

where (6.248a, b) applies for $m=1,2....$ and $a_0=1$. Thus, *the slope of a uniform (6.10a–c) cantilever beam under axial compression is given by (6.80; 6.83a, b)* ≡ *(6.84a, b):*

$$\zeta_4'(x)=\sum_{m=0}^{\infty}a_m G^{2m+1}\sin^{2m+1}(px)=\sum_{m=0}^{\infty}\zeta_{4,m}'(x),\tag{6.84a, b}$$

where: (i) the leading term $n=0$ is the linear slope (6.81a–c) ≡ *(6.68a); and (ii) the lowest-order non-linear correction $n=1$ is consistent with the approximation (6.23a).* The higher order terms omitted in (6.23b) generally affect the terms in (6.84b) beyond $n=0,1$ and change the coefficients (6.83b). All terms in (6.83b) are retained in the sequel to illustrate the method of calculating non-linear corrections of all orders. For example, the displacement can be obtained by integration of (6.84a, b) and thus consists of the lowest-order linear approximation plus non-linear corrections of all orders that are evaluated exactly next (subsection 6.1.11).

6.1.11 Linear Approximation and Non-Linear Corrections of All Orders

The exact displacement is given (6.85a) by a sum of terms (6.85b):

$$\zeta_4(x)=\sum_{n=0}^{\infty}\zeta_{4,m}(x):\qquad\zeta_{4,m}(x)\equiv a_m G^{2m+1}\int_0^x\sin^{2m+1}(p\xi)d\xi.\tag{6.85a, b}$$

The zero-order term is the linear approximation (6.86a–c):

$$\zeta_{4,0}(x)=a_0 G\int_0^x\sin(p\xi)d\xi=\frac{G}{p}\left[1-\cos(px)\right]$$

$$=\frac{2GL}{\pi}\left[1-\cos(px)\right]=A\left[1-\cos(px)\right]\tag{6.86a–e}$$

$$=2A\sin^2\left(\frac{px}{2}\right),$$

where (6.65b) [(6.81d)] were used to prove (6.86c) [(6.86d)] in agreement with (6.67a). The lowest-order non-linear correction is:

$$\zeta_{4,1}(x) = a_1 G^3 \int_0^x \sin^3(p\,\xi)\,d\xi = \frac{G^3}{2} \int_0^x \sin(p\xi)\left[1 - \cos^2(p\xi)\right]d\xi$$

$$= \frac{G^3}{2p}\left\{1 - \cos(px) + \frac{1}{3}\left[\cos^3(px) - 1\right]\right\}$$

$$= \frac{G^3}{6p}\left\{2 - \cos(px)\left[3 - \cos^2(px)\right]\right\}$$

$$= \frac{G^3}{12p}\left\{4 - \cos(px)\left[5 - \cos(2px)\right]\right\}$$

$$= \frac{G^3}{24p}\left[8 - 9\cos(px) + \cos(3px)\right]$$

$$= \frac{G^3}{12p}\left[9\sin^2\left(\frac{px}{2}\right) - \sin^2\left(\frac{3px}{2}\right)\right],$$

(6.87a–g)

where (6.83b; II.5.61c; II.5.88a) were used.

The two lowest order terms in (6.85a, b) have been evaluated explicitly in (6.86a–e) and (6.87a–g) corresponding to the lowest-order non-linear approximation (6.23a). To estimate the error of the approximation the higher order terms in (6.85b) may be considered. The expansion of the odd power of sine (II.5.79b) ≡ (6.88) as sum of sines of multiple angles is used to explicitly evaluate the *m*-th order:

$$\sin^{2m+1}(p\xi) = (-)^m\, 2^{-2m} \sum_{j=0}^m (-)^j \binom{2m+1}{j} \sin\left[(2m-2j+1)p\xi\right];\quad (6.88)$$

substituting (6.88) in the *m*-th order non-linear correction (6.85b) leads to:

$$\zeta_{4,m}(x) = a_m\, G^{2m+1} \int_0^x \sin^{2m+1}(p\xi)\,d\xi$$

$$= \frac{a_m}{p}\, G^{2m+1}(-)^m\, 2^{-2m} \sum_{j=0}^m (-)^j \binom{2m+1}{j} \frac{1 - \cos\left[(2m-2j+1)px\right]}{2m-2j+1}$$

$$= \frac{a_m}{p}\, G^{2m+1}(-)^m\, 2^{1-2m} \sum_{j=0}^m \frac{(-)^j}{2m-2j+1}\binom{2m+1}{j}\sin^2\left[\left(m-j+\frac{1}{2}\right)px\right];$$

(6.89a–e)

it can be confirmed (6.89b) with $m=0$ and $m=1$ leads respectively to (6.86b) and (6.87c). The maximum deflection at the tip $px=\pi/2$ is given by:

$$\zeta(L)=\frac{2}{p}\sum_{m=0}^{m}a_m\,G^{2m+1}\,(-)^m\,2^{-2m}\sum_{j=0}^{m}\frac{(-)^j}{2m-2j+1}\binom{2m+1}{j},\qquad(6.90)$$

that relates the constant G to the maximum deflection.

6.1.12 Comparison of Linear and Non-Linear Effects

The non-linear theory of buckling is illustrated next in the case of a cantilever beam (subsection 6.1.10), for which the linear approximation to the shape of the elastica (6.85a, b) is (6.86b) ≡ (6.91b) in the case of amplitude (6.91a) that satisfies (6.81a):

$$G=0.8:\qquad p\,\zeta_{4,0}(x)=0.8\big[1-\cos(px)\big]=1.6\sin^2\!\left(\frac{px}{2}\right);\qquad(6.91\text{a, b})$$

the dimensionless variables $p\zeta$ and px are used for plotting in Panel 6.2. The corresponding lowest-order non-linear correction (6.87f) is:

$$p\zeta_{4,1}=0.02133\big[8-9\cos(px)+\cos(3px)\big]=0.04266\left[9\sin^2\!\left(\frac{px}{2}\right)-\sin^2\!\left(\frac{3px}{2}\right)\right],$$
$$(6.92)$$

that is also plotted in Panel 6.1. The total non-linear deflection of the buckled cantilever beam to the lowest-order non-linear approximation (Panel 6.1) shows that the maximum deflection at (6.93a) is (6.93b) in the linear approximation:

$$px=\frac{\pi}{2}:\qquad p\zeta_{4,0}=0.8,\quad p\zeta_{4,1}=0.1707,\quad p(\zeta_{4,0}+\zeta_{4,1})=0.9707,\qquad(6.93\text{a–d})$$

to which the non-linear correction adds (6.93c) leading to the total value (6.93d). The linear approximation (6.91b) leads to a monotonic shape of the elastica (6.94b) over its whole length (6.94a):

$$0\le px\le\frac{\pi}{2}:\qquad\frac{d\zeta_{4,0}}{dx}=0.8\,\sin(px)>0;\qquad(6.94\text{a, b})$$

the lowest-order-non-linear correction (6.92) is also monotonic:

$$\frac{d\zeta_{4,1}}{dx}=0.064\big[3\sin(px)-\sin(3px)\big]>0,\qquad(6.95)$$

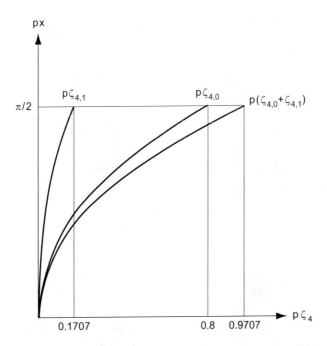

PANEL 6.2
The critical buckling load for a beam is the same in linear (non-linear) theory of small (large) deflection, but the shape of the buckled elastica, for example for a cantilever beam (Figure 6.3d), shows that non-linear effects increase the deflection.

and thus increases the deflection everywhere. The non-linear corrections of all higher orders (6.85a, b) are specified by (6.89a–e) including the maximum deflection at the tip (6.90); since they go beyond (6.23a) they are used only as order of magnitude estimates of the error of truncating the non-linear series after the first non-linear term. The second-order $m = 2$ non-linear correction (6.89e) would add a factor (6.83b) of order $3G^5/64 = 0.015$, which is a correction of less than 2% compared with (6.93d). This would be hardly visible in the plot on Panel 6.1 that is limited to the linear approximation (6.91b) plus the lowest-order non-linear correction (6.92). Thus, *(problem 191) the buckled shape of a cantilever beam is given by (6.85a; 6.89a–e) to all orders in the amplitude G, with the lowest-order non-linear approximation consisting of the linear approximation (6.86a–e) and lowest-order non-linear correction (6.87a–g); the higher-order terms go beyond the approximation (6.23a) and suggest as an order of magnitude that the lowest order non linear approximation is sufficient (6.91b; 6.92) in the case (6.91a) to obtain the shape of the elastica (Panel 6.2) with a 2% accuracy.* The lowest-order non-linear theory of the elastica of a buckled beam (subsection 6.1.4) is extended next from the cantilever beam (subsections 6.1.8–6.1.12) to other types of support (subsections 6.1.13–6.1.15) starting with the critical buckling loads.

6.1.13 Coincidence of Linear and Non-Linear Critical Buckling Loads

The critical buckling load for a cantilever beam was shown to coincide in the linear (6.64d) and lowest-order non-linear (6.79c) cases (6.65a–e). Two possible explanations are: (a) a cantilever beam can move at the free end; or (b) buckling is a linear phenomenon and thus its onset is not affected by non-linear effects. The choice between the two explanations (a) or (b) can be made by determining the critical buckling load of non-cantilever beams using the lowest-order non-linear theory and comparing with the linear theory. For a non-cantilever beam the simplification (6.74b) does not hold, and in (6.24) the argument of the square root is written:

$$2p^2 + \bar{B} + \bar{A}\eta - p^2\eta^2 = 2p^2 + \bar{B} + \frac{\bar{A}^2}{4p^2} - \left(p\eta - \frac{\bar{A}}{2p}\right)^2,$$
(6.96)

as the sum of a constant (6.97a) and the square of a variable (6.97b):

$$G^2 \equiv 2 + \frac{\bar{B}}{p^2} + \left(\frac{\bar{A}}{2p^2}\right)^2 : \qquad\qquad z = \eta - \frac{\bar{A}}{2p^2},$$
(6.97a, b)

leading to the integration:

$$p(x + \bar{C}) = \int \frac{d\eta}{\sqrt{G^2 - z^2}} = \frac{1}{G}\int \frac{dz}{\sqrt{1 - z^2/G^2}} = arc\sin\left(\frac{z}{G}\right).$$
(6.98a–c)

Inverting (6.98c) and using (6.97a, b) specifies the sine of the slope (6.99c) and (6.6a; 6.13b) the curvature and bending moment (6.99d), with amplitudes (6.99a, b):

$$H = \frac{\bar{A}}{2p^2}, \quad G^2 = 2 + \frac{\bar{B}}{p^2} + H^2: \quad \eta = H + G\sin\left[p(x + \bar{C})\right],$$
(6.99a–d)
$$M = -EIGp\cos\left[p(x + \bar{C})\right];$$

the three arbitrary constants $(\bar{A}, \bar{B}, \bar{C})$ may be replaced by $(H, G, \bar{C})$.

In the case of a beam clamped at both ends (6.26a, b) from (6.13a) follow the boundary conditions (6.100a, b) that imply (6.100c, d) by (6.99c).

$$\eta(0) = 0 = \eta(L): \qquad H + G\sin(p\bar{C}) = 0 = H + G\sin(p\bar{C} + pL).$$
(6.100a–d)

The compatibility of (6.100c, d) requires (6.101a) that implies (6.101b):

$$\sin(p\bar{C}) = \sin(p\bar{C} + pL): \qquad\qquad p_{1,n}L = 2n\pi.$$
(6.101a, b)

Thus the critical buckling load for a clamped beam (6.31b, c) is the same in the linear theory (6.31a) and in the lowest-order non-linear theory (6.101b) ≡ (6.31a). The curvature of the elastica (6.13b) is given (6.99c) by (6.102c):

$$k(0) = 0 = k(L): \qquad k(x) = pG\cos\left[p\left(x + \bar{C}\right)\right]; \qquad\qquad (6.102\text{a–c})$$

in the case of a beam pinned at both ends the vanishing of the curvature (6.102a, b) leads to (6.103a, b):

$$\cos\left(p\bar{C}\right) = 0 = \cos\left(p\bar{C} + pL\right): \qquad p_{3,n}L = n\pi, \qquad\qquad (6.103\text{a–c})$$

that are compatible for (6.103c). Thus, the critical buckling load for a pinned beam (6.39b, c) is the same in the linear (6.39a) and lowest-order non-linear theory (6.103c) ≡ (6.39a). This dismisses (supports) the conjecture (i) [(ii)] at the beginning of this subsection, showing that *the critical buckling load coincides (6.70a–d; 6.71a–d; 6.72a–d) in the linear and lowest-order non-linear theories because buckling is an instability triggered at linear level.* The coincidence of the critical buckling loads does not extend to the shape of the buckled elastica (subsection 6.9.14–6.9.15) because the square of the slope appears in the curvature (6.4a, b).

6.1.14 Non-Linear Effect on the Shape of the Buckled Elastica

The lowest-order non-linear approximation for the slope (6.23a) suggests (9.104a) including one order beyond the linear approximation for the shape (6.25) of the elastica:

$$\left[\eta(x)\right]^3 \ll 1: \qquad \zeta(x) = \int_0^x \eta(\xi)\left\{1 + \frac{1}{2}\left[\eta(\xi)\right]^2\right\}d\xi; \qquad\qquad (6.104\text{a, b})$$

the constant $\bar{D}$ can be omitted for zero displacement on one end (6.105a), and substitution of (6.99c) leads to (6.105b).

$$\zeta(0) = 0: \quad \zeta(x) = \int_0^x \left[H\left(1 + \frac{H^2}{2}\right) + G\left(1 + \frac{3H^2}{2}\right)\sin\left(p\xi + p\bar{C}\right) \right.$$

$$\left. + \frac{3HG^2}{2}\sin^2\left(p\xi + p\bar{C}\right) + \frac{G^3}{2}\sin^3\left(p\xi + p\bar{C}\right) \right]d\xi.$$

$$(6.105\text{a, b})$$

The change of variable (6.106a) leads to (6.106b):

$$\psi \equiv p\xi + p\bar{C}: \quad p\zeta(x) = \int_{p\bar{C}}^{px+p\bar{C}} \left[H\left(1 + \frac{H^2}{2} + \frac{3G^2}{4}\right) + G\left(1 + \frac{H^2}{2} + \frac{G^2}{2}\right)\sin\psi \right.$$

$$\left. -\frac{3HG^2}{4}\cos(2\psi) - \frac{G^3}{2}\sin\psi\cos^2\psi \right]d\psi$$

$$(6.106a, b)$$

In (6.106b) have been used some trigonometric relations to allow immediate integration:

$$\zeta(x) = H\left(1 + \frac{H^2}{2} + \frac{3G^2}{4}\right)x + \frac{G}{p}\left(1 + \frac{3H^2}{2} + \frac{G^2}{2}\right)\left[\cos(p\bar{C}) - \cos(px + p\bar{C})\right]$$

$$+ \frac{3HG^2}{8p}\left[\sin(2p\bar{C}) - \sin(2px + 2p\bar{C})\right] + \frac{G^3}{6p}\left[\cos^3(px + p\bar{C}) - \cos^3(p\bar{C})\right].$$

$$(6.107)$$

The shape of the elastica (6.107) involves the buckling parameter or eigenvalue and the constants $(G, H, \bar{C})$ with two relations arising from the boundary conditions.

In the case of the clamped beam (6.31b), the boundary condition (6.108a) substituted in (6.107) leads to the first relation (6.108b) between constants:

$$0 = \zeta(L): \qquad 0 = H\left(1 + \frac{H^2}{2} + \frac{3G^2}{4}\right); \qquad H + G\sin(p\bar{C}) = 0, \qquad (6.108a–c)$$

the second relation is one of (6.100c, d); for example, the simpler (6.100c) $\equiv$ (6.108c). The relations (6.108b, c) express two constants in terms of another. The pair of equations has two solutions other than the trivial case $G = 0 = H$, namely: (i) for (6.109a) from (6.108c) follows (6.109b); (ii) otherwise (6.108b) leads to (6.109c) and (6.108c) implies (6.109d):

$$H = 0: \quad \sin(p\bar{C}) = 0; \qquad G = -\frac{4}{3} - \frac{2H^2}{3}, \quad \csc(p\bar{C}) = \frac{4}{3H} + \frac{2H}{3}. \qquad (6.109a–d)$$

In the case of a pinned beam (6.39b), the same boundary condition (6.110a) $\equiv$ (6.108a) substituted in (6.107) leads to (6.110b):

$$\zeta(L) = 0: \quad 0 = H\left(1 + \frac{H^2}{2} + \frac{3G^2}{4}\right) + \frac{2G}{\pi}\left(1 + \frac{3H^2}{2} + \frac{G^2}{2}\right)\cos(p\bar{C}) - \frac{G^3}{3\pi}\cos^3(p\bar{C});$$

$$(6.110a, b)$$

the condition (6.103a) simplifies (6.110b) to (6.108b). Thus, *the shape [sine of the slope (6.13a)] of the buckled elastica in the lowest-order non-linear theory (6.23a) are given by (6.107) [(6.99c)] for [problem 192 (193)] a beam clamped (pinned) at the two ends, with critical buckling load (6.31a–c) [(6.39b–d)] with the three constants* $(G, H, \bar{C})$ *satisfying (6.109a, b) or (6.109c, d) [(6.103a; 6.108b)] and leaving one amplitude free.* The absence (presence) of non-linear effects on the critical buckling load (shape of the elastica) can be explained [subsection 6.1.13 (6.1.14)] in terms of the non-linear generation of harmonics (subsection 6.1.15).

6.1.15 Non-Linear Generation of Harmonics

In the simplest case of a cantilever beam (6.65a) there is (6.66a) a succession of **buckling harmonics** (6.111a) with increasing loads (6.111b, c):

$$\zeta_{4,n}(x) = A\left\{1 - \cos\left[\frac{\pi x}{L}\left(\frac{1}{2} + n\right)\right]\right\}, \quad -T_{4,n} = \frac{\pi^2 EI}{L^2}\left(\frac{1}{2} + n\right)^2 = -T_{4,1}\left(n + \frac{1}{2}\right)^2,$$

$$(6.111a\text{–}c)$$

with the critical buckling load (6.65c) being the lowest that corresponds to the **fundamental buckling mode** (6.67a) $\equiv$ (6.86a–e). The non-linear theory leads (6.85a) to the generation of harmonics (6.89a–c) of the fundamental, changing the shape of the buckled elastica but not the lowest critical buckling load. In the cases of clamped (pinned) beams (6.31a) [(6.39a)], there is (6.32e) [(6.40a)] also a succession of buckling harmonics (6.112a) [(6.113a)] with increasing loads (6.112b, c) [(6.113b, c)]:

$$\zeta_{1,n}(x) = A\left[1 - \cos\left(\frac{2\pi n x}{L}\right)\right], \quad -T_{1,n} = \frac{4\pi^2 EI n^2}{L^2} = -n^2 T_{1,1} \quad (6.112a\text{–}c)$$

$$\zeta_{3,n}(x) = A\sin\left(\frac{n\pi x}{L}\right), \quad -T_{3,n} = \frac{\pi^2 EI n^2}{L^2} = -n^2 T_{3,1}, \quad (6.113a\text{–}c)$$

with the critical buckling load being the lowest (6.31c) [(6.39c)] and corresponding to the fundamental buckling mode (6.32e) [(6.40a)].

For the clamped (pinned) beam (6.31b) [(6.39b)], the shape of the elastica (6.107) to the lowest non-linear order (6.109a, b) [(6.103a, 6.108b)] is given by (6.114a) [(6.114b)]

$$\zeta_1(x) = \frac{GL}{2\pi}\left(1 + \frac{G^2}{2}\right)\left[1 - \cos\left(\frac{2\pi x}{L}\right)\right] - \frac{G^3 L}{12\pi}\left[1 - \cos^3\left(\frac{2\pi x}{L}\right)\right], \quad (6.114a)$$

$$\zeta_3(x) = -\frac{GL}{\pi}\left(1 + \frac{3H^2}{2} + \frac{G^2}{2}\right)\sin\left(\frac{\pi x}{L}\right) + \frac{3HG^2 L}{8\pi}\sin\left(\frac{2\pi x}{L}\right) - \frac{G^3 L}{6\pi}\sin^3\left(\frac{\pi x}{L}\right).$$

$$(6.114b)$$

For the cantilever beam, the lowest-order non-linear approximation is (6.115d), the sum of (6.86b) and (6.87c):

$$\bar{A} = 0 = H, \sin\left(p\bar{C}\right) = 0: \quad \zeta_4(x) = \zeta_{4,0}(x) + \zeta_{4,1}(x)$$

$$= \frac{G}{p}\left[1 - \cos(px)\right] + \frac{G^3}{2p}\left[1 - \cos(px) + \frac{\cos^3(px) - 1}{3}\right]$$

$$= \frac{G}{p}\left(1 + \frac{G^2}{2}\right)\left[1 - \cos(px)\right] - \frac{G^3}{6p}\left[1 - \cos^3(px)\right],$$

(6.115a–f)

that coincides with the case (6.115f) ≡ (6.107) of clamping at $x = 0$ with the free end at $x = L$, using (6.74b) ≡ (6.115a), (6.99a) ≡ (6.115b), and (6.100c) ≡ (6.115c). *For a cantilever/pinned/clamped beam the linear buckling corresponds to a succession of increasing axial loads (6.111b, c; 6.113b, c; 6.112b, c) and corresponding harmonics (6.111a; 6.113a; 6.112a) for the buckled shape of the elastica; buckling first occurs for the smallest axial load corresponding to the fundamental buckled shape. The non-linear effect (problem 193) is to add harmonics to the fundamental, that: (i) does not change the critical buckling load, that remains the lowest; and (ii) does change the shape of the elastica through the addition of harmonics. The sum of the fundamental buckling mode and first harmonic is given by (6.115f)/(6.114b)/(6.114a) with an arbitrary amplitude G; the second amplitude is related to the first by (6.108b) in the case of clamped or pinned beams. The linear and non-linear buckling of uniform beams is summarized in the Table 6.1 for the four types of support; namely (i) clamped-clamped, (ii) clamped-pinned, (iii) pinned-pinned and (iv) clamped-free or cantilever.* The critical buckling loads and shapes of the elastica can be changed by point (distributed) springs [section 6.2 (6.3)] that may facilitate or oppose buckling.

6.2 Opposition or Facilitation of Buckling of Beams (Campos & Marta 2014)

It may be desirable to increase the resistance of a beam to buckling; that is, to increase the critical buckling load by using braces or springs to oppose the bending (Figure 6.4); this is a form of bracing that strengthens the beam to bear larger loads. Conversely, if the purpose is to demolish a structure more easily, the critical buckling load could be lowered using springs that favor bending (Figure 6.5). The springs could of the be translational (rotary) type that causes [subsection 6.2.1 (6.2.6)] a force (moment) proportional to the displacement (slope) and are applied: (i) at the tip for a cantilever beam [subsection 6.2.2 (6.2.7)]; or (ii–iv) at the middle for a clamped [subsection 6.2.3 (6.2.8)], pinned [subsection 6.2.4 (6.2.9)],

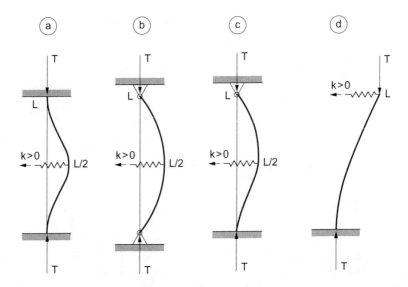

FIGURE 6.4
A translational spring may be used to oppose buckling; that is, increase the critical buckling load, by placing it for example at the tip (d) [middle (a, b, c)] of a cantilever (clamped and/or pinned) beam.

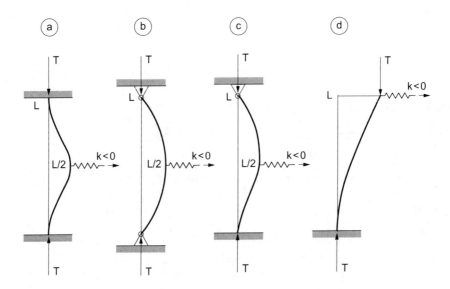

FIGURE 6.5
The buckling of a beam may be facilitated, that is the critical buckling reduced by reversing the position of the spring relative to Figure 6.4.

or clamped-pinned [subsection 6.2.5 (6.2.10)] beams. The relation between the resilience of the translational (rotary) spring and the critical buckling load is obtained (subsection 6.2.11) in all eight cases; it is analyzed in more detail for the cantilever beam (subsection 6.2.12): (i) starting with all the buckling modes in the absence of springs (subsection 6.2.13); (ii) proceeding to consider the effects of springs by analytical methods (subsection 6.2.14); then (iii) alternative graphical methods are presented for rotary (translational) springs [subsection 6.2.15 (6.2.16)]. These results apply to buckling modes of all orders (subsection 6.2.17), beyond the lowest critical buckling load.

6.2.1 Resilience Parameter for a Translational Spring

A translational spring with **translational resilience** k exerts a force proportional to the displacement (6.116) and if placed at the tip or free end balances the transverse force given by (6.15d) for the linear deflection of a uniform beam:

$$k\,\zeta(L) = EI\zeta'''(L) - T\zeta'(L). \tag{6.116}$$

The ratio to the constant (6.10b) beam stiffness of minus the constant (6.10a) compressive tension (the resilience of the linear spring) defines the square of the buckling parameter (6.10c) [cube of the **translational resilience parameter** (6.117a)], both with the dimensions of inverse length:

$$q^3 \equiv \frac{k}{EI}: \qquad\qquad \zeta'''(L) + p^2\,\zeta'(L) = q^3\,\zeta(L). \tag{6.117a, b}$$

The boundary condition (6.116) balancing (problem 194) the restoring force of a linear spring of resilience k against the linear transverse force of a uniform beam under tension (problem 194), can be written (6.117b), in terms of the buckling (6.10c) and resilience (6.117a) parameters, both with dimensions of inverse length.

6.2.2 Cantilever Beam with a Translational Spring at the Tip

The boundary conditions coincide with those for a cantilever beam with a free end (6.63a–c) ≡ (6.118a–c) except that the transverse force, instead of being zero (6.63d), is balanced by the restoring force of the translational spring (6.117b) ≡ (6.118d):

$$\zeta_4(0) = 0 = \zeta_4'(0), \qquad \zeta_4''(L) = 0, \qquad \zeta_4'''(L) + p^2\,\zeta_4'(L) = q^3\,\zeta_4(L).$$

$$\tag{6.118a–d}$$

The clamping boundary conditions at the base (6.118a, b) lead (6.18) to the linear transverse displacement (6.27c), to which are applied the boundary conditions (6.118c, d) at the tip, leading to:

$$
\begin{bmatrix}
\cos(pL) & \sin(pL) \\
q^3\left[1-\cos(pL)\right] & -p^3 + q^3\left[pL - \sin(pL)\right]
\end{bmatrix}
\begin{bmatrix}
C \\
D
\end{bmatrix}
= 0. \qquad (6.119)
$$

A non-trivial solution (6.29c) requires that (A, D) do not vanish simultaneously, and implies that the determinant of the matrix vanishes, leading to:

$$
p^3 \cos(pL) = q^3\left[pL \cos(pL) - \sin(pL)\right]; \qquad (6.120)
$$

this is the relation $T(k_t)$ between the critical buckling load (6.10c) and the resilience of the spring (6.117a).

The absence of a spring (6.121a) simplifies (6.120) to (6.121b) whose smallest root is (6.121c):

$$
q = 0: \qquad \cos(pL) = 0, \qquad pL = \frac{\pi}{2}, \qquad T_4(0) = -\frac{\pi^2}{4}\frac{EI}{L^2}, \qquad (6.121a\text{–}d)
$$

and specifies the critical buckling load (6.121d) in agreement with (6.65d). The critical buckling load (6.121d) is modified by the presence of the spring because (6.121c) is not a root of (6.120) if $q \neq 0$. In the presence of the spring, the critical buckling load is given by (6.120) ≡ (6.122):

$$
p^3 = q^3\left[pL - \tan(pL)\right]. \qquad (6.122)
$$

The critical buckling load (6.121d) is increased (6.123b) by a factor of four to that of a pinned beam (6.123a) ≡ (6.39c) corresponding to (6.10c) to (6.123c):

$$
T_4(k_a) = -\frac{\pi^2 EI}{L^2} = 4T_4(0): \qquad pL = \pi; \qquad q^3 = \frac{p^2}{L} = \frac{\pi^2}{L^3}, \qquad k_a = \frac{\pi^2 EI}{L^3}, \qquad (6.123a\text{–}e)
$$

(6.123c) corresponds (6.122) to (6.123d) the spring resilience (6.117a) given by (6.123e); that is, positive because the spring opposes bending. Conversely, the critical buckling load (6.121d) is reduced (6.124a) by a quarter to (6.124b) for (6.124c):

$$
T_4(k_b) = -\frac{\pi^2 EI}{16L^2} = \frac{T_4(0)}{4}; \qquad pL = \frac{\pi}{4}; \qquad (6.124a\text{–}c)
$$

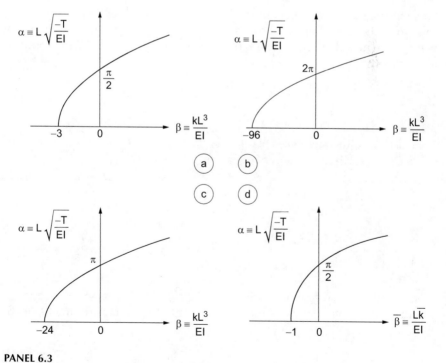

$$q^3 = \frac{p^3}{pL-1} = \frac{1}{16L^3}\frac{\pi^3}{\pi-4}, \qquad k_b = -\frac{\pi^3 EI}{16(4-\pi)L^3}, \qquad (6.124\text{d, e})$$

(6.124c) corresponds (6.122) to (6.124d) leading (6.117a) to a negative spring resilience (6.124e) showing that the spring favors the bending.

The relation between the buckling load and spring resilience (6.122) ≡ (6.125c) can be put into a dimensionless form (6.125a, b):

$$\alpha \equiv pL = L\sqrt{\frac{-T}{EI}}, \qquad \beta \equiv q^3 L^3 = \frac{kL^3}{EI}: \qquad \alpha^3 = \beta(\alpha - \tan\alpha), \qquad (6.125\text{a–c})$$

that is plotted in Panel 6.3a. Using the leading terms of the power series for the tangent (II.7.33b) ≡ (6.126a) implies (6.126b):

$$\tan\alpha = \alpha + \frac{\alpha^3}{3} + O(\alpha^5): \qquad \lim_{\alpha\to 0}\beta = \lim_{\alpha\to 0}\frac{\alpha^3}{\alpha-\tan\alpha} = -3. \qquad (6.126\text{a, b})$$

PANEL 6.3
A translational spring can be placed so as to oppose (favor) bending of a beam under compression [Figure 6.4 (6.5)] thus increasing (decreasing) the critical buckling load.

This proves that *(problem 195) the cantilever beam will buckle without an axial load (6.127a) corresponding to (6.126b) ≡ (6.127b, c):*

$$T_4(k_c)=0: \qquad \alpha=0, \qquad \beta=-3, \qquad k_c=-\frac{3EI}{L^3}, \qquad (6.127a\text{–}d)$$

if the spring resilience (6.117a) is (6.127d). The plot of (6.125c) in Panel 6.3a includes the preceding three cases (6.121a–d; 6.124a–e; 6.127a–d) as well as intermediate values, and concerns a cantilever beam. The shape of the elastica of the buckled, clamped-free beam with translational spring at the free end is given to within a multiplying constant by (6.128b):

$$D=-C\cot(pL): \qquad \zeta_4(x)=C\left[\cos(px)-1+\frac{px-\sin(px)}{\tan(pL)}\right], \qquad (6.128a,\,b)$$

that is obtained by substituting (6.128a) in (6.27c); the first line of (6.119) coincides with (6.128a). The same method applies to other cases of support, for example a beam clamped at both ends that is considered next (subsection 6.2.3).

6.2.3 Clamped Beam with a Translational Spring at the Middle

Since the beam is clamped at the end $x=0$, the equation of the elastica (6.27c) remains valid. The shape of the elastica is symmetric and thus the slope vanishes at the middle (6.129a) where the translational spring (6.117b) is applied (6.129b):

$$\zeta_1'\left(\frac{L}{2}\right)=0, \qquad \zeta_1'''\left(\frac{L}{2}\right)+p^2\,\zeta_1'\left(\frac{L}{2}\right)=q^3\,\zeta_1\left(\frac{L}{2}\right). \qquad (6.129a,\,b)$$

Substituting the shape of the elastica (6.27c) in the boundary conditions (6.129a, b) leads to the system of equations:

$$\begin{bmatrix} -\sin\left(\dfrac{pL}{2}\right) & \cos\left(\dfrac{pL}{2}\right)-1 \\ q^3\left[1-\cos\left(\dfrac{pL}{2}\right)\right] & -p^3+q^3\left[\dfrac{pL}{2}-\sin\left(\dfrac{pL}{2}\right)\right] \end{bmatrix}\begin{bmatrix} C \\ D \end{bmatrix}=0. \qquad (6.130)$$

The relation between the critical buckling load and spring resilience is specified by the vanishing of the determinant of the matrix in (6.130), leading to:

$$p^3\sin\left(\frac{pL}{2}\right)=q^3\left[\frac{pL}{2}\sin\left(\frac{pL}{2}\right)+2\cos\left(\frac{pL}{2}\right)-2\right]. \qquad (6.131)$$

The absence of spring (6.132a) simplifies (6.131) to (6.132b), whose smallest root is (6.132c), leading to the critical load buckling load (6.132d) ≡ (6.31c) for a clamped-clamped beam:

$$q=0: \qquad \sin\left(\frac{pL}{2}\right)=0, \quad p_{1,1}L=2\pi, \quad T_1(0)=-\frac{4\pi^2\,EI}{L^2}=16T_4(0), \qquad \text{(6.132a–e)}$$

that is 16 times (6.132e) that of the cantilever beam (6.121d).

The critical buckling load is reduced to (6.133a) a quarter (6.133b) as for a pinned beam (6.39c) for (6.133c):

$$T_{1d}(k_d)=-\frac{\pi^2\,EI}{L^2}=\frac{T_1(0)}{4}=T_3(0): \qquad\qquad pL=\pi; \qquad \text{(6.133a–c)}$$

$$q^3=\frac{2p^3}{\pi-4}=\frac{2\pi^3}{(\pi-4)L^3}, \qquad\qquad k_d=-\frac{2\pi^3\,EI}{(4-\pi)L^3}, \qquad \text{(6.133d, e)}$$

(6.133c) corresponds (6.131) to (6.133d) leading (6.117a) to a negative spring resilience (6.133e), implying that the spring favors bending.

Using (6.125a, b) the relation (6.131) between the critical buckling load (6.10c) and resilience of the spring (6.117a) can be put in the dimensionless form:

$$\alpha^3\sin\left(\frac{\alpha}{2}\right)=\beta\left[\frac{\alpha}{2}\sin\left(\frac{\alpha}{2}\right)+2\cos\left(\frac{\alpha}{2}\right)-2\right]. \qquad \text{(6.134)}$$

Using the power series (II.7.30a) ≡ (6.135a) [(II.7.23a) ≡ (6.135b)]:

$$\sin\left(\frac{\alpha}{2}\right)=\frac{\alpha}{2}-\frac{1}{3!}\left(\frac{\alpha}{2}\right)^3+O(\alpha^5), \qquad \text{(6.135a)}$$

$$\cos\left(\frac{\alpha}{2}\right)=1-\frac{1}{2}\left(\frac{\alpha}{2}\right)^2+\frac{1}{4!}\left(\frac{\alpha}{2}\right)^4+O(\alpha^6), \qquad \text{(6.135b)}$$

the term in square brackets in (6.134) scales for small α as:

$$\frac{\alpha^3}{\beta}\sin\left(\frac{\alpha}{2}\right)=\left(\frac{\alpha}{2}\right)^2\left(1-\frac{\alpha^2}{24}\right)+2\left(1-\frac{\alpha^2}{8}+\frac{\alpha^4}{384}\right)-2+O(\alpha^6)=-\frac{\alpha^4}{192}+O(\alpha^6),$$

$$\text{(6.136)}$$

implying the limit:

$$\lim_{\alpha \to 0} \beta = - \lim_{\alpha \to 0} \frac{192}{\alpha} \sin\left(\frac{\alpha}{2}\right) = -96. \tag{6.137}$$

Thus *buckling occurs (problem 196) in the absence of an axial load (6.138a) for a spring resilience (6.138b)*:

$$T_1(k_e) = 0: \qquad\qquad\qquad k_e = -\frac{96\, EI}{L^3}. \tag{6.138a, b}$$

The relation (6.134) between the critical buckling load (6.125a) and resilience of the spring (6.125b) is plotted in Panel 6.3b. The shape of the elastica of the buckled clamped-clamped beam with a linear spring at the middle is given to within a multiplying constant by (6.139b):

$$C = \left[\cot\left(\frac{pL}{2}\right) - \csc\left(\frac{pL}{2}\right) \right] D: \tag{6.139a}$$

$$\zeta_1(x) = D\left\{ \sin(px) - p(x) + \left[\cot\left(\frac{pL}{2}\right) - \csc\left(\frac{pL}{2}\right) \right] \left[\cos(px) - 1 \right] \right\}, \tag{6.139b}$$

that is obtained substituting (6.139a) in (6.27c); the first line of (6.130) coincides with (6.139a). The replacement of clamped by pinned supports leads to smaller critical buckling loads for the same spring resilience that are considered next (subsection 6.2.4).

6.2.4 Pinned Beam with a Translational Spring at the Middle

The boundary conditions at (6.36a, b) the pinned support at $x = 0$ applied to (6.18) relate (6.140a, b) the constants of integration in (6.18):

$$0 = \zeta_3(0) = A + C, \quad 0 = \zeta_3''(0) = -p^2 C, \tag{6.140a, b}$$

leading to the shape of the elastica:

$$\zeta_3(x) = Bx + D\sin(px). \tag{6.141}$$

The shape of the elastica is symmetric and thus the same boundary conditions (6.129a, b) with translational spring in the middle can be applied:

$$\begin{bmatrix} 1 & p\cos\left(\dfrac{pL}{2}\right) \\[3mm] p^2-\dfrac{q^3L}{2} & -q^3\sin\left(\dfrac{pL}{2}\right) \end{bmatrix}\begin{bmatrix} B \\[3mm] D \end{bmatrix}=0. \tag{6.142}$$

The vanishing of the determinant specifies the relation between the buckling load and the resilience of the spring:

$$p^3\cos\left(\frac{pL}{2}\right)=q^3\left[\frac{pL}{2}\cos\left(\frac{pL}{2}\right)-\sin\left(\frac{pL}{2}\right)\right]. \tag{6.143}$$

The absence of spring (6.144a) simplifies (6.142) to (6.144b) whose smallest positive root specifies (6.144c) the critical buckling load (6.144d) ≡ (6.39c) for a pinned-pinned beam:

$$q=0:\quad \cos\left(\frac{pL}{2}\right)=0,\quad p_{3,1}L=\pi,\quad T_3(0)=-\frac{\pi^2EI}{L^2}=4T_2(0)=\frac{1}{4}T_1(0),$$
$$\tag{6.144a–f}$$

that is four times larger (smaller) than in the clamped-free (6.144e) ≡ (6.121d) [clamped-clamped (6.144f) ≡ (6.132d)] case.

The critical buckling load (6.144d) is multiplied by a factor of four (6.145a) ≡ (6.31c) as for a free clamped beam for (6.145c):

$$T_3(k_f)=-\frac{4\pi^2EI}{L^2}=T_3(0):\quad pL=2\pi;\quad q^3=\frac{2p^2}{L}=\frac{8\pi^2}{L^3},\quad k_f=\frac{8\pi^2EI}{L^3},$$
$$\tag{6.145a–e}$$

corresponding (6.143) to (6.145d) to a spring resilience (6.145e) that is positive, implying that the spring opposes bending. The relation (6.143) between the critical buckling load (6.125a) and resilience of the spring (6.125b) can be put into the dimensionless form:

$$\alpha^3\cos\left(\frac{\alpha}{2}\right)=\beta\left[\frac{\alpha}{2}\cos\left(\frac{\alpha}{2}\right)-\sin\left(\frac{\alpha}{2}\right)\right]. \tag{6.146}$$

Using (6.135a, b) in the limit of small α the term in square brackets in (6.146) scales as:

$$\frac{\alpha^3}{\beta}\cos\left(\frac{\alpha}{2}\right)=\frac{\alpha}{2}\left(1-\frac{\alpha^2}{8}\right)-\frac{\alpha}{2}\left(1-\frac{\alpha^2}{24}\right)+O(\alpha^5)=-\frac{\alpha^3}{24}+O(\alpha^5). \tag{6.147}$$

This leads to the limit:

$$\lim_{\alpha \to 0} \beta = -\lim_{\alpha \to 0} 24 \cos\left(\frac{\alpha}{2}\right) = -24, \tag{6.148}$$

implying *that buckling occurs (problem 197) without an axial load (6.149a) for (6.149b) spring resilience (6.149c):*

$$T_3\left(k_g\right)=0: \qquad\qquad \beta=-24, \qquad k_g=-\frac{24EI}{L^2}, \tag{6.149a-c}$$

that favors bending, and in modulus is smaller (larger) than for the clamped-clamped (6.138b) [clamped-free (6.127d)] case. The relation (6.146) between the critical buckling load (6.125a) and the resilience of the spring (6.125b) is plotted in Panel 6.3c. The shape of the elastica of the buckled pinned-pinned beam with linear spring at the middle is given to within a multiplying constant by (6.150b):

$$B=-pD\cos\left(\frac{pL}{2}\right): \qquad \zeta_3(x)=D\left[\sin(px)-px\cos\left(\frac{pL}{2}\right)\right], \tag{6.150a, b}$$

that is obtained by substituting (6.150a) in (6.141): the first line of (6.142) coincides with (6.150a). The remaining combination of supports is the clamped-pinned beam considered next (subsection 6.2.5).

6.2.5 Clamped-Pinned Beam with Spring at the Middle

Since the shape is not symmetric the elastica (6.18) is given: (i) in the lower half by (6.27c) ≡ (6.151a) that satisfies the boundary conditions (6.26a, b) at the clamped end:

$$\zeta_3(x)=\begin{cases} A\left[1-\cos(px)\right]+D\left[\sin(px)-px\right] & \text{if} \quad 0\leq x\leq\frac{L}{2}; & (6.151a)\\[4mm] B(L-x)+C\sin\left[p(L-x)\right] & \text{if} \quad \frac{L}{2}\leq x<L, & (6.151b) \end{cases}$$

and (ii) in the upper half by (6.141) ≡ (6.151b) that meets the boundary conditions (6.140a, b) at the pinned end, replacing x by $L - x$. The four arbitrary constants are determined by four conditions at the matching point in the middle: (i–ii) continuity of the displacement and slope (6.152a, b):

$$\zeta_3\left(\frac{L}{2}-0\right)=\zeta_3\left(\frac{L}{2}+0\right), \qquad \zeta_3'\left(\frac{L}{2}-0\right)=\zeta_3'\left(\frac{L}{2}+0\right); \tag{6.152a, b}$$

$$\zeta_3''\left(\frac{L}{2}-0\right)=\zeta_3''\left(\frac{L}{2}+0\right), \qquad \zeta_3'''\left(\frac{L}{2}+0\right)-\zeta_3'''\left(\frac{L}{2}-0\right)=q^3\,\zeta_3\left(\frac{L}{2}\right), \tag{6.152c, d}$$

(iii) since there is no applied torque the curvature is also continuous (6.152c); and (iv) the transverse force has a jump (6.152d) due to the force of the spring. In the l.h.s of (6.152d), the ζ' term of the force can be omitted due to the continuity of the slope (6.152b) and on the r.h.s. of (6.152d) the displacement is unique by (6.152a). Substituting the shape of the elastica (6.151a, b) in the boundary conditions (6.152a–d) leads to the system of equations:

$$
\begin{bmatrix}
1-\cos\left(\dfrac{pL}{2}\right) & -\dfrac{L}{2} & -\sin\left(\dfrac{pL}{2}\right) & \sin\left(\dfrac{pL}{2}\right)-\dfrac{pL}{2} \\[2ex]
p\sin\left(\dfrac{pL}{2}\right) & 1 & -p\cos\left(\dfrac{pL}{2}\right) & p\cos\left(\dfrac{pL}{2}\right)-p \\[2ex]
\cos\left(\dfrac{pL}{2}\right) & 0 & \sin\left(\dfrac{pL}{2}\right) & -\sin\left(\dfrac{pL}{2}\right) \\[2ex]
p^{3}\sin\left(\dfrac{pL}{2}\right) & -q^{3}\dfrac{L}{2} & -q^{3}\sin\left(\dfrac{pL}{2}\right)-p^{3}\cos\left(\dfrac{pL}{2}\right) & p^{3}\cos\left(\dfrac{pL}{2}\right)
\end{bmatrix}
\begin{bmatrix} A \\[2ex] B \\[2ex] C \\[2ex] D \end{bmatrix}
= 0.
$$

$$(6.153)$$

The vanishing of the determinant of the matrix in (6.153) specifies (problem 198) the relation between the critical buckling load and the resilience of the spring for the clamped-pinned beam. The shape of the elastica of beam with linear spring at the middle is given to within a constant multiplying factor by (6.151a, b) where the four constants of integration can be expressed in terms of one using (6.153).

6.2.6 Force (Moment) Due to a Translational (Rotary) Spring

A linear (rotary) spring affects the critical buckling load by applying a force (moment) proportional to the displacement (slope); the same four combinations of support can be considered, namely clamped-free [subsection 6.2.2 (6.2.6)], clamped-clamped [subsection 6.2.3 (6.2.7)], pinned-pinned [subsection 6.2.4 (6.2.8)] and clamped-pinned [subsection 6.2.5 (6.2.9)]. If the linear spring is replaced by *(problem 199) a rotary spring, the free and boundary conditions (problem 199) are: (i) a bending moment (6.14d) proportional to the slope (6.154a) through the* **rotational resilience** $\bar{k}$ *of the spring; (ii) zero transverse force (6.14e) ≡ (6.154b):*

$$-EI\zeta''(L)= \bar{k}\,\zeta'(L), \qquad EI\zeta'''(L)-T\zeta'(L)=0. \qquad (6.154a, b)$$

The boundary conditions (6.154a, b) ≡ (6.155b, c) involve two parameters:

$$\bar{q}=\frac{\bar{k}}{EI}: \qquad \zeta''(L)+\bar{q}\,\zeta'(L)=0, \qquad \zeta'''(L)+p^{2}\,\zeta'(L)=0, \qquad (6.155a–c)$$

*namely the buckling parameter (6.10c) and the **rotational resilience parameter** (6.155a) defined as of the resilience of the rotary spring to the bending stiffness; both have the dimensions of inverse length.*

6.2.7 Rotary Spring at the Free End of a Cantilever Beam

The shape of the elastica (6.18) for a beam clamped (6.26a, b) at $x = 0$ is (6.27c). Substituting the shape (6.27c) of the elastica in the boundary conditions (6.155b, c) leads to the system of equations:

$$\begin{bmatrix} p^2 \cos(pL)+p\bar{q}\sin(pL) & p^2\sin(pL)-p\bar{q}\cos(pL)+p\bar{q} \\ 0 & 1 \end{bmatrix}\begin{bmatrix} C \\ D \end{bmatrix}=0.$$
(6.156)

The vanishing of the determinant of the matrix in (6.156) specifies the relation between the critical buckling load and resilience of the rotary spring:

$$p\cos(pL)=-\bar{q}\sin(pL).$$
(6.157)

In the absence of spring $\bar{q}=0$, this leads to the same critical buckling load (6.121a–d) as before.

The critical buckling load (6.121d) is multiplied by four to (6.158a) as for a free pinned beam (6.158c) by choosing (6.158c):

$$T_4\left(\bar{k}_a\right)=-\pi^2\frac{EI}{L^2}=4T_4(0)=T_3(0): \quad pL=\pi; \quad \bar{q}=\infty; \quad \bar{k}_a=\infty,$$
(6.158a–e)

this would require (6.155a) an infinite (6.158d) resilience (6.158e) of the rotary spring. The critical buckling load (6.121d) is divided by four (6.159a) for (6.159b):

$$T_1\left(\bar{k}_b\right)=-\frac{\pi^2 EI}{16L^2}, \quad pL=\frac{\pi}{4}; \quad \bar{q}=-p=-\frac{\pi}{4L}, \quad \bar{k}_b=-\frac{\pi EI}{4L},$$
(6.159a–e)

this corresponds (6.155a) to (6.155d) the resilience (6.155e) of the rotary spring. *The (problem 200) relation (6.157) between the critical buckling load (6.125a) and the resilience (6.155a) of the rotary spring (6.160a) is (6.160b):*

$$\bar{\beta}\equiv\bar{q}L=\frac{\bar{k}L}{EI}: \qquad\qquad \bar{\beta}=-\alpha\cot\alpha.$$
(6.160a, b)

The buckling in the absence of an axial load (6.161b) occurs (6.161a) for the resilience (6.161c) of the rotary spring:

$$\lim_{\alpha \to 0} \bar{\beta} = \lim_{\alpha \to 0} -\frac{\alpha}{\tan \alpha} = -1: \qquad T_4\left(\bar{k}_c\right) = 0, \qquad \bar{k}_c = -\frac{EI}{L}. \qquad \text{(6.161a–c)}$$

The relation (6.160b) between the critical buckling load (6.125a) and resilience of the spring (6.160a) is plotted in Panel 6.3d, including the cases (6.158a–d; 6.159a–d). The shape of the elastica of the buckled clamped-free beam with a rotary spring at the free end is given to within a multiplying constant by (6.162b):

$$D=0: \qquad\qquad \zeta_4(x) = C\left[\cos(px) - 1\right], \qquad \text{(6.162a, b)}$$

that is obtained by substituting (6.162a) in (6.27c); the second line of (6.156) coincides with (6.162a).

6.2.8 Rotary Spring at the Middle of a Clamped Beam

The rotary spring can cause a skew-symmetry that breaks the symmetry of the shape of the elastica of the buckled beam. Thus the shape of the elastica is given: (i) in the lower half by (6.27c) ≡ (6.163a) that meets the boundary condition (6.26a, b) of clamping at $x = 0$:

$$\zeta_1(x) = \begin{cases} A\left[1 - \cos(px)\right] + D\left[\sin(px) - px\right] & \text{if } 0 \le x \le \dfrac{L}{2}; \quad \text{(6.163a)} \\[2mm] B\left\{1 - \cos\left[p(L-x)\right]\right\} + C\left[\sin\left[p(L-x)\right] - p(L-x)\right] & \text{if } \dfrac{L}{2} \le x \le L, \quad \text{(6.163b)} \end{cases}$$

and (ii) in the upper half by (6.163b) that replaces x by $L - x$ to satisfy the clamping condition at $x = L$. At the matching point in the middle $x = L/2$: (i, ii) the displacement and slope are continuous (6.152a, b); (iii) since there is no transverse force the third derivative is also continuous (6.164a); and (iv) the bending moment has a jump (6.164b) due to the rotary spring:

$$\zeta'''\left(\frac{L}{2} - 0\right) = \zeta'''\left(\frac{L}{2} + 0\right), \qquad \zeta''\left(\frac{L}{2} + 0\right) - \zeta''\left(\frac{L}{2} - 0\right) = \bar{q}\,\zeta'\left(\frac{L}{2}\right). \qquad \text{(6.164a, b)}$$

Substituting (6.163a, b) in the matching conditions (6.152a, b; 6.164a, b) leads to:

$$
\begin{bmatrix}
1-\cos\left(\dfrac{pL}{2}\right) & \cos\left(\dfrac{pL}{2}\right)-1 & \dfrac{pL}{2}-\sin\left(\dfrac{pL}{2}\right) & \sin\left(\dfrac{pL}{2}\right)-\dfrac{pL}{2} \\[2mm]
p\sin\left(\dfrac{pL}{2}\right) & -p\sin\left(\dfrac{pL}{2}\right) & -p-p\cos\left(\dfrac{pL}{2}\right) & -p+p\cos\left(\dfrac{pL}{2}\right) \\[2mm]
-\sin\left(\dfrac{pL}{2}\right) & \sin\left(\dfrac{pL}{2}\right) & \cos\left(\dfrac{pL}{2}\right) & -\cos\left(\dfrac{pL}{2}\right) \\[2mm]
p^2\cos\left(\dfrac{pL}{2}\right)+p\,\bar{q}\sin\left(\dfrac{pL}{2}\right) & -p^2\cos\left(\dfrac{pL}{2}\right) & p^2\sin\left(\dfrac{pL}{2}\right) & -p^2\sin\left(\dfrac{pL}{2}\right)-p\bar{q}+p\bar{q}\cos\left(\dfrac{pL}{2}\right)
\end{bmatrix}
\begin{bmatrix} A \\ B \\ C \\ D \end{bmatrix} = 0,
$$

$$(6.165)$$

The relation (problem 201) between the critical buckling load (6.125a) and the resilience of the rotary spring (6.160a) is specified for the clamped-clamped beam by the vanishing of the determinant of the matrix (6.165). The shape of the elastica of a buckled clamped-clamped beam with a rotary spring in the middle is given to within a multiplying constant by (6.163a, b), where all four constants of integration can be expressed in terms of one of them using (6.165).

6.2.9 Pinned Beam with Rotary Spring at the Middle

The symmetry under buckling is again violated by the skew-symmetry of the rotary spring, and the shape of the elastica is given: (i) in the lower half by (6.141) ≡ (6.166a) that meets the pinning boundary conditions at $x = 0$:

$$
\zeta_3(x) =
\begin{cases}
Bx + D\sin(px) & \text{if} \quad 0 \le x \le \dfrac{L}{2}\,; & (6.166a) \\[4mm]
A(L-x) + C\sin\big[\,p(L-x)\,\big] & \text{if} \quad \dfrac{L}{2} \le x \le L, & (6.166b)
\end{cases}
$$

and (ii) in the upper half (6.166b) substituting x by $L - x$. Substituting the shape of the elastica (6.166a, b) in the matching conditions (6.152a, b; 6.164a, b) leads to the system of equations:

$$
\begin{bmatrix}
-\dfrac{L}{2} & \dfrac{L}{2} & -\sin\left(\dfrac{pL}{2}\right) & \sin\left(\dfrac{pL}{2}\right) \\[2mm]
1 & 1 & -p\cos\left(\dfrac{pL}{2}\right) & p\cos\left(\dfrac{pL}{2}\right) \\[2mm]
0 & 0 & -\cos\left(\dfrac{pL}{2}\right) & \cos\left(\dfrac{pL}{2}\right) \\[2mm]
0 & -\bar{q} & p^2\sin\left(\dfrac{pL}{2}\right) & -p^2\sin\left(\dfrac{pL}{2}\right)-p\bar{q}\cos\left(\dfrac{pL}{2}\right)
\end{bmatrix}
\begin{bmatrix} A \\ B \\ C \\ D \end{bmatrix} = 0. \qquad (6.167)
$$

The relation (problem 202) between the critical buckling load (6.125a) and resilience of the rotary spring (6.160a) is specified for the pinned-pinned beam by the vanishing of the determinant of the matrix in (6.167). The shape of the elastica of a buckled pinned-pinned beam with a rotary spring in the middle is given to within a multiplying constant by (6.166a, b) where the four constants of integration can be expressed in terms of one of them using (6.167).

6.2.10 Clamped-Pinned Beam with a Rotary Spring

The shape of the elastica is not symmetric because: (i) the clamping and pinning boundary conditions are distinct and lead to an unsymmetric shape of the elastica; and (ii) the rotary spring in the middle violates symmetry by adding skew-symmetry. The shape of the elastica is given by (6.151a) in the lower and (6.151b) in the upper half. The matching conditions at the location $x = L/2$ of the rotary spring are (6.152a, b; 6.164a, b). Substituting the former (6.151a, b) in the latter (6.152a, b; 6.164a, b) leads to the system of equations:

$$
\begin{bmatrix}
1 - \cos\left(\dfrac{pL}{2}\right) & -\dfrac{L}{2} & -\sin\left(\dfrac{pL}{2}\right) & \sin\left(\dfrac{pL}{2}\right) - \dfrac{pL}{2} \\
p\sin\left(\dfrac{pL}{2}\right) & 1 & -p\cos\left(\dfrac{pL}{2}\right) & -p + p\cos\left(\dfrac{pL}{2}\right) \\
-\sin\left(\dfrac{pL}{2}\right) & 0 & \cos\left(\dfrac{pL}{2}\right) & -\cos\left(\dfrac{pL}{2}\right) \\
-p^2\cos\left(\dfrac{pL}{2}\right) & \bar{q} & -p^2\sin\left(\dfrac{pL}{2}\right) - p\bar{q}\cos\left(\dfrac{pL}{2}\right) & p^2\sin\left(\dfrac{pL}{2}\right)
\end{bmatrix}
\begin{bmatrix} A \\ B \\ C \\ D \end{bmatrix} = 0.
$$

(6.168)

The relation (problem 203) between the critical buckling load (6.125a) and the resilience of the rotary spring (6.160a) for a clamped-pinned beam is specified by the roots of the determinant of the matrix (6.168). The shape of the elastica of a buckling clamped-pinned beam with a rotary spring at the middle is given to within a multiplying constant by (6.151a, b) where the four constants of integration can be expressed in terms of one of them using (6.168).

6.2.11 Combinations of Four Supports and Two Types of Springs

The effect of a translational (rotary) spring on the buckling of a beam [subsections 6.2.1(6.2.6)] has been considered for the four classical combinations of support: (i) clamped-free [subsection 6.2.2. (6.2.7)]; (ii) clamped-clamped [subsection 6.2.3 (6.2.8)]; (iii) pinned-pinned [subsection 6.2.4 (6.2.9)]; and (iv) clamped-pinned [subsection 6.2.5 (6.2.10)]. The spring was placed at the tip in the case (i) and at the middle in the remaining cases (iii–iv). For each of the eight combinations was obtained: (i) the relation between the critical buckling load and the resilience of the spring; and (ii) the resulting shape of the buckled elastica taking into account the effect of the linear or rotary spring.

Of the eight cases, four are simplest (Table 6.2), leading to plots of the relation between the critical buckling load and the resilience of the spring: (a, d) the cantilever or clamped-free beam with translational (rotary) spring at the tip [Panel 6.3a(d)]; and (b, c) the clamped-clamped (pinned-pinned) beam with a linear spring at the middle [Panel 6.3b(c)]. The linear or rotary spring can be placed so as to oppose (favor) bending [Figure 6.4 (6.5)] thus increasing (decreasing) the critical buckling load. Table 6.2 indicates in the four simplest cases (a–d) the value of the resilience of the spring that causes buckling without an axial load.

The buckling relation between the critical axial load (6.125a) and the resilience of a translational (6.125b) or rotary (6.160a) spring has been obtained in all eight cases of: (i–iii) clamped-clamped (6.165), pinned-pinned (6.167), and clamped-pinned (6.168) beam with a rotary spring in the middle; (iv–v) the cantilever beam with a translational (6.125c) or rotary (6.157) spring at the tip; (vi–viii) clamped-clamped (6.134), pinned-pinned (6.146), and clamped-pinned (6.153) beam with a translational spring in the middle. In cases iv, v, vi, and vii the relation between axial tension and spring resilience was illustrated respectively in Panels 6.3a, d, b, and c near the critical spring resilience that leads to buckling without axial load. The relation between axial load and spring resilience is considered next not only for the first but also for all buckling modes (subsections 6.2.12–6.2.13) for the case of a cantilever beam with a translational or rotary (subsection 6.2.13) spring at the tip (subsections 6.2.14–6.2.17).

TABLE 6.2

Resilience of the Spring that Causes Buckling without an Axial Load for the Four Simplest Cases

Case	Relation	Beam	Spring	Resilience
a	Panel 6.3a	cantilever	linear	$k = -\dfrac{3EI}{L^3}$
b	Panel 6.3b	clamped-clamped	linear	$k = -\dfrac{96EI}{L^3}$
c	Panel 6.3c	pinned-pinned	linear	$k = -\dfrac{24EI}{L^3}$
d	Panel 6.3d	cantilever	rotary	$k = -\dfrac{EI}{L^3}$

Note: It is possible to cause buckling without an axial compression by using translational or rotational springs (Figures 6.3–6.4).

6.2.12 Buckling Modes for a Cantilever Beam

The buckling relation specifying the critical axial buckling load (6.125a) for a cantilever beam is (6.160b) ≡ (6.169):

$$\frac{\tan\alpha}{\alpha} = -\frac{1}{\bar\beta} \equiv \bar{s},$$ (6.169)

for a rotary spring (6.160a), and (6.125c) ≡ (6.170):

$$\frac{\tan\alpha}{\alpha} = 1 - \frac{\alpha^2}{\beta} \equiv s,$$ (6.170)

for a translational spring (6.125b), both cases with the spring at tip. In the case of a pinned-pinned beam with a linear spring in the middle, the buckling relation (6.146) ≡ (6.171):

$$\frac{\tan(\alpha/2)}{\alpha/2} = 1 - \frac{2\alpha^2}{\beta} = 1 - \frac{8}{\beta}\left(\frac{\alpha}{2}\right)^2,$$ (6.171)

is similar to (6.170) with the substitutions $\alpha \to \alpha/2$ and $\beta \to \beta/8$. Since the case (6.171) is reducible to (6.170), only the latter will be considered in the sequel. *In the absence (problem 204) of either translational (6.172a) or rotary (6.172b) spring, respectively (6.170) and (6.169) both imply (6.172c) that there is an infinity of buckling modes (6.172d):*

$$\beta = 0 \quad \text{or} \quad \bar\beta = 0: \qquad \tan\alpha = \infty \quad \Rightarrow \quad \alpha_n = n\pi - \frac{\pi}{2},$$ (6.172a–d)

with (6.173a) leading (6.125a; 6.172d) ≡ (6.173b) to the critical buckling loads (6.10c) ≡ (6.173c):

$$n = 1,2,3,...: \quad p_{4,n}L = \alpha_n, \quad T_{4,n} = -EI\left(p_{4,n}\right)^2 = -\frac{\pi^2 EI(2n-1)^2}{4L^2}.$$ (6.173a–c)

From either (6.128b) or (6.162b) follows the shape (6.174a) and slope (6.174b) of the modes:

$$\zeta_{4,n}(x) = A_n\left\{1 - \cos\left[\left(n - \frac{1}{2}\right)\left(\frac{\pi x}{L}\right)\right]\right\},$$ (6.174a)

$$\zeta'_{4,n}(x) = \frac{\pi A_n(2n-1)}{2L}\sin\left[\left(n - \frac{1}{2}\right)\frac{\pi x}{L}\right],$$ (6.174b)

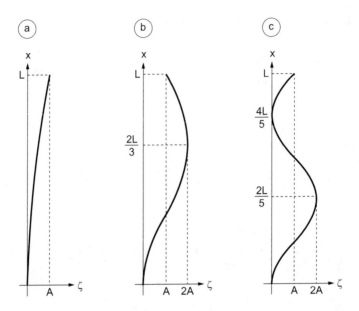

PANEL 6.4
The critical buckling load corresponds to the first bending mode of the beam under compression; for example, a cantilever beam (Figure 6.4d). Higher-order modes correspond to larger axial compression loads and lead to shapes with more zeros or nodes.

corresponding to:

$$\zeta_{4,n}(L) = A_n\,, \qquad \zeta'_{4,n}(L) = \frac{\pi A_n}{2L}(-)^{n+1}(2n-1), \qquad \text{(6.174c, d)}$$

the deflection (6.174c) and slope (6.174d) at the free end. The first three modes of buckling of a cantilever beam (Panel 6.4) are considered next (subsection 6.2.13).

6.2.13 First Three Modes of Buckled Cantilever Beam

The first buckling mode (6.175a) of a cantilever beam (6.175b) under compression without spring support (Panel 6.4a) in the linear case corresponds to (6.65b) ≡ (6.175b) the critical load (6.67a) ≡ (6.175c) and displacement (6.174a) ≡ (6.175d) and slope (6.174b) ≡ (6.175e):

$$n = 1, \quad p_{4,1}L = \frac{\pi}{2}, \quad T_{4,1} = -\frac{\pi^2 E I}{4L^2}:$$

$$\text{(6.175a–e)}$$

$$\zeta_{4,1}(x) = A_1\left[1 - \cos\left(\frac{\pi x}{2L}\right)\right], \quad \zeta'_{4,1}(x) = \frac{\pi A_1}{2L}\sin\left(\frac{\pi x}{2L}\right),$$

implying (Panel 6.4a) a deflection of the elastica increasing monotonically from the clamped to the free end.

The second mode (6.176a) corresponds (6.176b) to the critical buckling load (6.176c):

$$n = 2, \quad p_{4,2} L = \frac{3\pi}{2}, \quad T_{4,2} = -\frac{9\pi^2 EI}{4L^2}:$$

$$\zeta_{4,2}(x) = A_2 \left[1 - \cos\left(\frac{3\pi x}{2L}\right) \right], \quad \zeta'_{4,2}(L) = \frac{3\pi A_2}{2L} \sin\left(\frac{3\pi x}{2L}\right),$$

$$(6.176a\text{–}e)$$

corresponding to the displacement (6.174a) ≡ (6.176d) and slope (6.174b) ≡ (6.176b). The slope vanishes (6.177a) at the height (6.177b) corresponding to the maximum displacement (6.177c) that is twice that at the tip (6.177d):

$$\zeta'_{4,2}(L) = 0: \quad x_1 = \frac{2L}{3}, \quad \zeta_{4,2\max} = \zeta_{4,2}(x_1) = 2A_2 = 2\zeta_{4,2}(L); \quad \zeta'_{4,2}(L) = -\frac{3\pi A_2}{2L},$$

$$(6.177a\text{–}e)$$

thus the slope is negative (6.177e) at the tip showing that the displacement of the elastica for the second buckling mode (Panel 6.4b) is not monotonic and has one inflexion.

The third (6.178a) buckling mode corresponds (6.178b) to the critical buckling load (6.178c) and displacement (6.174a) ≡ (6.178d) and slope (6.174b) ≡ (6.178e):

$$n = 3: \quad p_{4,3} = \frac{5\pi}{2}, \quad T_{4,n} = -\frac{25\pi^2 EI}{9L^2}:$$

$$\zeta_{4,3}(x) = A_3 \left[1 - \cos\left(\frac{5\pi x}{2L}\right) \right], \quad \zeta'_{4,3}(x) = \frac{5\pi A_3}{2L} \sin\left(\frac{5\pi x}{2L}\right).$$

$$(6.178a\text{–}e)$$

The slope vanishes (6.179a) at two points with the lower (6.179b) [higher (6.175c)] corresponding to the maximum (6.179d) [zero (6.179e)] displacement:

$$\zeta'_{4,3}(x_{2,3}) = 0: \quad x_{2,3} = \frac{2L}{5}, \frac{4L}{5}, \quad \zeta_{4,3}\left(\frac{2L}{5}\right) = 2A_3 = \zeta_{\max}, \quad \zeta_{4,3}\left(\frac{4L}{5}\right) = 0.$$

$$(6.179a\text{–}e)$$

The displacement at the tip is unchanged (6.180a) for any mode whereas the slope (6.180b) increases in modulus (6.180c) with alternating sign (6.180d):

$$\zeta_{4,3}(L) = A_3, \quad \zeta'_{4,3}(L) = \frac{5\pi A_3}{2L}, \quad \frac{3\pi A_2}{2L} = -\zeta'_{4,2}(L), \quad \frac{\pi A_1}{2L} = \zeta'_{4,1}(L),$$

$$(6.180a\text{–}d)$$

implying the existence of two inflexions (Panel 6.4c) for the third buckling mode.

Thus *(problem 205) the first or fundamental buckling mode (6.65b) ≡ (6.175b)*
of a uniform cantilever beam under compression without spring support leads to
the displacement (6.67a) ≡ (6.175d) and slope (6.68a) ≡ (6.175e) of the elastica cor-
responding (Panel 6.4a) to a monotonically increasing deflection from the clamped
based to the free tip; that is, no inflexions. The second (third) buckling mode,
corresponding to 9(25) times larger critical buckling load (6.176c) ≡ (6.181a)
[(6.178c) ≡ (6.181b)]:

$$T_{4,2} = -EI\left(p_{4,2}\right)^2 = -\frac{9\pi^2 EI}{4L^2} = 9T_4, \tag{6.181a}$$

$$T_{4,3} = -EI\left(p_{4,3}\right)^2 = -\frac{25\pi^2 EI}{4L^2} = 25T_4, \tag{6.181b}$$

have displacement (6.176d; 6.177c, d) [(6.178d; 6.179b–e)] and slope (6.176e; 6.177e)
[(6.178e; 6.180b)] implying that the elastica has one (two) inflexions [Panel 6.4b (c)].
Likewise the n-th buckling mode (6.173a–c) would lead to n inflexions of the elastica.
The shape of the modes (6.174a, b) and the values (6.174c, d) are changed in
the presence of the translational (rotary) spring since (6.172d; 6.173b) are longer roots of (6.170) [(6.169)]. The roots are considered next, first analytically
(subsection 6.2.14) and then graphically (subsections 6.2.15–6.2.16).

6.2.14 Infinite Roots for the Critical Buckling Load

The buckling relations for the cantilever beam with a rotary (6.169) or linear
(6.170) spring at the tip both involve the circular tangent whose MacLaurin
series (II.7.22c) ≡ (6.182b):

$$|\alpha| < \frac{\pi}{2}: \qquad \tan\alpha = \frac{1}{\alpha}\sum_{n=1}^{\infty}(-)^n\frac{1-2^{2n}}{(2n)!}B_{2n}\left(2\alpha\right)^{2n}, \tag{6.182a, b}$$

is valid for (II.7.22a) ≡ (6.182a) and involves the Bernoulli numbers B_{2n} of
which the first four are (II.7.32c–e; II.7.36c) ≡ (6.183a–d):

$$B_0 = 1, \qquad B_2 = \frac{1}{6}, \qquad B_4 = -\frac{1}{30}, \qquad B_6 = \frac{1}{42}. \tag{6.183a–d}$$

Substituting (6.182b) in (6.169) gives the series:

$$-\frac{1}{\beta} = \sum_{n=1}^{\infty}(-)^n\frac{1-2^{2n}}{(2n)!}B_{2n}\,2^{2n}\alpha^{2n-2} = 1+\frac{\alpha^2}{3}+\frac{2}{15}\alpha^4 + O\left(\alpha^6\right) = G\prod_{n=1}^{\infty}(\alpha-\alpha_n),$$
$$\tag{6.184}$$

that agrees with (6.126a) and (6.161a) at lowest order; $G \neq 0$ in (6.184) whose roots specify the critical axial loads for all the buckling modes of a cantilever beam with a rotary spring at the tip; in the case of a translational spring (6.182b) is substituted in (6.170) leading to:

$$-\frac{1}{\beta} = \frac{\tan\alpha - \alpha}{\alpha^3} = \frac{1}{\alpha^3}\sum_{n=2}^{\infty}(-)^n\frac{1-2^{2n}}{(2n)!}B_{2n}\,2^{2n}\,\alpha^{2n-1}$$

$$(6.185)$$

$$= \frac{1}{3} + \frac{2}{15}\alpha^2 + O(\alpha^4) = H\prod_{n=1}^{\infty}(\alpha - \alpha_n),$$

that agrees with (6.126b) to lowest order, and where $H \neq 0$. The roots of (6.185) [(6.184)] can be calculated approximately by truncating the series and specify the critical buckling load (6.125a) for a cantilever beam with a translational (6.125b) [rotary (6.160a)] spring at the tip. They can be visualized graphically by a method applied next, first to the case of a rotary (subsection 6.2.15) and then to the case of a translational (subsection 6.2.16) spring opposing or favoring the buckling of the cantilever beam.

6.2.15 Rotary Spring Favoring or Opposing Buckling

The buckling relation for the cantilever beam with a rotary spring (6.169) involves the circular tangent that is plotted in Panel 6.1, showing where it equals its variable, represented by the diagonal of the quadrant. The smallest roots of (6.186a) are recorded (6.186b–d) for future use:

$$\tan\theta_n = \theta_n: \qquad \theta_1 = 4.494, \qquad \theta_2 = 7.725, \qquad \theta_3 = 10.904, \qquad (6.186a\text{--}d)$$

where the smallest (6.186a) $\equiv$ (6.48a) coincides with the lowest critical buckling load for a clamped-pinned beam without spring support (II.7.22a) $\equiv$ (6.182b). The ratio of the circular tangent to its variable, represented by the function $\bar{s}$ in (6.169), is plotted in Panel 6.5 and the roots for the critical buckling load are the intersections with the horizontal lines of constant spring resilience, leading (Table 6.3) to six cases: (I) in the absence of rotary spring $\beta = 0$ the roots for $\bar{s} = -\infty$ are (6.172d); (II) if the rotary spring opposes bending $\beta > 0$ then $\bar{s} < 0$ the roots lie in the range $n\pi - \pi/2 < \alpha_n < n\pi$, implying an increase in the critical buckling load; (III) for an infinitely strong spring opposing bending $\beta = \infty$ then $\bar{s} = 0$ the critical buckling loads are $\alpha_n = n\pi$; (IV) if the rotary spring weakly favors bending $0 > \beta > -1$ then $0 < \bar{s} < 1$ the critical buckling load still increases $n\pi < \alpha_n < \theta_n$ where θ_n is the n-th root of (6.186a); (V) for a spring with transition resilience $\beta = -1$ then $\bar{s} = 1$ a new root α_0 appears, leading to buckling without an axial load, in agreement with (6.161a–c); and (VI) for a stronger rotary spring favoring bending $\beta < -1$ then $\bar{s} > 1$ the critical buckling load increases, $0 < \alpha_0 < \pi/2$ and $\theta_n < \alpha_n < n\pi + \pi/2$.

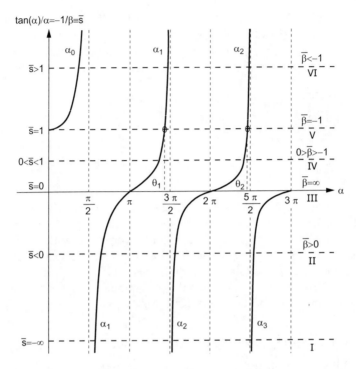

PANEL 6.5

Roots of the critical buckling load (6.113a) versus the resilience of the rotary spring (6.148a) at the tip of a cantilever beam (6.157).

TABLE 6.3

Critical Buckling Load for Cantilever Beam with Rotary Spring

		Opposing Bending		Favoring Bending		
Spring	**None**	**Finite**	**Infinite**	**Weak**	**Transition**	**Strong**
Case	**I**	**II**	**III**	**IV**	**V**	**VI**
Resilience	$\bar{\beta} = 0$	$\bar{\beta} > 0$	$\bar{\beta} = \infty$	$0 > \bar{\beta} > -1$	$\bar{\beta} > -1$	$\bar{\beta} < -1$
$\bar{s} = -\dfrac{1}{\beta}$	$s = -\infty$	$s < 0$	$s = 0$	$0 < s < 1$	$s = 1$	$s > 1$
Lowest root	$\alpha_1 = \dfrac{\pi}{2}$	$\dfrac{\pi}{2} < \alpha_1 < \pi$	$\alpha_1 = \pi$	$\pi < \alpha_1 < \theta_1$	$\alpha_0 = 0$	$0 < \alpha_0 < \dfrac{\pi}{2}$
Other roots	$\alpha_n = n\pi - \dfrac{\pi}{2}$	$n\pi - \dfrac{\pi}{2} < \alpha_n < n\pi$	$\alpha_n = n\pi$	$n\pi < \alpha_n < \theta_n$	$\alpha_n = \theta_n$	$\theta_n < \alpha_n < n\pi + \dfrac{\pi}{2}$

$$\alpha \equiv pL \equiv L\sqrt{-\frac{T}{EI}}; \qquad \beta \equiv \bar{q}L \equiv \frac{\bar{K}_r L}{EI}; \qquad n = 1,2,3,\dots$$

Note: The critical buckling load for a beam acted by a spring depends on the resilience of the spring; for example, for a cantilever beam with a rotary spring at the tip (Figure 6.4d and 6.5d).

Panel 6.3d corresponds (problem 206) to the top left of Panel 6.5 where (i) the root α_0 is the lowest-order buckling mode for a rotary spring favoring bending; and (ii) the root α_1 is the lowest-order buckling mode for a rotary spring opposing bending. For a given critical buckling load α, there is only one possible buckling mode: (i) with a rotary spring favoring bending if $n\pi < \alpha_n < n\pi + \pi/2$ with $n = 0,1,2,...$; (ii) for a rotary spring opposing bending if $n\pi - \pi/2 < \alpha < n\pi$ with $n = 1,2,3...$, and (iii) there is a jump from one mode to the next for $\alpha = n\pi$. For a given spring resilience $\bar{\beta}$, an infinity of buckling modes with increasing critical buckling load are possible: (i) for a rotary spring favoring bending, the modes are α_n with $n = 0,1,2,...$; (ii) for a rotary spring opposing bending for α_n with $n = 1,2,3,....$ The preceding conclusions are modified for a translational spring at the tip of a cantilever beam because (6.169) is replaced by (6.170) where: (i) the l.h.s. is the same; and (ii) the r.h.s. depends not on β but also on α. Thus Panel 6.5 is replaced next (subsection 6.2.16) by Panels 6.6 and 6.7 for the translational spring. Both the rotary and translational spring have a transition resilience with different value (subsection 6.2.17).

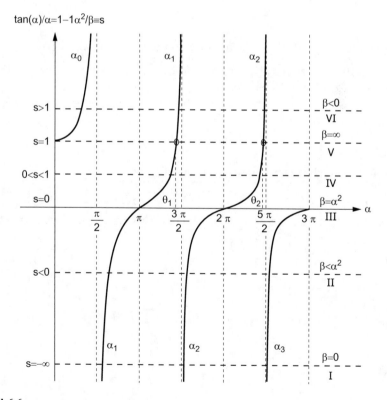

PANEL 6.6
Roots of the critical buckling load (6.113a) versus the resilience of a translational spring (6.113b) at the tip of a cantilever beam (6.158).

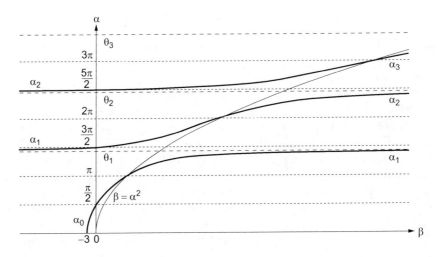

PANEL 6.7

Alternate form of Panel 6.6 with modified axis, namely α vertically and $s = 1 - \alpha^2/\beta$ replaced by β horizontally.

6.2.16 Transition Resilience for Buckling without an Axial Load

The buckling relation (6.170) for a cantilever beam with a spring at the tip is analyzed in Panel 6.6 by comparing the ratio of the circular tangent to its variable lines with the curves for s with the roots α_n as intersections, leading (Table 6.4) to six cases: (I) in the absence of spring $\beta = 0$ then $s = -\infty$ the roots

TABLE 6.4

Critical Buckling Load for Cantilever Beam with Translational Spring

		Opposing Bending				Favoring Bending Strong
Spring	None	Finite	Infinite	Weak	Transition	
Case	I	II	III	IV	V	VI
Resilience	$\beta = 0$	$\beta > 0$	$\beta = \infty$	$\beta > \alpha^2 > 0$	$\beta = \infty$	$\beta < 0$
$s = 1 - \dfrac{\alpha^2}{\beta}$	$s = -\infty$	$s < 0$	$s = 0$	$0 < s < 1$	$s = 1$	$s > 1$
Lowest root	$\alpha_1 = \dfrac{\pi}{2}$	$\dfrac{\pi}{2} < \alpha_1 < \pi$	$\alpha_1 = \pi$	$\pi < \alpha_1 < \theta_1$	$\alpha_0 = 0$	$0 < \alpha_0 < \dfrac{\pi}{2}$
Other roots	$\alpha_n = n\pi - \dfrac{\pi}{2}$	$n\pi - \dfrac{\pi}{2} < \alpha_n < n\pi$	$\alpha_n = n\pi$	$n\pi < \alpha_n < \theta_n$	$\alpha_n = \theta_n$	$\theta_n < \alpha_n < n\pi + \dfrac{\pi}{2}$

$$\alpha \equiv pL \equiv L\sqrt{-\frac{T}{EI}}; \qquad \beta \equiv qL^3 \equiv \frac{kL^3}{EI}; \qquad n = 1,2,3,.....$$

Note: As in Table 6.3, the critical buckling load of a cantilever beam with a translational spring at the tip depends on the resilience of the spring.

are (6.172d), of which the $\alpha_1 = \pi/2$ corresponds to the critical buckling load (6.121c); (II) for a weak spring opposing bending $\beta < \alpha^2$ then $s < 0$ and the roots lie in the interval $n\pi - \pi/2 < \alpha_n < n\pi$ corresponding to higher critical buckling loads; (III) for a critical spring resilience:

$$\beta = \alpha^2 \quad \Leftrightarrow \quad q = p^2/L \quad \Leftrightarrow \quad s = 0, \qquad (6.187\text{a--c})$$

the roots are $\alpha_n = n\pi$; (IV) for a strong spring still opposing bending $0 < \beta > \alpha^2$ then $0 < s < 1$ and the roots lie in the range $n\pi < \alpha_n < \theta_n$, where θ_n is a root of (6.186a) corresponding to a further increase in the critical buckling load that can never exceed $p_n L < \theta_n$; (V) an infinitely strong spring, $\beta = \infty$ or $s = 1$ causes buckling with zero axial load because a new root α_0 appears, and the remaining roots are $\alpha_n = \theta_n$ for the higher-order buckling modes; and (VI) a spring favoring bending $\beta < 0$ or $s > 1$ leads to a lowest-order buckling mode with $0 < \alpha_0 < \pi/2$ and higher-order buckling modes with $\theta_n < \alpha_n < n\pi + \pi/2$. Panel 6.5 (6.6) and Table 6.3 (6.4) for the cantilever beam with a rotary (translational) spring at the tip look similar, but there is an important difference: (i) in Panel 6.5 the horizontal lines $\bar{\beta} = \text{const}$ do not depend on α; while (ii) in Panel 6.6 the horizontal lines $1 - \alpha^2/\beta = \text{const}$ depend both on β and α. In the case (ii) Panel 6.6 is transformed to Panel 6.7 separating α and β along the two axis.

For (i) a translational spring (problem 207) opposing bending of a cantilever beam the roots of (6.170) specifying (6.125a, b) the critical buckling loads all start at $\alpha_n = n\pi - \pi/2$ with $n = 1, 2, 3, \ldots$. and the critical buckling load increases with the resilience of the spring $\beta > 0$ passing through $\alpha_n = n\pi$ for $\beta = (\alpha_n)^2$ and reaching an asymptotic $\beta \to \infty$ maximum $\alpha_n = \theta_n$ where θ_n is the n-th root of (6.186a); (ii) for a translational spring favoring bending, $\beta < 0$ the roots α_n start at $\alpha_n = n\pi + \pi/2$ with $n = 1, 2, 3, \ldots$. and as $|\beta| = -\beta$ increases, the critical buckling load decreases to the asymptotic $\beta \to -\infty$ limit $\alpha_n = \theta_{n-1}$, where θ_{n-1} is the $(n - 1)$-th root of (6.186a); (iii) thus there is a jump of 2π the same root between a translational spring opposing and favoring bending. Another difference is that for a translational spring favoring bending, there is an additional lowest-order root α_0 that (i) allows buckling without an axial load $\alpha_0 = 0$ for $\beta = -3$ in agreement with (6.127a--d); and (ii) for $-3 < \beta < 0$, the critical buckling load increases in the range $0 < \alpha_0 < \pi/2$. Panel 6.3c corresponds to the bottom left of Panel 6.7, that includes all buckling modes. For a given critical buckling load α, there is only one mode: (i) for $n\pi - \pi/2 < \alpha < \theta_n$, it corresponds to a linear spring opposing bending; (ii) for $\theta_n < \alpha < n\pi + \pi/2$, it corresponds to a translational spring favoring bending, with $n = 1, 2, 3, \ldots$. in both cases; and (iii) for a translational spring favoring bending, there is an additional lower-order mode $0 < \alpha_0 < \pi/2$. For a given resilience of the spring there is an infinity of buckling modes α_n: (i) with $n = 1, 2, 3, \ldots$. for a translational spring opposing bending; and (ii) with $n = 0, 1, 2, \ldots$. for a translational spring favoring bending.

6.2.17 Strengthening a Structure or Facilitating Its Demolition

In all the preceding cases of buckling of a beam with any combination of supports and translational or rotary spring at tip or middle, the roots α_n determine the buckled shape (problem 208). For the cantilever beam with a rotary spring at the tip the roots α_n of (6.184) specify the buckled shape (6.188):

$$\zeta_{4,n}(x) = A\left[1 - \cos\left(\alpha_n \frac{x}{L}\right)\right],\tag{6.188}$$

and the deflection at the tip (6.189a) may not be the maximum:

$$\zeta_{4,n}(L) = A\left[1 - \cos(\alpha_n)\right], \qquad \qquad \zeta_n'(L) = A\frac{\alpha_n}{L}\sin(\alpha_n),\tag{6.189a, b}$$

nor does the slope at tip (6.170b) have to be zero. Expressions for the shape and slope of the buckled cantilever beam with a translational spring at the tip can be obtained by substituting in (6.128b) the roots of (6.185).

Table 6.2 relates to Panel 6.3 that shows the relation between the critical axial buckling load and the resilience of the spring near the critical case of buckling without axial load. For all possible combinations of axial buckling load and spring resilience, the buckling relation is less simple as shown in detail for a cantilever beam (subsection 6.2.14) with rotary (subsection 6.2.15) or translational (subsection 6.2.16) spring at the tip. The analysis in this case was made for all buckling modes without (subsections 6.2.12–6.2.13) and with (subsection 6.2.14) spring. The first three modes without spring are illustrated in Panel 6.4, and the effect of the springs was demonstrated analytically (subsection 6.2.14) and graphically (subsections 6.2.15–6.2.16). A common baseline graph (Panel 6.1) illustrates the relation critical axial load and spring resilience for a cantilever beam in the cases of rotary (Panel 6.5 and Table 6.3) and translational (Panels 6.6–6.7 and Table 6.4) springs.

The present theory can be used in all eight cases in two ways: (i) the direct problem of determining the critical buckling load for a given resilience of the springs; and (ii) the inverse problem of selecting the resilience of the spring so that the critical buckling load takes a desired value. The desired value of the critical buckling load may be: (α) an increase to resist buckling under higher axial load by using a spring that opposes bending, thus increasing the load-bearing capability of a structure or its safety margin; (β) a decrease to demolish a structure by buckling using a smaller axial load and a spring that favors buckling collapse as an alternative to explosive demolition or tedious disassembly.

6.3 Beam under Traction/Compression with Attractive/Repulsive Springs

The buckling of a beam has been considered first under a compressive axial tension (section 6.1) without springs; then localized translational or rotary springs were added (section 6.2) to oppose (facilitate) buckling in the case of attractive (repulsive) springs pulling toward (pushing away) from the undeflected position. Next the case of axial traction is added (section 6.3), retaining the translational springs this time distributed continuously along the whole length of the beam. Thus is considered the linear bending of a uniform beam allowing (subsection 6.3.1) all four combinations of: (i) axial compression or traction; and (ii) attractive or repulsive translational springs distributed transversely along its length. This corresponds to the solution of an unforced linear fourth-order biquadratic differential equation with constant coefficients (subsection 6.3.2) leading (Table 6.5) to ten cases, of which four are degenerate, two special, and four general. The four degenerate cases are: (i/ii) axial compression (section 6.1) [traction (subsection 6.3.3)] without springs leading to (excluding) buckling; (iii/iv) a bar (chapter III.4) that is a beam without axial tension and with attractive (repulsive) springs [subsection 6.3.4 (6.3.5)]. The two special cases (V–VI) balance attractive springs against an axial tension that [subsection 6.3.6 (6.3.7)] may be a compression (traction). The four general cases (vii–ix) are (subsections 6.3.8–6.3.10) an axial traction or compression dominating an attractive or repulsive spring, and (x) an attractive spring dominating the tension (subsection 6.3.11). For all cases I to X, buckling is possible (impossible) if (subsection 6.3.12) the combined tension-resilience buckling load (subsection 6.3.13) is negative (real positive or complex). The elastic stability of a beam under axial traction or compression supported on attractive or repulsive spring (subsection 6.3.1) is determined in the absence of forcing (subsections 6.3.2–6.3.13); the forcing specifies the deflection by external transverse loads, such as a uniform shear stress (subsection 6.3.14) corresponding to the weight of the uniform beam in a constant gravity filed.

6.3.1 Beam Supported on Attractive or Repulsive Springs

Consider (Figure 6.6) linear (6.14a) $\equiv$ (6.190a) deflection of a beam by a shear stress (6.14e): (i) in the presence of an axial traction $T > 0$ or compression $T < 0$; (ii) adding (6.190b) a distributed translational spring with **differential resilience** k' that is attractive (repulsive) for $k' > 0 (k' < 0)$ in the sense that it pulls toward (pushes away from) the undeflected position:

$$\zeta'^2 \ll 1: \qquad \left(EI\zeta''\right)'' - \left(T\zeta'\right)' + k'\,\zeta = f(x). \qquad (6.190a, b)$$

TABLE 6.5

Ten Cases of a Beam under Compression or Traction Continuously Supported on Translational Springs

Case	Subsection	Conditions	Critical Load
I	6.1.6	$T < 0 = k'$	$\alpha \dfrac{EI}{L^2} = -T$
II	6.3.3	$T > 0 = k'$	×
III	6.3.4	$T = 0 < k'$	×
IV	6.3.5	$T = 0 > k'$	$\alpha^2 \dfrac{EI}{L^4} = -k'$
V	6.3.6	$T < 0, T^2 = 4k'EI$	$\alpha \dfrac{EI}{L^2} = -\dfrac{T}{2} = \sqrt{k'EI}$
VI	6.3.7	$T > 0, T^2 = 4k'EI$	×
VII	6.3.8	$T^2 > 4k'EI, T > 0 < k'$	×
VIII	6.3.9	$T^2 > 4k'EI, T < 0 < k'$	$\alpha \dfrac{EI}{L^2} = -\dfrac{T + \sqrt{T^2 - 4k'EI}}{2}$
IX	6.3.10	$T^2 > 4k'EI, k' < 0$	$\alpha \dfrac{EI}{L^2} = -\dfrac{T + \sqrt{T^2 - 4k'EI}}{2}$
X	6.3.11	$T^2 < 4k'EI$	×

× - cases in which buckling is not possible. In all other cases the shape, slope, and curvature of the buckled beam is given in Table 6.1

T - axial tension
k'- differential resilience of the distributed translational spring
E - Young modulus of the material
I - moment of inertia of the cross-section
$\alpha = 4\pi^2$ = clamped beam
$\alpha = 2.08^2 \pi^2$ = clamped-pinned beam
$\alpha^2 = \pi^2$ pinned beam
$\alpha = \dfrac{\pi^2}{4}$ = cantilever beam

Note: A beam under traction or compression supported continuously on translation springs (Figure 6.6) leads to 10 cases for the occurrence or non-occurrence of buckling.

Extending the definition of **uniform beam** to include, besides constant tension (6.10a) ≡ (6.191a) and bending stiffness (6.10b) ≡ (6.172b), also constant differential spring resilience (6.191c) simplifies (6.190b) to (6.191d):

$$T, EI, k' = const: \qquad \zeta'''' - p^2 \operatorname{sgn}(T)\ \zeta'' + r^4 \operatorname{sgn}(k')\,\zeta = f(x), \qquad (6.191a–d)$$

where: (i) appear the **stiffness (differential resilience) parameter** (6.192a) [(6.193a)] that has the dimension of inverse length and equals the square

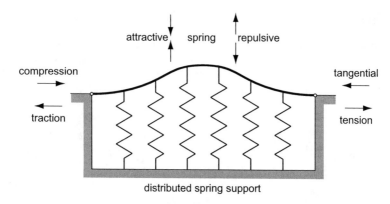

FIGURE 6.6
A beam under axial traction or compression may be acted upon by a discrete spring
(Figures 6.4–6.5) or continuously supported on springs (Figure 6.6) leading to 10 cases of occur-
rence or non-occurrence of buckling (Table 6.5).

(quartic) root of the modulus of the axial tension (resilience of the spring)
divided by the bending stiffness (6.9a):

$$p = \left| \frac{T}{EI} \right|^{1/2} : \qquad \operatorname{sgn}(T) = \begin{cases} +1 & \text{for} \quad T > 0: \quad \text{traction,} \\ -1 & \text{for} \quad T < 0: \quad \text{compression,} \end{cases} \qquad (6.192\text{a–c})$$

$$r = \left| \frac{k'}{EI} \right|^{1/4} : \qquad \operatorname{sgn}(k') = \begin{cases} +1 & \text{for} \quad k' > 0: \quad \text{attractive} \\ -1 & \text{for} \quad k' < 0: \quad \text{repulsive;} \end{cases} \qquad (6.193\text{a–c})$$

(ii) there are four combinations of two cases; namely, axial tension that is a
traction (6.192b) [compression (6.192c)] and attractive (6.193b) [repulsive (6.193c)]
spring. The buckling parameter (6.192a) agrees with (6.10c) for a compression
$T < 0$ in the section 6.1. The resilience of the spring k_k (k') has a different meaning since: (i) it represents a translational spring applied at a point (Figures 6.3–
6.4) [distributed over the length of the beam (Figure 6.6)]; (ii) it appears in the
boundary condition (6.116) [balance of transverse forces (6.193b)]; (iii) its product
by the displacement equals the transverse force (6.194a) [shear stress (6.194b)]:

$$\{F(x), f(x)\} = \{k, k'\} \zeta(x): \qquad k'(x) = \frac{dk}{dx}, \qquad (6.194\text{a–c})$$

(iv) the relation (6.6c) implies that the distributed resilience is the longitudinal derivative of the point resilience (6.194c); and (v) the distinct cubic
(quartic) power in (6.117a) [(6.191d)] ensures that in both cases the resilience
parameter (6.117a) [(6.193a)] has the dimensions of inverse length.

6.3.2 Biquadratic Differential Equation with Constant Coefficients

It has been shown that *(problem 209) the linear (6.190a) displacement of a uni-form beam (6.191a–c) under axial tension (6.192a–c) and supported on linear springs (6.193a–c) is specified (problem 209) in the absence of shear stress (6.195a) by a linear unforced fourth-order differential equation with constant coefficients (6.195b):*

$$f(x) = 0: \quad \left\{ P_4\left(\frac{d}{dx}\right) \right\} \zeta(x) = 0: \quad P_4(D) = D^4 - p^2 \operatorname{sgn}(T)D^2 + r^4 \operatorname{sgn}(k'),$$

$$(6.195a–c)$$

whose characteristic polynomial (6.195c) ≡ (6.196a) ≡ (6.196b):

$$P_4(D) = \left(D^2 - b_+\right)\left(D^2 - b_-\right) = (D - a_{++})(D - a_{+-})(D - a_{-+})(D - a_{--}), \quad (6.196a, b)$$

has roots specified by (6.197a, b):

$$2b_\pm = p^2 \operatorname{sgn}(T) \pm \sqrt{p^4 - 4r^4 \operatorname{sgn}(k')}, \quad a_{\pm\pm} = \pm\sqrt{b_\pm}. \quad (6.197a, b)$$

The general integral of (6.195a, b) is:

$$\zeta(x) = A\exp(a_{++}x) + B\exp(a_{+-}x) + C\exp(a_{-+}x) + D\exp(a_{--}x), \quad (6.198)$$

where (A, B, C, D) are arbitrary constants determined by boundary conditions and the roots (6.196a, b) are assumed to be distinct; the case of coincident roots requires modification (subsections 1.3.6–1.3.10). A pinned beam is chosen as the detailed example (subsections 6.2.3–6.2.11) followed by extension to the other three classical combinations of supports as boundary conditions (subsections 6.2.12–6.2.13). The roots (6.196a, b) lead to ten cases I–X of solution (Table 6.5). The first (second) case I (II) without spring and with compression (traction) leads to buckling (subsection 6.1.6) [excludes any deflection (subsection 6.3.3)].

6.3.3 Beam under Traction without Spring Support

A beam (problem 210) without spring support (6.199a) under an axial traction (6.199b) has no deflection (6.199d) in the absence of shear stresses (6.199c):

II: $k' = 0,$ $T > 0,$ $f(x) = 0:$ $\zeta_{II}(x) = 0.$ $(6.199a–d)$

This is physically obvious because tractions straighten the beam. It can be proved mathematically from (6.195a–b) ≡ (6.200a–c):

$$r = 0, \operatorname{sgn}(T) = 1: \qquad 0 = \zeta'''' - \frac{|T|}{EI}\zeta'' = \zeta'''' - p^2\,\zeta'', \qquad \text{(6.200a–c)}$$

$$P_4(D) = D^2\left(D^2 - p^2\right): \qquad \{b_+, b_-\} = \{p^2, 0\}, \quad \{a_{\pm+}, a_{\pm-}\} = \{\pm p, 0\}, \qquad \text{(6.200d–f)}$$

so that the characteristic polynomial (6.195c) ≡ (6.196a, b) ≡ (6.200d) has double roots (6.197a, b) ≡ (6.200e, f) that are real and symmetric. The corresponding general integral for the displacement is:

$$\zeta_{II}(x) = A + Bx + C\cosh(px) + D\sinh(px), \qquad \text{(6.201)}$$

that is similar to the buckling case (6.18), replacing circular with hyperbolic functions; the replacement of oscillatory by monotonic functions excludes buckling as shown next. The pinning boundary conditions (6.36a, b) ≡ (6.202a, c) at the first support lead to (6.202b, d):

$$0 = \zeta_{II}(0) = A + C; \qquad 0 = \zeta_{II}''(0) = C: \qquad \zeta_{II}(x) = Bx + D\sinh(px). \qquad \text{(6.202a–e)}$$

and the corresponding shape of the elastica (6.202e) is similar to (6.37c), replacing circular by hyperbolic functions. The pinned boundary conditions at the second support (6.36c, d) ≡ (6.203b, c) lead to (6.202d, e):

$$p \neq 0: \quad 0 = \zeta_{II}''(L) = p^2 D\sinh(pL), \quad 0 = \zeta_{II}(L) = BL: \quad B = 0 = D, \quad \zeta_{II}(x) = 0,$$
$$\text{(6.203a–h)}$$

that for (6.203a) imply (6.203f, g) and hence no deflection (6.203h) ≡ (6.199d). A similar conclusion of absence of deflection can be expected in the case III without axial tension and with attractive spring (subsection 6.3.4).

6.3.4 Bar Continuously Supported on Attractive Springs

*A **bar**, that is a beam without axial tension (6.204a), supported along its entire length (problem 211) by linear attractive springs (6.204b) does not deflect (6.204d) in the absence of shear stresses (6.204c):*

$$\text{III:} \qquad T = 0, \quad k' > 0, \quad f(x) = 0: \quad \zeta_{III}(x) = 0. \qquad \text{(6.204a–d)}$$

Again, this is physically obvious because the attractive springs keep the bar in the undeflected position. It can be proved mathematically from (6.195a) that in this case (6.195a–c) $\equiv$ (6.205a–c):

$$p = 0, \operatorname{sgn}(k') = 1: \qquad 0 = \zeta'''' + \frac{|k'|}{E\,I}\zeta = \zeta'''' + r^4\,\zeta, \qquad (6.205a-c)$$

$$P_4(D) = D^4 + r^4: \qquad b_\pm = \sqrt{-r^4} = \pm i\,r^2, \qquad a_{\pm\pm} = r\frac{\pm 1 \pm i}{\sqrt{2}}, \qquad (6.205d-f)$$

so that the characteristic polynomial (6.195c) $\equiv$ (6.196a, b) $\equiv$ (6.205d) has roots (6.197a, b) $\equiv$ (6.205d, e) where the square (quartic) roots (I.10.38b) $\equiv$ (6.206a–c) of −1 were used:

$$-1 = e^{\pm i\pi}, \qquad \sqrt[2]{-1} = \pm i = e^{\pm i\pi/2} = e^{\pm i\pi/2 + i 2\pi}, \qquad (6.206a, b)$$

$$\sqrt[4]{-1} = \sqrt[2]{\pm i} = e^{\pm i\pi/4}\,e^{\pm i\pi/4 + i\pi} = \frac{\pm 1 \pm i}{\sqrt{2}}. \qquad (6.206c)$$

The general integral for the displacement is:

$$\bar{r} \equiv \frac{r}{\sqrt{2}}: \quad \zeta_{III}(x) = e^{\bar{r}x}\left[A\cos(\bar{r}x) + B\sin(\bar{r}x)\right] + e^{-\bar{r}x}\left[C\cos(\bar{r}x) + D\sin(\bar{r}x)\right]. \tag{6.207}$$

The pinning boundary conditions at the first support (6.36a, b) $\equiv$ (6.208a, c) lead to (6.208b, d):

$$0 = \zeta_{III}(0) = A + C; \qquad 0 = \zeta_{III}''(0) = 2\bar{r}^2(B - D):$$
$$\zeta_{III}(x) = 2A\cos(\bar{r}\,x)\sinh(\bar{r}\,x) + 2B\sin(\bar{r}\,x)\cosh(\bar{r}\,x), \tag{6.208a-e}$$

substitution of (6.208a, b) in (6.207) specifies the displacement (6.208e). When substituting (6.207) in (6.208b) were used:

$$\left[e^{\pm \bar{r}x}\cos(\bar{r}\,x)\right]'' = \mp 2\bar{r}^2\,e^{\pm \bar{r}x}\sin(\bar{r}\,x), \tag{6.209a}$$

$$\left[e^{\pm \bar{r}x}\sin(\bar{r}\,x)\right]'' = \pm 2\bar{r}^2\,e^{\pm \bar{r}x}\cos(\bar{r}\,x). \tag{6.209b}$$

The pinning boundary conditions at the other end (6.36c, d) ≡ (6.210a, b) lead to (6.210c):

$$\zeta_{III}(L)=0=\zeta_{III}''(L):\quad \begin{bmatrix} \cos(\bar{r}L)\sinh(\bar{r}L) & \sin(\bar{r}L)\cosh(\bar{r}L) \\ -\sin(\bar{r}L)\cosh(\bar{r}L) & \cos(\bar{r}L)\sinh(\bar{r}L) \end{bmatrix}\begin{bmatrix} A \\ B \end{bmatrix}=0,$$

(6.210a–c)

where were used:

$$\left[\cos(\bar{r}x)\sinh(\bar{r}x)\right]''=-2\,\bar{r}^2\sin(\bar{r}x)\cosh(\bar{r}x),\qquad (6.211a)$$

$$\left[\sin(\bar{r}x)\cosh(\bar{r}x)\right]''=2\bar{r}^2\cos(\bar{r}x)\sinh(\bar{r}x).\qquad (6.211b)$$

The determinant of the matrix in (6.187c) is given by:

$$\begin{aligned}E_{III}&=\cos^2(\bar{r}L)\sinh^2(\bar{r}L)+\sin^2(\bar{r}L)\cosh^2(\bar{r}L)\\&=\sinh^2(\bar{r}L)+\sin^2(\bar{r}L)\left[\cosh^2(\bar{r}L)-\sinh^2(\bar{r}L)\right]\\&=\sinh^2(\bar{r}L)+\sin^2(\bar{r}L),\end{aligned}$$

(6.212)

that cannot vanish (6.213b) for (6.213a):

$$r\neq 0:\qquad E_{III}\neq 0,\qquad A=0=B,\qquad \zeta_{III}(x)=0,\qquad (6.213a\text{–}e)$$

and hence (6.210c) implies (6.213c, d) and by (6.208e) zero displacement (6.213e) ≡ (6.204d). This conclusion will change in the case IV a bar supported on repulsive springs (subsection 6.3.5) that push it away from the undeflected position.

6.3.5 Bar Supported on Translational Repulsive Springs

In this case IV still in the absence of axial tension (6.204a) ≡ (6.214a), changing attractive (6.204b) to repulsive (6.214b) springs leads (6.214c, d) to different roots (6.197a, b) ≡ (6.214f, g) of the characteristic polynomial (6.195c) ≡ (6.196a, b) ≡ (6.214e):

$$\text{IV:}\qquad T=0,\qquad k'<0:\qquad 0=\zeta''''-\frac{|k'|}{EI}\zeta=\zeta''''-r^4\zeta,\qquad (6.214a\text{–}d)$$

$$P_4(D)=D^4-r^4:\qquad b_\pm=\sqrt{r^4}=\pm r^2,\qquad a_{\pm\pm}=\pm r,\pm ir,\qquad (6.214e\text{–}g)$$

and the corresponding deflection (6.215) is:

$$\zeta_{IV}(x) = A\cos(rx) + B\sin(rx) + C\cosh(rx) + D\sinh(rx). \qquad (6.215)$$

The pinned boundary conditions at the first end (6.36a, b) ≡ (6.216a, c) lead to (6.216b, d) and hence (6.216e, f):

$$0 = \zeta_{IV}(0) = A + C, \quad 0 = \zeta_{IV}''(0) = r^2(C - A):$$
$$A = 0 = C, \quad \zeta_{IV}(x) = B\sin(rx) + D\sinh(rx), \qquad (6.216a\text{–}g)$$

that simplifies (6.215) to (6.216g). The pinned boundary conditions at the other end (6.36c, d) ≡ (6.217a, b) lead to (6.217c):

$$\zeta_{IV}(L) = 0 = \zeta_{IV}''(L): \qquad \begin{bmatrix} \sin(rL) & \sinh(rL) \\ -\sin(rL) & \sinh(rL) \end{bmatrix} \begin{bmatrix} B \\ D \end{bmatrix} = 0. \qquad (6.217a\text{–}c)$$

A non-trivial solution (6.218a) corresponds to a vanishing determinant (6.218c) that is possible for (6.218b) if (6.218d) holds:

$$(B, D) \neq (0, 0), \quad r \neq 0: \quad E_{IV} = 2\sin(rL)\sinh(rL) = 0, \quad \sin(rL) = 0, \quad r_{3n}L = n\pi; \qquad (6.218a\text{–}d)$$

thus there is a **critical spring resilience** (6.219a) for buckling (6.219b):

$$r_{3,1} = \frac{\pi}{L}, \quad k_3' = -EI\left|r_{3,1}\right|^4 = -\frac{\pi^4 EI}{L^4}. \qquad (6.219a, b)$$

Substituting (6.219a) in (6.217c) implies (6.220a) so that the shape of the buckled bar (6.216g) is (6.220b):

$$D = 0: \qquad \zeta_{IV}(x) = B\sin(r_{3,1}x) = B\sin\left(\frac{\pi x}{L}\right), \qquad (6.220a, b)$$

which is the same (6.220b) ≡ (6.40a) as for a beam without springs and with an axial compression (6.221d):

$$\gamma \equiv \frac{\pi^2}{L^2}: \qquad -\left(\frac{T}{EI}\right)^2 = \gamma^2 = \frac{k'}{EI}, \qquad T^2 \leftrightarrow -k'EI. \qquad (6.221a\text{–}d)$$

It has been shown that *(problem 212) the linear (6.190a) displacement (6.40a, b), slope (6.41a–d) and bending moment (6.42a, b) of a uniform (6.191a–c) pinned (6.36a–d) beam apply equally (6.221a) to the buckling (deflection) by an axial compression (6.221b) [repulsive spring (6.221c)]. It follows that from the point of view of buckling of a beam (a) an axial compression without spring is equivalent to (b) a repulsive spring without axial tension if they are related by (6.221d). In the opposite case of axial traction (attractive spring) there is no deflection.* The cases I(II) of axial compression (traction) alone [subsection 6.1.6 (6.3.4)] and cases III (IV) of attractive (repulsive) spring alone [subsection 6.3.4 (6.3.3)], are followed by cases V–X of the two combined; the simplest are the cases V (VI) of balance [subsection 6.3.6 (6.3.7)] of an axial compression (traction) with an attractive (repulsive) spring.

6.3.6 Beam with Axial Compression Balanced by Attractive Spring

The **tension-spring balance** is defined by (6.222a) ≡ (6.222b):

$$p^4 = 4r^4 \quad \leftrightarrow \quad T^2 = 4k'EI > 0, \quad b_\pm = \frac{p^2}{2}\,\mathrm{sgn}(T), \quad a_{\pm\pm} = \pm\sqrt{-\frac{p^2}{2}\,\mathrm{sgn}(T)},$$

$$(6.222\text{a–d})$$

that leads to the roots (6.197a, b) ≡ (6.222c, d) of the characteristic polynomial (6.195c) ≡ (6.196a, b) ≡ (6.222e, f):

$$P_4(D) = D^4 - 4r^2\,\mathrm{sgn}(T)D^2 + r^4\,\mathrm{sgn}(k') = D^4 - p^2\,\mathrm{sgn}(T)D^2 + \frac{p^4}{4}\,\mathrm{sgn}(k').$$

$$(6.222\text{e, f})$$

In the case V of axial compression (6.223b) with tension-spring balance (6.222b) ≡ (6.223a) leading to (6.195a–c) ≡ (6.223c, d):

$$V: \quad T^2 = 4EIk' > 0, \quad T < 0: \quad 0 = \zeta'''' + \frac{|T|}{EI}\zeta'' + \frac{|k'|}{EI}\zeta = \zeta'''' + p^2\zeta' + r^4\zeta,$$

$$(6.223\text{a–d})$$

the roots (6.197a, b) ≡ (6.222c, d) of the characteristic polynomial (6.195c) ≡ (6.196a, b) ≡ (6.222e, f) are double (6.224a) imaginary conjugates (6.224b):

$$b_\pm = -\frac{p^2}{2}, \quad a_{\pm\pm} = \pm i\frac{p}{\sqrt{2}} \equiv \pm i\bar{p}: \quad \zeta_{\bar{V}}(x) = (A + Bx)\cos(\bar{p}x) + (C + Dx)\sin(\bar{p}x),$$

$$(6.224\text{a–d})$$

where the notation (6.224c) is used in the displacement of the elastica (6.224d). The pinned boundary conditions (6.36a, b) ≡ (6.225a, c) at one end lead to (6.225b, d):

$$0 = \zeta_V(0) = A, \quad 0 = \zeta_V''(0) = 2\bar{p}D: \quad \zeta_V(x) = C\sin(\bar{p}x) + Bx\cos(\bar{p}x),$$
$$(6.225a\text{–}e)$$

that simplify (6.224b) to (6.225e). The pinned boundary conditions at the other end (6.36c, d) ≡ (6.226a, b) lead to (6.226c):

$$\zeta(L) = 0 = \zeta_V''(L): \quad \begin{bmatrix} \sin(\bar{p}L) & L\cos\bar{p}L \\ \bar{p}\sin\bar{p}L & \bar{p}L\cos(\bar{p}L) + 2\sin(\bar{p}L) \end{bmatrix} \begin{bmatrix} C \\ B \end{bmatrix} = 0.$$
$$(6.226a\text{–}c)$$

A non-trivial solution exists (6.227a) if the determinant of the matrix in (6.226c) is zero (6.227c) for (6.227b):

$$(C,B) \neq (0,0), \bar{p} \neq 0: \quad E_v = 2\sin^2(\bar{p}L) = 2\sin^2\left(\frac{pL}{\sqrt{2}}\right) = 0, \quad p_{3,1}L = \pi\sqrt{2} = r_{3,1}L\sqrt{2},$$
$$(6.227a\text{–}e)$$

leading: (i) to (6.227d) for the stiffness parameter; (ii) by (6.222a) to (6.227e) for the resilience parameter; (iii) the corresponding (6.192a, c; 6.227d) critical buckling compression is (6.227f):

$$T = -EI(p_{3,1})^2 = -\frac{2\pi^2 EI}{L^2}; \quad k' = EI(r_{3,1})^4 = \frac{\pi^4 EI}{L^4}, \quad (6.227f, g)$$

(iv) the corresponding (6.193a, b; 6.227e) critical buckling resilience is (6.227g); and (v) the values (6.227f, g) are consistent with (6.222b). This extends the preceding results (subsection 6.3.4) to the following statement (*problem 213*): *the linear (6.190a) displacement (6.40a, b), slope (6.41a–d), and bending moment (6.42a, b) of a uniform (6.191a–c) pinned (6.36a–d) beam apply equally in the: (i) case I of buckling under axial compression alone (subsection 6.1.6); (ii) case IV of deflection by equivalent (6.221c) ≡ (6.228a) repulsive springs (subsection 6.3.4); (iii) case V of balanced axial compression and attractive spring (6.222b):*

$$p_{3,1} \to p_{3,1}\sqrt{2}, \quad T \to 2T, \quad T^2 = 4k'EI, \quad (6.228a\text{–}c)$$

multiplies the buckling parameter (6.227d) by $\sqrt{2}$ in (6.228a), thus multiplies the axial compression by 2 in (6.228b), leading to (6.228c) that is four times (6.221d) *because the axial compression must overcome an attractive spring to buckle the beam: and (iv) the case VI of balanced axial traction and attractive springs leads to no deflection as shown next (subsection 6.3.7).*

6.3.7 Beam with Axial Traction Balanced by Attractive Springs

Case VI concerns the balance of axial tension and spring resilience (6.222b) opposite to (6.223a–d) case V, in the sense of an axial traction (6.229b) and attractive springs (6.229a) leading to (6.195a–c) ≡ (6.229c, d):

$$\text{VI:} \quad T^2 = 4k'EI > 0, \quad T > 0: \quad 0 = \zeta'''' + \frac{|T|}{EI}\zeta'' + \frac{T^2}{4EI}\zeta = \zeta'''' - p^2\,\zeta'' + \frac{p^4}{4}\zeta.$$

(6.229a–d)

The characteristic polynomial (6.195c) ≡ (6.196a, b) ≡ (6.230a, b) in case V has double roots (6.197a, b) ≡ (6.230c, d):

$$P_4(D) = D^4 + p^2 D + \frac{p^2}{4} = D^2 + 2r^2 D^2 + r^4: \quad b_{\pm} = \frac{p^2}{2}, \quad a_{\pm\pm} = \pm\frac{p}{\sqrt{2}} = \pm\bar{p},$$

(6.230a–d)

and the corresponding displacement of the elastica is:

$$\zeta_{VI}(x) = (A + Bx)\cosh(\bar{p}x) + (C + Dx)\sinh(\bar{p}x).$$ (6.231)

The pinned boundary conditions (6.36a, b) ≡ (6.232a, c) at one end lead to (6.232b, d):

$$0 = \zeta_{VI}(0) = A, \quad 0 = \zeta''_{IV}(0) = 2\bar{p}D: \quad \zeta(x) = C\sinh(\bar{p}x) + Bx\cosh(\bar{p}x),$$

(6.232a–e)

that simplify (6.231) to (6.232e). The remaining boundary conditions at the other end (6.36c, d) ≡ (6.233a, b) lead to (6.233c):

$$\zeta_{VI}(L) = 0 = \zeta''_{IV}(L): \quad \begin{bmatrix} \sinh(\bar{p}L) & L\cosh(\bar{p}L) \\ \bar{p}\sinh(\bar{p}L) & \bar{p}L\cosh(\bar{p}L) + 2\sinh(\bar{p}L) \end{bmatrix} \begin{bmatrix} C \\ B \end{bmatrix} = 0.$$

(6.233a–c)

The determinant (6.234b) of the matrix in (6.233c) does not vanish for non-zero traction (6.234a), leading (6.234c, d) to:

$$p \neq 0: \quad E_{VI} = 2\sinh^2(\bar{p}L) \neq 0, \quad C = 0 = B, \quad \zeta_{VI}(x) = 0, \quad (6.234a–c)$$

and hence (6.234e) to the absence of deflection. It that been shown that *(problem 214) for a linear (6.190a) uniform (6.191a–c) beam pinned (6.36a–d) at both ends in the absence (6.195a) of shear stresses (6.235c) the tension-spring balance (6.229a) with axial traction (6.229b) leads to the absence of deflection (6.235d) for an axial traction (6.235a) combined with repulsive (6.235b) spring:*

$$0 < T, \qquad T^2 = 4k'EI, \qquad f(x) = 0: \qquad \zeta_{VI}(x) = 0. \qquad \text{(6.235a–d)}$$

This should be expected because in the case II (III) of axial traction without spring (attractive spring without axial tension), there is no deflection (6.199a–d) [(6.204a–d)] and the combination [subsection 6.3.2 (6.3.3)] must also lead to no deflection (subsection 6.3.7). So far we have considered: (i) the cases I to IV of axial compression (traction) alone [subsection 6.1.6 (6.3.3)] or attractive (repulsive) spring alone [subsection 6.3.4 (6.3.5)]; (ii) the cases V (VI) of axial compression (traction) balanced by an attractive spring [subsection 6.3.6 (6.3.7)]. The remaining four cases concern [case(s) X (VII–IX)] unbalanced tension-spring with [subsection (s) 6.3.11 (6.3.8–6.3.10)] predominance of spring resilience (axial tension).

6.3.8 Beam with Axial Traction Dominating Attractive Spring

In the general case of unbalanced tension-resilience (6.236a), the characteristic polynomial (6.195c) ≡ (6.196a, b) has roots (6.197b) ≡ (6.236b) specified by (6.192a; 6.193a; 6.197a) ≡ (6.236c):

$$T^2 \neq 4k'EI: \qquad a_\pm \equiv \pm\sqrt{b_\pm}, \qquad 2EIb_\pm = T \pm \sqrt{T^2 - 4k'EI}. \qquad \text{(6.236a–c)}$$

The cases VII–IX concern predominance of axial tension over spring resilience (6.237a) and in the case VII of *(problem 215) axial traction (6.237b) and attractive springs (6.237c) lead to no deflection (6.237e) in the absence of transverse loads (6.237d):*

$$\text{VII:} \qquad T^2 > 4k'EI, \quad T > 0, \quad k' > 0, \quad f(x) = 0: \qquad \zeta_{VII}(x) = 0. \qquad \text{(6.237a–e)}$$

In the case (6.237a–c) corresponding to (6.195a–c) ≡ (6.238a, b), the roots of the characteristic polynomial (6.197a, b) ≡ (6.238c–f) are two real symmetric pairs:

$$0 = \zeta'''' - \frac{|T|}{EI}\zeta'' + \frac{|k'|}{EI}\zeta = \zeta'''' - p^2\zeta'' + r^4\zeta, \qquad \text{(6.238a, b)}$$

$$s^2 \equiv \left|p^4 - 4r^4\right|^{1/2} < p^2: \qquad b_\pm = \frac{p^2 \pm s^2}{2} > 0, \quad a_{\pm\pm} = \pm\frac{1}{\sqrt{2}}\left|p^2 \pm s^2\right|^{1/2} \equiv \pm a_\pm.$$

$$\text{(6.238c–f)}$$

The corresponding displacement is:

$$\zeta_{VII}(x) = A\cosh(a_+x) + B\sinh(a_+x) + C\cosh(a_-x) + D\sinh(a_-x), \qquad (6.239)$$

The pinning boundary conditions (6.36a, b) ≡ (6.240a, c) lead to (6.240b, c):

$$0 = \zeta_{VII}(0) = A + C, \qquad 0 = \zeta_{VII}''(0) = a_+^2 A + a_-^2 C; \qquad b_+ \neq b_-, \quad a_+ \neq a_-,$$
$$(6.240a\text{-}f)$$

since (6.237a) implies (6.240e, f), (6.241a, b) follows, simplifying (6.239) to (6.241c):

$$A = 0 = C: \qquad \zeta_{VII}(x) = B\sinh(a_+x) + D\sinh(a_-x). \qquad (6.241a\text{-}c)$$

The second set of pinning boundary conditions (6.36c, d) ≡ (6.242a, b) leads to (6.242c):

$$\zeta_{VII}(L) = 0 = \zeta_{VII}''(L): \qquad \begin{bmatrix} \sinh(a_+L) & \sinh(a_-L) \\ a_+^2\sinh(a_+L) & a_-^2\sinh(a_-L) \end{bmatrix} \begin{bmatrix} B \\ D \end{bmatrix} = 0.$$
$$(6.242a\text{-}c)$$

The determinant of the matrix in (6.242c) is not zero (6.243a, b):

$$a_+ \neq a_-: \quad E_{VII} = \left(a_-^2 - a_+^2\right)\sinh(a_-L)\sinh(a_+L) \neq 0, \quad B = 0 = D, \quad \zeta_{VII}(x) = 0,$$
$$(6.243a\text{-}e)$$

implying (6.243c, d) and hence (6.241a) no deflection (6.243e) ≡ (6.237e). If the spring is kept attractive (subsection 6.3.7) and traction is changed to compression (case VIII), buckling is possible (subsection 6.3.9).

6.3.9 Beam with Axial Compression Dominating Attractive Springs

In the case VIII of predominant (6.244a) axial compression (6.244b) with attractive springs (6.244c) leading to (6.195a–c) ≡ (6.244d, e), the roots (6.197a, b) ≡ (6.238c; 6.244f, g) of the characteristic polynomial (6.195c) ≡ (6.196a, b) are double conjugate imaginary:

$$\text{VIII:} \qquad T^2 > 4k'EI, \quad T < 0, \quad k' > 0: \quad 0 = \zeta'''' - \frac{|T|}{EI}\zeta'' + \frac{k'}{EI}\zeta, \qquad (6.244a\text{-}d)$$

$$0 = \zeta'''' + p^2\zeta'' + r^4\zeta, \qquad b_\pm = \frac{-p^2 \pm s^2}{2} < 0, \qquad a_{\pm\pm} = \pm i a_\pm. \qquad (6.244e\text{-}g)$$

The corresponding displacement is:

$$\zeta_{VIII}(x) = A\cos(a_+x) + B\sin(a_+x) + C\cos(a_-x) + D\sin(a_-x). \qquad (6.245)$$

The pinned boundary conditions (6.36a, b) $\equiv$ (6.246a, c) lead to (6.246b, d):

$$0 = \zeta_{VIII}(L) = A + C, \qquad\qquad 0 = \zeta_{VIII}''(L) = -a_+^2 A - a_-^2 C; \qquad (6.246a\text{–}d)$$

using (6.240f) from (6.246b, d) follows (6.247a, b), simplifying (6.245) to (6.247c):

$$A = 0 = C: \qquad\qquad \zeta_{VIII}(x) = B\sin(a_+x) + D\sin(a_-x). \qquad\qquad (6.247a\text{–}c)$$

The second set of pinning boundary conditions (6.36c, d) $\equiv$ (6.248a, b) lead to (6.248c):

$$\zeta_{VIII}(L) = 0 = \zeta_{VIII}''(L): \qquad \begin{bmatrix} \sin(a_+L) & \sin(a_-L) \\ a_+^2\sin(a_+L) & a_-^2\sin(a_-L) \end{bmatrix} \begin{bmatrix} B \\ D \end{bmatrix} = 0. \qquad (6.248a\text{–}c)$$

Buckling is possible (6.249a) if the determinant of the matrix in (6.248c) vanishes (6.249b):

$$(B,D) \neq (0,0): \qquad E_{VIII} = \left(a_+^2 - a_-^2\right)\sin(a_+L)\sin(a_-L) = 0, \qquad (6.249a, b)$$

and that is the case if one of the equivalent conditions (6.250a, b) holds:

$$\sin(a_{\pm}L) = 0, \qquad a_+L = n\pi; \qquad a_-L = \pi, \qquad (6.250a\text{–}c)$$

the smallest root in (6.250b) is (6.250c) corresponding to:

$$\frac{\pi^2 EI}{L} = EI(a_-)^2 = EIb_- = -\frac{T + \sqrt{T^2 - 4k'EI}}{2}, \qquad (6.251)$$

where (6.238c, d; 6.192a, 6.193a) were used. The condition (6.250c) $\equiv$ (6.252a) in (6.248c) leads to (6.252b):

$$a_-L = \pi: \qquad B = 0, \qquad \zeta_{VIII}(x) = D\sin(a_-L) = D\sin\left(\frac{\pi x}{L}\right), \qquad (6.252a\text{–}d)$$

and the shape of the elastica (6.247c) simplifies to (6.252c) $\equiv$ (6.252d) $\equiv$ (6.40a). It has been shown that *(problem 216) the displacement (6.40a, b), slope (6.41a–d) and bending moment (6.42a, b) apply to the linear buckling of a uniform beam in the case VIII of dominant (6.244a) axial compression (6.244b) with an attractive spring (6.244c). The cases of dominant axial tension include besides the case VII (VIII) of traction (compression) with attractive spring [subsection 6.3.8) (6.3.9)] and the case IX of a repulsive spring (subsection 6.3.10).*

6.3.10 Beam with Axial Tension Dominating Repulsive Springs

The case IX of dominant axial tension (6.253a) with a repulsive spring (6.253b) leads to (6.195a–c) ≡ (6.253c, d)

$$\text{IX:} \quad T^2 > 4k'EI, \quad k' < 0: \quad 0 = \zeta'''' - \frac{|T|}{EI}\text{sgn}(T)\zeta'' - \frac{|k'|}{EI}\zeta, \quad (6.253\text{a–c})$$

$$\zeta'''' - p^2\,\text{sgn}(T)\,\zeta'' - r^4\zeta = 0. \quad (6.253\text{d})$$

In this case IX the characteristic polynomial (6.195c) ≡ (6.196a, b) has roots (6.197a) ≡ (6.254b) where (6.254a) implies (6.254c, d):

$$t^2 \equiv \left|p^2 + 4r^2\right|^{1/2} > p^2, \quad 2b_\pm = \frac{p^2 \pm t^2}{2}, \quad b_+ > 0 > b_-, \quad a_{+\pm} = \pm a_+, \quad a_{-\pm} = \pm i a_-,$$

$$(6.254\text{a–f})$$

and hence (6.254c) a real and symmetric (6.254e) and (6.254d) an imaginary symmetric (6.254f) pair of roots. The corresponding displacement is:

$$\zeta_{IX}(x) = A\cosh(a_+x) + B\sinh(a_+x) + C\cos(a_-x) + D\sin(a_-x). \quad (6.255)$$

The similarity of (6.255) and (6.215), replacing $a_\pm$ by r, suggests that buckling is possible, as is confirmed next. The pinned boundary conditions (6.36a, b) ≡ (6.256a, c) lead to (6.256b, d):

$$0 = \zeta_{IX}(L) = A + C, \quad 0 = \zeta''_{IX}(0) = a_+^2 A - a_-^2 C; \quad (6.256\text{a–d})$$

using (6.240f) from (6.256b, d) follows (6.257a, b), simplifying the displacement (6.255) to (6.257c):

$$A = 0 = C: \quad \zeta(x) = B\sinh(a_+x) + D\sin(a_-x). \quad (6.257\text{a–c})$$

The second set of pinning boundary conditions (6.36c, d) ≡ (6.258a, b) lead to (6.2589c):

$$\zeta_{IX}(L) = 0 = \zeta_{IX}''(L): \qquad \begin{bmatrix} \sinh(a_+L) & \sin(a_-L) \\ a_+^2 \sinh(a_+L) & -a_-^2 \sin(a_-L) \end{bmatrix} \begin{bmatrix} B \\ D \end{bmatrix} = 0. \qquad (6.258a\text{--}c)$$

Buckling is possible (6.259a) if the determinant of the matrix in (6.258c) vanishes (6.259b):

$$(B,D) \neq (0,0): \qquad E_{IX} = \left(a_+^2 + a_-^2\right)\sinh(a_+L)\sin(a_-L) = 0, \quad \sin(a_- L) = 0. \qquad (6.259a\text{--}c)$$

leading to (6.259c) ≡ (6.250c) the same results (6.251; 6.252a–d). It has been shown that *(problem 217) the displacement (6.40a, b), slope (6.41a–d), and bending moment (6.42a, b) apply to the linear buckling of a uniform beam in the case IX of repulsive spring (6.253b) with dominant axial tension (6.253a) that may be either a traction or a compression in (6.251).* The only case X remaining is that of axial tension dominated by the resilience of the springs that must be attractive (subsection 6.3.11).

6.3.11 Beam with Attractive Springs Dominating the Axial Tension

In the case X of axial tension dominated by the springs (6.260a), the latter must be attractive (6.260b), leading to (6.195a–c) ≡ (6.260c, d):

$$X: \qquad 4k'EI > T^2, \qquad k' > 0: \quad 0 = \zeta'''' - \frac{|T|}{EI}\operatorname{sgn}(T)\zeta'' + \frac{|k'|}{EI}\zeta, \qquad (6.260a\text{--}c)$$

$$0 = \zeta'''' - p^2 \operatorname{sgn}(T)\zeta'' + r^4\zeta. \qquad (6.260d)$$

The characteristic polynomial (6.195c) ≡ (6.196a, b) has roots (6.197a, b; 6.238a) ≡ (6.261b) because (6.260a) implies (6.261a):

$$p^4 < 4r^2: \qquad b_\pm = \frac{p^2 \pm is^2}{2} = w^2 e^{2i\phi}; \qquad a_{\pm\pm} = \pm w e^{\pm i\phi} = \pm w\left(\cos\phi \pm i\sin\phi\right). \qquad (6.261a\text{--}d)$$

The roots (6.261b) may be put into the form (6.261c), leading to (6.261d) where: (i) from (6.261a; 6.238c) follows (6.262a) implying (6.262b):

$$s^4 = 4r^4 - p^4: \qquad w^4 = |b_\pm|^2 = \frac{p^4 + s^4}{4} = r^4 = \frac{k'}{EI}, \qquad (6.262a, b)$$

$$2\phi = \pm \arg(b_\pm) = arc\tan\left(\frac{s^2}{p^2}\right) = arc\tan\left(\sqrt{\frac{4r^4}{p^4}-1}\right) = arc\tan\left(\sqrt{\frac{4k'EI}{T^2}-1}\right).$$

$$(6.262c)$$

The roots (6.261d) correspond to the displacement:

$$\zeta_X(x) = \exp(xw\cos\phi)\left[A\cos(xw\sin\phi) + B\sin(xw\sin\phi)\right]$$

$$(6.263)$$

$$+ \exp(-xw\cos\phi)\left[C\cos(xw\sin\phi) + D\sin(xw\sin\phi)\right].$$

The similarity of (6.263) and (6.207) suggests that buckling is not possible as is proved next.

The pinned boundary conditions (6.36a, b) ≡ (6.264a, c) lead to (6.264b, d):

$$0 = \zeta_X(0) = A + C, \quad 0 = \zeta_X''(0) = (A+C)w^2\cos(2\phi) + (B-D)w^2\sin(2\phi),$$

$$(6.264a, b)$$

where were used:

$$\left[\exp(\pm xw\cos\phi)\cos(xw\sin\phi)\right]''$$

$$= w^2\exp(\pm xw\cos\phi)\left\{(\cos^2\phi - \sin^2\phi)\cos(xw\sin\phi) \mp 2\cos\phi\sin\phi\sin(xw\sin\phi)\right\}$$

$$= w^2\exp(\pm xw\cos\phi)\left[\cos(2\phi)\cos(xw\sin\phi) \mp \sin(2\phi)\sin(xw\sin\phi)\right]$$

$$= w^2\exp(\pm xw\cos\phi)\cos(2\phi \pm xw\sin\phi),$$

$$(6.265a)$$

$$\left[\exp(\pm xw\cos\phi)\sin(xw\sin\phi)\right]''$$

$$= w^2\exp(\pm xw\cos\phi)\left\{(\cos^2\phi - \sin^2\phi)\sin(xw\sin\phi) \pm 2\cos\phi\sin\phi\cos(xw\sin\phi)\right\}$$

$$= w^2\exp(\pm xw\cos\phi)\left[\cos(2\phi)\sin(xw\sin\phi) \pm \sin(2\phi)\cos(xw\sin\phi)\right]$$

$$= w^2\exp(\pm xw\cos\phi)\sin(xw\sin\phi \pm 2\phi).$$

$$(6.265b)$$

From (6.264b, d) follow (6.266a, b), that simplify (6.263) to (6.266c):

$$A = -C, B = D: \quad \zeta_X(x) = 2A\sinh(xw\cos\phi)\cos(xw\sin\phi)$$

$$(6.266a–c)$$

$$+ 2B\cosh(xw\cos\phi)\sin(xw\sin\phi),$$

that is equivalent to (6.266c) ≡ (6.267c):

$$\{u,v\} \equiv w\{\cos\phi, \sin\phi\}: \quad \zeta_X(x) = 2A\sinh(xu)\cos(xv) + 2B\cosh(xu)\sin(xv).$$
$$(6.267a\text{--}c)$$

using the notation (6.267a, b).

The second set of pinning boundary conditions (6.36c, d) ≡ (6.268a, b) leads to (6.268c):

$$\zeta_X(L) = 0 = \zeta_X''(L) = 0: \quad \begin{bmatrix} \sinh(uL)\cos(vL) & \cosh(uL)\sin(vL) \\ D_1 & D_2 \end{bmatrix}\begin{bmatrix} A \\ B \end{bmatrix} = 0,$$
$$(6.268a\text{--}c)$$

where:

$$D_1 = \left(u^2 - v^2\right)\sinh(uL)\cos(vL) - 2uv\cosh(uL)\sin(vL), \quad (6.269a)$$

$$D_2 = \left(u^2 - v^2\right)\cosh(uL)\sin(vL) + 2uv\sinh(uL)\cos(vL). \quad (6.269b)$$

The determinant of the matrix in (6.268c) is given by:

$$u \neq 0 \neq v: \quad E_X = D_2\sinh(uL)\cos(vL) - D_1\cosh(uL)\sin(vL)$$
$$= 2uv\left[\sinh^2(uL)\cos^2(vL) + \cosh^2(uL)\sin^2(vL)\right]$$
$$= 2uv\left\{\sinh^2(uL) + \sin^2(vL)\left[\cosh^2(uL) - \sinh^2(uL)\right]\right\}$$
$$= 2uv\left[\sinh^2(uL) + \sin^2(vL)\right] > 0;$$
$$(6.270a\text{--}c)$$

since it is not zero, (6.268c) implies (6.271a, b) so that (6.267c) that there is no deflection (6.271f):

$$X: \quad A = 0 = B, \quad 4k'EI > T^2, \quad k' > 0, \quad f(x) = 0: \quad \zeta_X(x) = 0. \quad (6.271a\text{--}f)$$

Thus *(problem 218) a linear (6.190a) uniform (6.191a–c) beam supported on attractive springs (6.271d) that dominate the axial tension (6.271c) has no deflection (6.271f) in the absence of shear stresses (6.271e).* The ten cases of linear uniform beam with axial compression or traction supported on attractive or repulsive linear springs are compared next (subsection 6.3.12).

6.3.12 Generalized Critical Buckling Condition

The ten preceding cases (subsections 6.3.2–6.3.11) are listed in Table 6.5 for the pinned beam, together with the cantilever beam that leads to the same results replacing π^2 by $\pi^2/4$ as in the passage from (6.39a–d) to (6.65a–e); the passage to a clamped (clamped-pinned) beam would replace π^2 by $4\pi^2$ (2.046 π^2) as in (6.31a–c) [(6.48a–c)]. The preceding results may be summarized as follows *(problem 219): a linear (6.190a) uniform (6.191a–c) beam (6.190b) in the absence of transverse loads (6.199c) has* **critical buckling condition:**

$$\frac{EI}{L^2}\left\{4\pi^2, 2.046\pi^2, \pi^2, \frac{\pi^2}{4}\right\}$$

$$\equiv -\bar{T} \equiv -T, \quad -|k'EI|^{1/2}, \quad -\frac{T}{2}, \quad -\frac{T+|T^2-4|k'|EI|^{1/2}}{2}, \quad -\frac{T+|T^2+4|k'|EI|^{1/2}}{2},$$

(6.272)

where: (i) the l.h.s. corresponds to clamped (6.31a–c) $\equiv$ (6.273a), clamped-pinned (6.48a–c) $\equiv$ (6.273b), pinned (6.39a–d) $\equiv$ (6.273c), and cantilever (6.65a–c) $\equiv$ (6.273d) beams:

$$-\frac{\bar{T}L^2}{EI} = \begin{cases} 4\pi^2 & \text{for clamped,} & (6.273a) \\ 2.042\pi^2 & \text{for clamped-pinned,} & (6.273b) \\ \pi^2 & \text{for pinned,} & (6.273c) \\ \dfrac{\pi^2}{4} & \text{for cantilever;} & (6.273d) \end{cases}$$

(ii) on the r.h.s. to the case I of compression without springs (6.274a), case IV of repulsive springs without axial tension (6.274b), case V of axial compression balanced by attractive spring (6.274c), case VIII of axial compression dominating attractive springs (6.274d), and case IX of axial tension dominating repulsive springs (6.274e):

$$\bar{T} = \frac{T+\sqrt{T^2-4k'EI}}{2} < 0: \begin{cases} \text{I:} & T<0=k', \quad \bar{T}=T; & (6.274a) \\ \text{IV:} & T=0>k', \quad \bar{T}=|k'EI|^{1/2}; & (6.274b) \\ \text{V:} & T<0, \quad k'=\dfrac{T^2}{4EI}>0, \quad \bar{T}=\dfrac{T}{2}; & (6.274c) \\ \text{VIII:} & T^2>4k'EI, \quad T<0<k', \quad 2\bar{T}=T+|T^2+4|k'|EI|^{1/2}; & (6.274d) \\ \text{IX:} & T^2>4k'EI, \quad k'<0, \quad 2\bar{T}=T+|T^2+4|k'|EI|^{1/2}; & (6.274e) \end{cases}$$

*are the five cases with buckling specified by the **effective axial tension** $\bar{T}$ that is negative, implying a predominance of axial compression $T < 0$ and/or repulsive springs $k' < 0$.* The effective axial tension, that acts as a combined tension-spring buckling load, also indicates when buckling is not possible (subsection 6.3.13).

6.3.13 Combined Tension-Spring Buckling Load

Buckling is not possible because the effective axial tension is: (i) positive in the case II of axial traction without spring (6.274f), case VI of axial traction balanced by attractive spring (6.274g), and case VII of axial traction dominating attractive spring (6.274h); and (ii) not real, that is complex in the case III of attractive spring without axial tension (6.274i) and case X of attractive spring dominating axial tension (6.274j):

$$\bar{T} > 0 \begin{cases} \text{II:} & T > 0 = k', & \bar{T} = T; & (6.274f) \\[2mm] \text{VI:} & T^2 = 4k'EI > 0, & \bar{T} = T; & (6.274g) \\[2mm] \text{VII:} & T^2 > 4k'EI, \ k' < 0, & 2\bar{T} = T + \left| T^2 + 4|k'|EI \right|^{1/2} & (6.274h) \end{cases}$$

$$\bar{T} \notin |R \begin{cases} \text{III:} & T = 0 < k', & \bar{T} = \pm i \left| k'EI \right|^{1/2}, & (6.274i) \\[2mm] \text{X:} & T^2 < 4k'EI, & 2\bar{T} = T \pm i \left| 4k'EI - T^2 \right|^{1/2}. & (6.274j) \end{cases}$$

*The effective axial tension is defined (problem 220) by the **combined tension-spring buckling load** (6.274a–e) ≡ (6.275a):*

$$\bar{T} = \frac{T + \sqrt{T^2 - 4k'EI}}{2}: \quad \text{buckling} \begin{cases} \text{possible:} & \bar{T} < 0, \\[2mm] \text{impossible:} & \bar{T} > 0 \text{ or } \bar{T} \notin |R, \end{cases} \quad (6.275a\text{–}c)$$

showing that buckling is possible (6.275b) [impossible (6.275c)] in the cases where the combined tension-resilience buckling load is negative (6.274a–e) [positive (6.274f–h) or not real (6.274i, j)]. In all cases (6.274a–e) when buckling is possible (problem 220) the displacement, slope, and curvature of the elastica are determined by the boundary conditions alone; that is, coincide with the case of linear buckling under compression without springs (section 6.1). Thus the shape of the buckled beam depends only on the supports: (i) clamped (6.32e) ≡ (6.276a);

(ii) pinned (6.40a) ≡ (6.276b); (ii) clamped-pinned (6.50b) ≡ (6.276c); or (iv) cantilever (6.67a) ≡ (6.276d):

$$\zeta(x) = A \times \begin{cases} 1 - \cos\left(\dfrac{2\pi x}{L}\right) \equiv \zeta_1(x) & \text{for clamping,} & (6.276a) \\[2ex] \sin\left(\dfrac{\pi x}{L}\right) \equiv \zeta_2(x) & \text{for pinning,} & (6.276b) \\[2ex] a\left(1 - \dfrac{x}{L}\right) + \sin\left(\dfrac{ax}{L}\right) - a\cos\left(\dfrac{ax}{L}\right) & \text{for clamping-pinning,} & (6.276c) \\[2ex] 1 - \cos\left(\dfrac{\pi x}{2L}\right) & \text{for cantilever,} & (6.276d) \end{cases}$$

where A is an arbitrary constant, and the value (6.48a) appears in the clamped-pinned case. A beam without transverse loads has been considered for: (i) linear and non-linear buckling in the absence of spring support (section 6.1); and (ii/iii) linear buckling in the presence of point translational or rotary springs (section 6.2) [distributed continuous translational springs (section 6.3)]. The beam with transverse loads can be considered without (with) spring support [section III.4.6 (subsection 6.3.14)].

6.3.14 Deflection by a Uniform Shear Stress

The linear (6.190a) bending (6.191d) of a uniform beam (6.191a–c) can (subsection 6.3.1) be considered in the: (i) absence of forcing (6.195a–c) to assess elastic stability (subsections 6.3.2–6.3.13); or (ii) presence of forcing (6.190b) to determine the deflection under external transverse loads. The simplest (Figure 6.7) is a uniform shear stress, for example corresponding (6.277b) to a uniform beam with mass density ρ per unit length in a uniform gravity field with acceleration g:

$$\zeta_* = \frac{\rho g}{k'}: \qquad\qquad EI\zeta'''' - T\zeta'' + k'\zeta = f = \rho g; \qquad\qquad (6.277a, b)$$

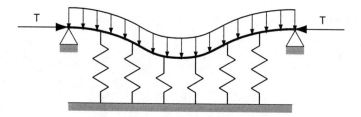

FIGURE 6.7
The buckling (Figures 6.3–6.6) considers a beam under axial compression without transverse loads, leading to a "free" shape. The free shape is added to the forced deflection by a transverse load like the weight.

a particular integral is (6.277a). In the case VII of axial traction (6.237b) ≡ (6.278b) dominating (6.237a) ≡ (6.278a) attractive springs (6.237c) ≡ (6.278c) there is no buckling (subsection 6.3.8) and the complete integral of (6.277b) adds (6.277a) to (6.239) leading to (6.278d).

$$T^2 > 4k'EI, \quad T > 0, \quad k' > 0:$$

$$\zeta(x) = \zeta_{VII}(x) + \zeta_* = \frac{\rho g}{k'} + A\cosh(a_+x) + B\sinh(a_+x) + C\cosh(a_-x) + D\sinh(a_-x).$$

$$(6.278a\text{–}d)$$

The boundary conditions (6.36a, b) ≡ (6.279a, c) for a pinned beam lead to a dissimilar (6.279b) ≠ (6.240b) [similar (6.279d) ≡ (6.240d)] condition on the coefficients since only the former (not the latter) is affected by the forcing (6.277a, b):

$$0 = \bar{\zeta}(0) = \frac{\rho g}{k'} + A + C, \qquad\qquad 0 = \bar{\zeta}''(0) = a_+^2 A + a_-^2 C. \qquad (6.279a\text{–}d)$$

The system of equations (6.279a, b) ≡ (6.280b) has non-zero determinant (6.280a):

$$E_0 \equiv a_-^2 - a_+^2 \neq 0: \qquad \begin{bmatrix} 1 & 1 \\ a_+^2 & a_-^2 \end{bmatrix}\begin{bmatrix} A \\ C \end{bmatrix} = \begin{bmatrix} -\dfrac{\rho g}{k'} \\ 0 \end{bmatrix}, \qquad (6.280a, b)$$

and can be solved (6.281a, b) to determine two constants of integration:

$$k'(a_+^2 - a_-^2)\{A, C\} = \rho g\{a_-^2, -a_+^2\}. \qquad (6.281a, b)$$

Substitution of (6.281a, b) in (6.278d) leads to:

$$k'(a_+^2 - a_-^2)\bar{\zeta}(x) = \rho g\{a_+^2[1 - \cosh(a_-x)] - a_-^2[1 - \cosh(a_+x)]\}$$

$$+ k'(a_+^2 - a_-^2)[B\sinh(a_+x) + D\sinh(a_-x)]. \qquad (6.282)$$

that: (i) satisfies (6.279a, c); and (ii) leaves two constants of integration (B, D) undetermined.

The constants of integration (A, C) $[(B, D)]$ are determined by the pinned boundary conditions (6.279a, c) [(6.283a, b)] at $x = 0(x = L)$:

$$\bar{\zeta}(L) = 0 = \bar{\zeta}''(L): \quad k'\left(a_+^2 - a_-^2\right)\begin{bmatrix} \sinh(a_+L) & \sinh(a_-L) \\ a_+^2 \sinh(a_+L) & a_-^2 \sinh(a_-L) \end{bmatrix}\begin{bmatrix} B \\ D \end{bmatrix}$$

$$= \rho g \begin{bmatrix} a_-^2\{1 - \cosh(a_+ L)\} - a_+^2\{1 - \cosh(a_-L)\} \\ a_+^2 a_-^2\{\cosh(a_-L) - \cosh(a_+ L)\} \end{bmatrix}.$$

$$(6.283a\text{–}c)$$

The determinant of the matrix on the l.h.s. of (6.283c) is non-zero (6.243a): (i) excluding buckling in the absence of transverse loads (subsection 6.3.8); (ii) in the presence of transverse loads (subsection 6.3.14) specifies the constants of integration (B, D) in (6.282):

$$E_{VII} k'\left(a_+^2 - a_-^2\right)\begin{bmatrix} B \\ D \end{bmatrix} = \rho g \begin{bmatrix} a_-^2 \sinh(a_- L) & -\sinh(a_- L) \\ -a_+^2 \sinh(a_+ L) & \sinh(a_+ L) \end{bmatrix}$$

$$\times \begin{bmatrix} a_-^2\{1 - \cosh(a_+ L)\} - a_+^2\{1 - \cosh(a_- L)\} \\ a_+^2 a_-^2\{\cosh(a_- L) - \cosh(a_+ L)\} \end{bmatrix},$$

$$(6.284)$$

using in (6.284) the inverse matrix of that in (6.283c).

Thus the constants of integration (B, D) are given by (6.284) ≡ (6.285a, b):

$$B\sinh(a_+L) = \frac{\rho g\, a_-^2}{k'\left(a_+^2 - a_-^2\right)}\left[1 - \cosh(a_+L)\right], \quad (6.285a)$$

$$D\sinh(a_-L) = -\frac{\rho g\, a_+^2}{k'\left(a_+^2 - a_-^2\right)}\left[1 - \cosh(a_- L)\right]. \quad (6.285b)$$

Substitution of (6.285a, b) in (6.282) specifies the shape of the elastica:

$$k'\frac{a_+^2 - a_-^2}{\rho g}\, \bar{\zeta}(x) = a_+^2\left[1 - \cosh(a_-x) - \frac{1 - \cosh(a_-L)}{\sinh(a_-L)}\sinh(a_- x)\right]$$

$$(6.286)$$

$$- a_-^2\left[1 - \cosh(a_+x) - \frac{1 - \cosh(a_+L)}{\sinh(a_+L)}\sinh(a_+ x)\right],$$

that satisfies the differential equation (6.277b) with the boundary conditions (6.279a, c; 6.283a, b). It has been shown that *(problem 221) the shape of the elastica of a uniform beam (6.191a–c) under linear deflection (6.190a) by a uniform shear stress (6.190b) like the weight in a constant gravity field (6.277b) is given by (6.286) under the assumptions that: (i) the axial traction (6.278b) dominates (6.278a) the attractive springs (6.278c); and (ii) the beam is pinned at both ends (6.279a, c; 6.283a, b).* Four cases of beams without spring support and with distinct boundary conditions and transverse loads are considered (problems 222–225) in the example 10.10. The deformations of a straight elastic rod consist of: (i) torsion under an axial moment (subsections II.6.4–II.6.8); (ii) bending under transverse loads (chapter III.4) with possible buckling under axial loads (section 6.1) that may additionally be combined with transverse springs (sections 6.2–6.3); and (iii) axial loads, that is compressions or tractions alone (section 6.4).

6.4 Axial Traction/Compression of a Straight Bar

The simplest problem of elasticity is the axial deformation of a bar, which is analogous to: (i) the transverse deflection of a strings (6.4.1); or (ii) steady heat conduction between parallel walls (subsection 6.4.2). The case of non-uniform loads is analogous to elastic strings (chapter III.2); the case of inhomogeneous material may be considered for various profiles (subsection 6.4.3) such as linear (section I.32.9) [quadratic (section 6.4.4)].

6.4.1 Analogy with the Deflection of an Elastic String

The simplest problem of elasticity; that is, entirely one-dimensional, is the traction $T > 0$ (compression $T < 0$) of a bar [Figure 6.8a(b)]. In both cases, the balance of the **longitudinal force** F and **stress** T at the ends (Figure 6.9) leads to (6.287a) ≡ (6.287b):

$$0 = F\,dx + T + dT - T: \qquad\qquad -F = \frac{dT}{dx} = T', \qquad\qquad (6.287a, b)$$

that is, the one-dimensional form of the force-stress balance (II.4.39a–d) in a medium at rest. The **longitudinal displacement** (6.288a) leads to an **extension (contraction)**; that is, an increase (decrease) in length if (6.288b) is positive (negative):

$$\vec{u} = \vec{e}_x\, u(x): \qquad (ds)^2 - (dx)^2 = (dx + du)^2 - (dx)^2 \equiv 2S(dx)^2, \qquad (6.288a–c)$$

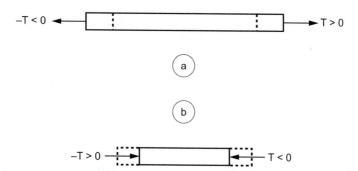

FIGURE 6.8
Besides bending (Figures 6.1–6.7), another deformation of a straight rod is extension (a) [contraction (b)] under traction (compression).

corresponding (6.288c) ≡ (6.289a) to a positive (negative) **exact strain** in the non-linear case:

$$S = \frac{\left(1+u'\right)^2 - 1}{2} = u' + \frac{u'^2}{2}; \qquad u'^2 \ll 1: \qquad S = u', \qquad \text{(6.289a–c)}$$

in the linear case (6.289b) of **small strain**, the strain is the spatial derivative of the displacement (6.289c). The stress in an **elastic material** is proportional by the **Hooke (1678) law** to the strain (6.290a) through the **Young modulus** E:

$$T = ES; \qquad u'^2 \ll 1: \qquad -F = \left(ES\right)' = \left(Eu'\right)', \qquad \text{(6.290a–d)}$$

in the linear case (6.289b) ≡ (6.290b) the displacement (6.288a) satisfies (6.287b; 6.290a; 6.289c) ≡ (6.290c, d). *The equation for the axial deformation of a bar (6.290d) is analogous (problem 226) to the linear (6.291a) transverse deflection of an elastic string (6.291b)* ≡ *(III.2.11c) corresponding to a beam (6.14f) without E I = 0 bending stiffness:*

$$\zeta'^2 \ll 1: \quad -f = \left(T\zeta'\right)'; \quad \vec{e}_y\,\zeta = \vec{u} \quad \leftrightarrow \quad \vec{e}_x\,u = \vec{u}, \quad T \leftrightarrow E, \quad f \leftrightarrow F.$$

$$\text{(6.291a–e)}$$

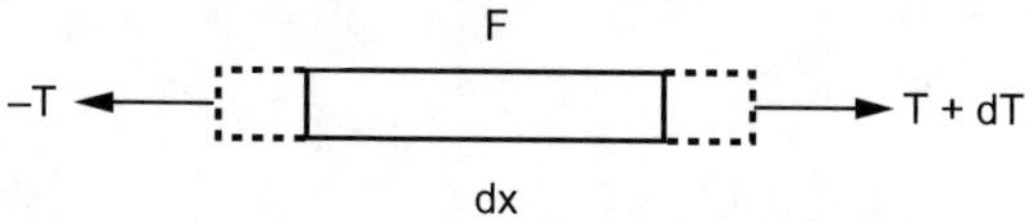

F

$-T \longleftarrow$ [ ] $\longrightarrow T + dT$

dx

FIGURE 6.9
The extension (contraction) of a rod under traction (compression) are [Figure 6.8a (b)] both cases of longitudinal deformation in contrast with transversal deformation or bending (Figures 6.1–6.7).

The longitudinal deformation (transverse deflection) of an elastic bar (6.290d)
[string (6.291b)], both in the linear case of small strain (6.290b) [slope (6.291a)], are
analogous replacing: (i) the transverse ζ by the longitudinal u displacement (6.291c);
(ii) the tension T of the string by the Young modulus E of the material (6.289d); and
(iii) the longitudinal force F by the shear stress f that is the transverse force per unit
length (6.6c).

6.4.2 Analogy with Steady Heat Conduction

The heat sources Q in a region are balanced by the heat flux J out of the
region in the case (6.292a) of steady heat conduction:

$$Q = J'; \qquad \chi > 0: \qquad J = -\chi\theta', \qquad (6.292a\text{--}c)$$

in the one-dimensional form (6.292a) of the heat equation (I.32.3) the heat
flux is given by the **Fourier law (1818)** as proportional (I.32.4b) $\equiv$ (6.292c) to
the **temperature** θ gradient θ', in the direction of decreasing temperature,
since the **thermal conductivity** χ is positive (6.292b) $\equiv$ (I.32.4a). Substituting
(6.292c) in (6.292a) leads to (6.293a):

$$Q = -\left(\chi\theta'\right)': \qquad \theta \leftrightarrow u, \qquad \chi \leftrightarrow E, \qquad Q \leftrightarrow F, \qquad (6.293a\text{--}d)$$

showing the *analogy (problem 227) between steady heat conduction (6.293a) [the*
axial deformation of a rod (6.290d)] replacing: (i) the temperature θ by (6.293b) the
displacement u; (i) the thermal conductivity by (6.293c) the Young modulus E; and
(iii) the heat source Q by (6.293d), the longitudinal force F.

6.4.3 Linear/Non-Linear Deformation of Homogeneous/
Inhomogeneous Media

The solution is similar for the three analogous linear problems of: (a) axial
deformation of an elastic rod (6.290d); (b) transverse deflection of an elastic
string (6.291b); and (c) one-dimensional steady heat conduction (6.293a). It is
therefore sufficient to proceed with one of the problems (a), for which *(prob-*
lem 228) the longitudinal force applied to a bar causes a stress (6.287b) independent
of the material (6.294a):

$$T(0) - \int_0^x F(\xi)d\xi = T(x) = E(x)S(x) = E(x)u'(x); \qquad (6.294a\text{--}c)$$

$$u(x) = u_0 + xT(0) - \int_0^x \frac{1}{E(\eta)} \int_0^\eta F(\xi)d\xi, \qquad (6.294d)$$

the strain (6.294b) and the displacement (6.294c) ≡ (6.294d) depend on the Young modulus of the material. In the case of an homogeneous material that has a constant Young modulus (6.295a), the displacement (6.290d) satisfies (6.295b):

$$E = const: \quad u'' = -\frac{F}{E}; \quad F = const, \quad u(0) = 0 = u(L): \quad u(x) = \frac{F}{2E}x(L-x).$$

$$(6.295a\text{–}f)$$

If the force is also constant (6.295c) and the rod is fixed at the two ends (6.295d, e), the displacement at all positions is given by (6.295f). The result (6.295a–f) is proved as follows: (i) the general integral of (6.295b) with E, F constant (6.295a, c) is (6.295g) where (C_1, C_2) are arbitrary constants of integration:

$$u(x) = -\frac{Fx^2}{2E} + C_1 x + C_2: \quad 0 = u(0) = C_2, \quad 0 = u(L) = -\frac{FL^2}{2E} + C_1 L.$$

$$(6.295g\text{–}k)$$

(ii) the constants of integration are determined by the boundary conditions that the rod is fixed at both ends (6.295h, j) leading to (6.295i, k); and (iii) substitution of (6.295i, k) in (6.295g) proves (6.295f). This result can be generalized to: (i) non-linear deflection with large strain (notes III.4.5–III.4.7); and (ii) the linear case for an inhomogeneous medium whose properties depend on position. The case of a thermal conductivity a linear function of position was considered before (section I.32.9); a distinct but analogous problem is a Young modulus, a quadratic function of position, and is considered next (subsection 6.4.4).

6.4.4 Axial Contraction/Extension of an Inhomogenous Bar

A **graded material** is an inhomogeneous material whose properties vary in one direction, for example a non-uniform rod. In the case of a uniform force (6.296a), the profile of the Young modulus specifies the stress (6.296b) and strain (6.296c):

$$F = const: \quad -Fx + C = T = ES = Eu',$$

$$(6.296a\text{–}c)$$

to within a constant C. For a quadratic profile (Figure 6.10) of the Young modulus (6.297a) the longitudinal displacement is specified by (6.296b) ≡ (6.297b):

$$E(x) = E_0 + (E_1 - E_0)\frac{x^2}{L^2}: \quad u(x) - u(0) = \int_0^x \frac{C - F\xi}{E_0 + (E_1 - E_0)\xi^2/L^2}\, d\xi.$$

$$(6.297a, b)$$

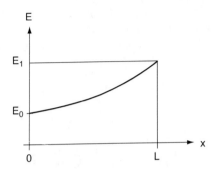

FIGURE 6.10
The extension (contraction) of a straight rod [Figure 6.8a (b)] under traction (contraction) depends on the Young modulus that is a function of position for an inhomogeneous material.

The change of variable (6.298a, b) performs the integration in (6.297b) ≡ (6.298c) in terms of the argument of the circular tangent (II.7.124a) and natural logarithm (II.3.33a):

$$\eta \equiv a\frac{\xi}{L}, \ a \equiv \left|\frac{E_1}{E_0} - 1\right|^{1/2} : \ u(x) - u(0) = \frac{L}{E_0 a^2} \int_0^{ax/L} \frac{Ca - FL\eta}{1+\eta^2} d\eta$$

$$= \frac{L}{E_0 a^2}\left[Ca \, arc\tan\eta - \frac{FL}{2}\log\left(1+\eta^2\right)\right]_0^{ax/L} \qquad (6.298a–c)$$

$$= \frac{CL}{E_0 a} arc\tan\left(a\frac{x}{L}\right) - \frac{FL^2}{2E_0 a^2}\log\left(1 + a^2\frac{x^2}{L^2}\right).$$

Substituting (6.298b) in (6.298c) specifies the displacement (6.299b):

$$u(0) = 0: \qquad u(x) = \frac{CL}{\sqrt{E_0(E_1 - E_0)}} arc\tan\left(\frac{x}{L}\sqrt{\frac{E_1}{E_0} - 1}\right)$$

$$\qquad\qquad\qquad\qquad (6.299a, b)$$

$$- \frac{FL^2}{2(E_1 - E_0)}\log\left[1 + \frac{x^2}{L^2}\left(\frac{E_1}{E_0} - 1\right)\right],$$

assuming that the rod is fixed at one end (6.299a).

The remaining constant of integration is determined (6.300b) by the condition (6.300a) that the bar is fixed at the other end:

$$u(L) = 0: \qquad FL\log\left(\frac{E_1}{E_0}\right) = 2C\sqrt{\frac{E_1}{E_0} - 1} \ arc\tan\left[\sqrt{\frac{E_1}{E_0} - 1}\right]. \qquad (6.300a, b)$$

Solving (6.300b) for C and substituting in (6.299b) specifies the longitudinal displacement:

$$u(x) = \frac{FL^2}{2(E_1 - E_0)} \left\{ -\log\left[1 + \left(\frac{E_1}{E_0} - 1\right)\frac{x^2}{L^2}\right] \right.$$

$$\left. + \frac{\log(E_1/E_0)}{\arctan\left(\sqrt{E_1/E_0 - 1}\right)} \arctan\left(\frac{x}{L}\sqrt{\frac{E_1}{E_0} - 1}\right) \right\},$$

(6.301)

that satisfies the boundary conditions (6.299a; 6.300a) and the differential equation (6.290d; 6.297a)$\equiv$(6.302a, b):

$$-F = \left\{ \left[E_0 + (E_1 - E_0)\frac{x^2}{L^2}\right]u' \right\}' = \left[E_0 + (E_1 - E_0)\frac{x^2}{L^2}\right]u'' + 2\frac{E_1 - E_0}{L^2}x u'.$$

(6.302a, b)

Thus *a rod under axial tension (6.290d) made of an inhomogeneous material with Young modulus (6.297a) and fixed at both ends (6.299a; 6.300a) has (problem 229) a displacement (6.301) that: (i) satisfies the differential equation (6.302a, b); and (ii–iii) leads to the stress (6.303a) [strain (6.303a)]:*

$$T(x) = \left[E_0 + (E_1 - E_0)\frac{x^2}{L^2}\right]S(x) = -Fx + \frac{FL}{2\sqrt{E_1/E_0 - 1}}\frac{\log(E_1/E_0)}{\arctan\sqrt{E_1/E_0 - 1}},$$

(6.303a, b)

as follows from (6.290a; 6.297a) $\equiv$ (6.303a) [(6.296b; 6.300b) $\equiv$ (6.303b)].

6.5 In-Plane Loads in a Flat Plate

A pair of one(two)-dimensional analogues [section 6.4 (6.5)] are axial (in-plane) loads in a bar (plate). The Hooke law of linear elasticity relating the stress and strain tensors (subsection 6.5.1) applies to tractions, compressions, and shears for a thin plate (subsection 6.5.2) [plane elasticity (subsection 6.5.3)], with the difference that the normal stress (strain) is zero (subsection 6.5.2). This is equivalent to a substitution of material parameters in the differential equation satisfied by the displacement vector (subsection 6.5.4) in the presence of arbitrary external forces. If the external forces are constant or absent, the components of the stress tensor derive from a scalar stress function (subsection 6.5.5) that satisfies a biharmonic equation forced by the dilatation. Three examples of in-plane stresses in a plate concern the effect of: (i) a torque applied in a circular area (subsection 6.5.6); (ii) a circular hole in the presence of stresses at infinity (subsections 6.5.7–6.5.8); and (iii) a disk under axial compression (subsection 6.5.9). The solution of (i, ii) [(iii)] uses the differential equation satisfied by the stress function (displacement vector); the stress function is specified in (i) [(ii)] using real (complex) variables. Thus the three examples illustrate three methods (chapter II.4) of solution of problems in plane elasticity: (a, b) the stress function using real (complex) coordinates [subsection(s) 6.5.6. (6.5.7–6.5.8)] as a solution of a biharmonic equation; and (c) the balance of force and stresses expressed as a differential equation for the displacement vector (subsection 6.5.9).

6.5.1 Linear Relation between Stresses and Strains in Elasticity

The one-dimensional relation (6.290a) between stress and strain in linear elasticity (6.290b) is extended to three dimensions, also in the linear approximation (6.304a), by the **direct Hooke law** (6.304b):

$$\left(S_{ij}\right)^2 \ll 1: \qquad\qquad T_{ij} = \frac{E}{1+\sigma}\left(S_{ij} + \frac{\sigma}{1-2\sigma}S_{kk}\,\delta_{ij}\right), \qquad\qquad (6.304a, b)$$

involving: (i) the **Poisson ratio** σ as moduli of elasticity as well as the Young modulus E; (ii) the strain tensor (II.4.12a–d) $\equiv$ (6.304c) that equals half the symmetric derivative of the displacement vector; (iii) the repeated index, which implies a summation (6.304d) in the strain tensor (6.304c) and corresponds to the trace of the matrix (6.304e) and specifies the **volume change** (6.304f):

$$2S_{ij} = \partial_i u_j + \partial_j u_i: \qquad S_{kk} \equiv \sum_{k=1}^{3} S_{kk} = S_{xx} + S_{yy} + S_{zz} \equiv D_3 = \nabla.\vec{u}, \qquad (6.304c\text{–}g)$$

that equals the divergence of the displacement vector (6.304g); and (iv) the **unit or identity matrix** (6.305b, c) in three-dimensions (6.305a), whose trace is (6.305d):

$$i,j = 1,2,3: \qquad \delta_{ij} \equiv \begin{cases} 0 & \text{if } i \neq j, \\ \\ 1 & \text{if } i = j, \end{cases} \qquad \delta_{ii} \equiv \prod_{i=1}^{3} \delta_{ii} = 3. \qquad (6.305a\text{–}d)$$

The stress T_{ij} (strain S_{ij}) tensors are both symmetric (6.306a, b), and the six independent components of the stresses are specified in terms of the six independent components of the strains by the direct Hooke law (6.304b) consisting of two sets of three equations:

$$T_{ij} = T_{ji}, \qquad S_{ij} = S_{ji}: \qquad \{T_{xy}, T_{xz}, T_{yz}\} = \frac{E}{1+\sigma}\{S_{xy}, S_{xz}, S_{yz}\}, \qquad (6.306a\text{–}e)$$

stating that: (i) the shear stresses are proportional (6.306c–e) ≡ (II.4.76a) to the shear strains; and (ii) the normal stresses, that is tractions and compressions:

$$T_{xx} = \frac{E}{1+\sigma}\left(S_{xx} + \frac{\sigma}{1-2\sigma}D_3\right) = \frac{E}{(1+\sigma)(1-2\sigma)}\left[(1-\sigma)S_{xx} + \sigma(S_{yy} + S_{zz})\right],$$
$$(6.307a)$$

$$T_{yy} = \frac{E}{1+\sigma}\left(S_{yy} + \frac{\sigma}{1-2\sigma}D_3\right) = \frac{E}{(1+\sigma)(1-2\sigma)}\left[(1-\sigma)S_{yy} + \sigma(S_{xx} + S_{zz})\right],$$
$$(6.307b)$$

$$T_{zz} = \frac{E}{1+\sigma}\left(S_{zz} + \frac{\sigma}{1-2\sigma}D_3\right) = \frac{E}{(1+\sigma)(1-2\sigma)}\left[(1-\sigma)S_{zz} + \sigma(S_{xx} + S_{yy})\right],$$
$$(6.307c)$$

involve: (ii-1) the normal strains, that is extensions and contractions; also (ii-2) the volume changes (6.307a–c) ≡ (II.4.76b, c).

The **pressure** p is defined as minus the mean value of the three normal stresses:

$$-3p \equiv T_{xx} + T_{yy} + T_{zz} = T_{ii} = \frac{E}{1+\sigma}\left(1 + \frac{3\sigma}{1-2\sigma}\right)S_{ii} = \frac{E}{1-2\sigma}D_3, \qquad (6.308)$$

and is related (6.304b) to the volume change (6.304c) by (6.308). Substitution of (6.308) ≡ (6.309a) ≡ (6.309b):

$$p = -\frac{E}{3(1-2\sigma)}D_3, \qquad S_{kk} = \frac{1-2\sigma}{E}T_{kk}, \qquad T_{ij} = \frac{E}{1+\sigma}S_{ij} + \frac{\sigma}{1+\sigma}T_{kk}\delta_{ij},$$
$$(6.309a\text{–}c)$$

in (6.304b) leads (6.309c) ≡ (6.310) to the **inverse Hooke law** specifying the strains in terms of the stresses:

$$S_{ij} = \frac{1+\sigma}{E}T_{ij} - \frac{\sigma}{E}T_{kk}\delta_{ij}. \qquad (6.310)$$

The inverse Hooke law (6.310) has two sets of three independent components, namely: (i) the preceding set (6.306c–e) of shear strains and stresses; and (ii) the inverse (6.311a–c) of (6.307a–c) for normal strains and stresses:

$$S_{xx} = \frac{1+\sigma}{E} T_{xx} + \frac{\sigma}{3E} p = \frac{1}{E} T_{xx} - \frac{\sigma}{E}\left(T_{yy} + T_{zz}\right), \tag{6.311a}$$

$$S_{yy} = \frac{1+\sigma}{E} T_{yy} + \frac{\sigma}{3E} p = \frac{1}{E} T_{xx} - \frac{\sigma}{E}\left(T_{xx} + T_{zz}\right), \tag{6.311b}$$

$$S_{zz} = \frac{1+\sigma}{E} T_{zz} + \frac{\sigma}{3E} p = \frac{1}{E} T_{zz} - \frac{\sigma}{E}\left(T_{xx} + T_{yy}\right), \tag{6.311c}$$

where (6.310; 6.308) were used to obtain (6.311a–c) ≡ (II.4.78b, c). Thus *(problem 230) in linear elasticity (6.304a) the stresses are specified by the strains (viceversa) by the direct (6.304b) ≡ (6.306c–e; 6.307a–c) [inverse (6.310) ≡ (6.306c–e; 6.311a–c)] Hooke law, that implies the relation (6.309a) between the pressure (6.308) and volume change (6.304c).* The intermediate cases between one-dimensional (6.290a, b) and three-dimensional (6.304a–c) elasticity are the two, two-dimensional cases, namely: (a) in-plane stresses in a thin plate (subsection 6.5.2); and (b) plane elasticity (subsection 6.5.3).

6.5.2 Thin Elastic Plate without Transverse Load

One case of two-dimensional elasticity is **in-plane stresses** in a thin elastic plane not subject to a stress force (6.312a) on the surfaces with normals (6.312b); thus three components of the stress tensor vanish (6.312c–e):

$$0 = T_i = T_{ij}\, n_j\,, \qquad \vec{n} = \pm \vec{e}_z: \qquad 0 = T_{xz} = T_{yz} = T_{zz}. \tag{6.312a–e}$$

Since the plate is thin it may be assumed that the out-of-plane stresses (6.312c–e) are negligible compared with the in-plane stresses $\left(T_{xx}, T_{yy}, T_{xy}\right)$. The neglect of out-of-plane shear (6.312c, d) [normal (6.312e)] stresses implies by the Hooke law (6.306d, e) [(6.307c)] that the out-of-plane shear (normal) strains vanish (6.313a, b) [do not vanish (6.313c):

$$S_{xz} = 0 = S_{yz}\,, \qquad S_{zz} = -\frac{\sigma}{1-\sigma}\left(S_{xx} + S_{yy}\right). \tag{6.313a–c}$$

From (6.313c) it follows that in-plane extensions (contractions) imply that the plate becomes thinner (thicker). The in-plane shear stress is given

by (6.306c) ≡ (6.314c) and substitution of (6.313c) in (6.307a, b) specifies the
in-plane normal stresses (6.314a, b):

$$\left\{ T_{xx}, T_{yy} \right\} = \frac{E}{1-\sigma^2} \left\{ S_{xx} + S_{yy}\,\sigma, S_{yy} + \sigma\,S_{xx} \right\}, \qquad T_{xy} = \frac{E}{1+\sigma} S_{xy}. \qquad (6.314\text{a–c})$$

Thus, *for a thin elastic plate not subject to transverse loads (problem 231): (i) the
out-of-plane stresses (6.312c–e) are negligible compared with the in-plane stresses
(6.314a–c); and (ii) the out-of-plane shear strains vanish (6.313a, b) and the out-
of-plane normal strain is determined by the in-plane normal strains (6.313c).* The
comparison with plane elasticity (chapter II.4) follows (subsection 6.5.3).

6.5.3 Comparison with Stresses and Strains in Plane Elasticity

The second case of two-dimensional elasticity is **plane elasticity** (chapter II.4) for which the zero out-of-plane stresses (6.312c–e) are replaced by
zero out-of-plane strains (6.315a–c):

$$0 = \hat{S}_{xz} = \hat{S}_{yz} = \hat{S}_{zz}, \qquad \hat{T}_{xz} = 0 = \hat{T}_{yz}, \qquad (6.315\text{a–e})$$

implying (6.306d, e) zero out-of-plane shear stresses (6.315d, e). The plane
elasticity (in-plane stresses in a thin plate without transversal loads) are: (i)
similar in the vanishing out-of-plane shear stresses (6.315d, e) ≡ (6.312c, d)
and strains (6.315a, b) ≡ (6.313a, b); and (ii) differ in the vanishing of the out-
of-plane normal stress (6.312e) [strain (6.315c)]. In the case of plane elasticity
(6.315c), the in-plane normal (6.307a, b) stresses are given by (6.316a, b):

$$\left\{ \hat{T}_{xx}, \hat{T}_{yy} \right\} = \frac{\hat{E}}{\left(1+\hat{\sigma}\right)\left(1-2\hat{\sigma}\right)} \left\{ \left(1-\hat{\sigma}\right)\hat{S}_{xx} + \hat{\sigma}\,\hat{S}_{yy}, \left(1-\hat{\sigma}\right)\hat{S}_{yy} + \hat{\sigma}\,\hat{S}_{xx} \right\}, \qquad (6.316\text{a, b})$$

and the in-plane shear stresses by (6.306c) ≡ (6.317a):

$$\hat{T}_{xy} = \frac{\hat{E}}{1+\hat{\sigma}} \hat{S}_{xy}; \qquad \hat{T}_{zz} = \hat{\sigma}\left(\hat{T}_{xx} + \hat{T}_{yy} \right), \qquad (6.317\text{a, b})$$

the absence of out-of-plane normal strain (6.315c) implies (6.311c) the existence of an out-of-plane normal stress (6.317b); the tractions (compressions)
in the plane require an out-of-plane traction (compression) to prevent the
appearance of an out-of-plane normal strain. Thus, *in (problem 232) plane elasticity (chapter II.4): (i) the out-of-plane (in-plane) strains are zero (6.315a–c) [non-
zero]; (ii) the in-plane (out-of-plane) shear stress (stresses) does not vanish (6.317a)
[do vanish(6.315d, e)]; and (iii) the out-of-plane normal stress (6.317b) is determined
by the in-plane normal stresses (6.316a, b).*

The stress-strain relations for plane elasticity (6.316a, b; 6.317a, b) and for in-plane stresses in a thin plate not subject to transversal forces (6.313c; 6.314a–c) coincide with the substitutions (problem 233) of Young moduli $\hat{E}$ $\leftrightarrow$ E *and Poisson ratio* $\hat{\sigma}$ $\leftrightarrow$ σ *given by:*

$$\sigma = \frac{\hat{\sigma}}{1-\hat{\sigma}}, \qquad\qquad E = \frac{\hat{E}}{1-\hat{\sigma}^2}, \qquad (6.318a, b)$$

since: (i) comparing the terms in curly brackets in (6.314a, b) ≡ (6.316a, b) implies (6.318a); (ii) the factors out of brackets in (6.314a, b) ≡ (6.316a, b) [(6.314c) ≡ (6.317a)] imply (6.319a) (6.319b):

$$\frac{E}{1-\sigma^2} = \frac{\hat{E}(1-\hat{\sigma})}{(1+\hat{\sigma})(1-2\hat{\sigma})}, \qquad\qquad \frac{E}{1+\sigma} = \frac{\hat{E}}{1+\hat{\sigma}}; \qquad (6.319a, b)$$

(iii) substituting (6.318a) in (6.319b) leads to (6.319c) ≡ (6.318b):

$$E = \hat{E}\frac{1+\sigma}{1+\hat{\sigma}} = \frac{\hat{E}}{1+\hat{\sigma}}\left(1+\frac{\hat{\sigma}}{1-\hat{\sigma}}\right) = \frac{\hat{E}}{1-\hat{\sigma}^2}; \qquad (6.319c)$$

and (iv) substitution of (6.318a, b) in (6.319a) leads to an identity:

$$\frac{E}{1-\sigma^2} = \frac{\hat{E}}{1-\hat{\sigma}^2}\left[1-\left(\frac{\hat{\sigma}}{1-\hat{\sigma}^2}\right)^2\right]^{-1} = \frac{\hat{E}}{1-\hat{\sigma}^2}\frac{(1-\hat{\sigma})^2}{(1-\hat{\sigma})^2-\hat{\sigma}^2} = \frac{\hat{E}}{1-2\hat{\sigma}}\frac{1-\hat{\sigma}}{1+\hat{\sigma}}.$$
$$(6.319d)$$

As for plane elasticity (subsection II.4.4.2), in the case of in-plane stresses in a thin plate not subject to transverse loads, the displacement vector satisfies a second-order differential equation (subsection 6.5.4).

6.5.4 Second-Order Differential Equation for the Displacement Vector

The balance of forces and stresses (II.4.38a, b) for a static plate is given by (6.320c, d):

$$\frac{d\vec{F}}{dV} = \frac{1}{h}\frac{d\vec{F}}{dA} = \frac{\vec{f}}{h}: \qquad \partial_x T_{xx} + \partial_y T_{xy} + \frac{f_x}{h} = 0 = \partial_x T_{xy} + \partial_y T_{yy} + \frac{f_y}{h}, \qquad (6.320a{-}d)$$

where $\vec{f}$ is the force (6.230b) per unit area dA, which divided by the thickness of the plate h becomes (6.320a) the force per unit volume dV. The displacement vector in the plane (6.321a) leads: (i) to the strains (II.4.12a–c) ≡ (6.304c) ≡ (6.321b–d):

$$\vec{u} = u_x\,\vec{e}_x + u_y\,\vec{e}_y: \quad S_{xx} = \partial_x\,u_x, \quad S_{yy} = \partial_y\,u_y, \quad 2S_{xy} = \partial_x\,u_y + \partial_y\,u_x; \qquad (6.321a\text{–}d)$$

and (ii) by (6.314a–c) to the stresses (6.322a–c):

$$\left\{ T_{xx}, T_{yy} \right\} = \frac{E}{1-\sigma^2}\left\{ \partial_x\,u_x + \sigma\partial_y\,u_y\,,\, \partial_y\,u_y + \sigma\partial_x\,u_x \right\},$$

$$T_{xy} = \frac{E}{2(1+\sigma)}\left(\partial_x\,u_y + \partial_y\,u_x \right). \tag{6.322a–c}$$

Substitution of (6.322a–c) in (6.320c, d) leads to two second-order differential equations (6.323a, b):

$$-\frac{2(1-\sigma^2)}{Eh}\,f_x = 2\partial_{xx}\,u_x + (1+\sigma)\partial_{xy}\,u_y + (1-\sigma)\partial_{yy}\,u_x$$

$$= (1-\sigma)\left(\partial_{xx}\,u_x + \partial_{yy}\,u_x \right) + (1+\sigma)\partial_x\left(\partial_x\,u_x + \partial_y\,u_y \right), \tag{6.323a}$$

$$-\frac{2(1-\sigma^2)}{Eh}\,f_x = 2\partial_{yy}\,u_y + (1+\sigma)\partial_{xy}\,u_x + (1-\sigma)\partial_{xx}\,u_y$$

$$= (1-\sigma)\left(\partial_{yy}\,u_y + \partial_{xx}\,u_y \right) + (1+\sigma)\partial_y\left(\partial_x\,u_x + \partial_y\,u_y \right), \tag{6.323b}$$

satisfied by the two components of the displacement vector.

Using the divergence (III.6.30) ≡ (6.324a), gradient (III.6.23b) ≡ (6.324b), and Laplacian (III.6.44) ≡ (6.324c) in two-dimensional Cartesian coordinates:

$$\nabla.\vec{u} \equiv \partial_x\,u_x + \partial_y\,u_y, \qquad \nabla \equiv \vec{e}_x\,\partial_x + \vec{e}_y\,\partial_y, \qquad \nabla^2 = \partial_{xx} + \partial_{yy}, \qquad (6.324a\text{–}c)$$

the pair of second-order differential equations (6.323a, b) for the components of the displacement can be written as a single vector equation (6.325a):

$$-\frac{2(1-\sigma^2)}{Eh}\,\vec{f} = (1-\sigma)\nabla^2\vec{u} + (1+\sigma)\nabla(\nabla.\vec{u}), \tag{6.325a}$$

$$= 2\nabla(\nabla.\vec{u}) - (1-\sigma)\nabla\wedge(\nabla\wedge\vec{u}), \tag{6.325b}$$

$$= 2\nabla^2\,\vec{u} + (1+\sigma)\nabla\wedge(\nabla\wedge\vec{u}), \tag{6.325c}$$

and the alternative forms (6.325b, c) use the identity (III.6.48a) ≡ (6.326b) involving the curl (6.326a) in two-dimensional Cartesian coordinates:

$$\nabla \wedge \vec{u} \equiv \vec{e}_z \left(\partial_x u_y - \partial_y u_x \right): \qquad \nabla^2 \vec{u} = \nabla \left(\nabla . \vec{u} \right) - \nabla \wedge \left(\nabla \wedge \vec{u} \right). \qquad (6.326a, b)$$

Thus *(6.325a–c) are (problem 234) three equivalent forms (6.324a–c; 6.326a, b) of the second-order differential equation satisfied by the displacement vector (6.321a) for an elastic plate of small thickness h subject only to in-plane surface forces (6.320a, b). The corresponding strains (stresses) are (6.321b–d; 6.327) [(6.322a–c)]:*

$$S_{zz} = -\frac{\sigma}{1+\sigma} \left(\partial_x u_x + \partial_y u_y \right) = -\frac{\sigma}{1+\sigma} \left(\nabla . \vec{u} \right), \qquad (6.327)$$

where (6.327) follows from (6.313c; 6.321b, c; 6.324a). In the absence of surface forces, the second-order differential equation for the displacement vector can be replaced (subsection 6.5.5) by a fourth-order differential equation for a scalar stress function.

6.5.5 Biharmonic Equation for the Stress Function

Like in plane elasticity (chapter II.4), in the case of constant surface forces (II.4.39a–d) ≡ (6.328b, c):

$$\vec{f} = \text{costant}: \qquad \partial_x T_{xx} + \partial_y T_{xy} = -f_x, \quad \partial_x T_{yx} + \partial_y T_{yy} = -f_y, \qquad (6.328a–c)$$

is satisfied (6.329b–d) by a three times differentiable (6.329a) **stress function:**

$$\Theta \in D^3 \left(| R^2 \right): \quad \left\{ T_{xx}, T_{yy}, T_{xy} \right\} = \left\{ \partial_{yy} \Theta, \partial_{xx} \Theta, -\partial_{xy} \Theta - y f_x - x f_y \right\}. \qquad (6.329a–d)$$

as can be checked from:

$$\partial_x T_{xx} + \partial_y T_{xy} = \partial_{xyy} \Theta - \partial_{yxy} \Theta - f_x = -f_x, \qquad (6.329f)$$

$$\partial_x T_{xy} + \partial_y T_{yy} = -\partial_{xxy} \Theta - f_y + \partial_{yxx} \Theta = -f_y. \qquad (6.329g)$$

The stress function (6.329b–d) satisfies (6.322a, b), a Poisson equation:

$$\nabla^2 \Theta \equiv \partial_{xx} \Theta + \partial_{yy} \Theta = T_{xx} + T_{yy} = \frac{E}{1-\sigma} \left(\partial_x u_x + \partial_y u_y \right)$$

$$= \frac{E}{1-\sigma} \left(\nabla . \vec{u} \right) \equiv \frac{E}{1-\sigma} D_2 = \frac{E}{1-2\sigma} D_3, \qquad (6.330a)$$

forced by the **area change** D_2 that is related to the volume change (6.304c) by (6.330b):

$$D_3 \equiv S_{xx} + S_{yy} + S_{zz} = \left(S_{xx} + S_{yy}\right)\left(1 - \frac{\sigma}{1-\sigma}\right) = \frac{1-2\sigma}{1-\sigma}D_2, \quad (6.330b)$$

where (6.313c) was used; this is similar to the stress function in plane elasticity that satisfies a **isotropic Poisson equation** (II.4.105a, c) $\equiv$ (6.331a):

$$\nabla^2 \Theta = \frac{\hat{E}}{\left(1+\hat{\sigma}\right)\left(1-2\hat{\sigma}\right)}\left(\nabla.\vec{u}\right) = \frac{\hat{E}}{\left(1+\hat{\sigma}\right)\left(1-2\hat{\sigma}\right)}D_2, \quad (6.331a)$$

with the transformation of coefficients from (6.330a) to (6.331a) given by:

$$\frac{E}{1-\sigma} = \frac{\hat{E}}{1-\hat{\sigma}^2}\left(1-\frac{\hat{\sigma}}{1-\hat{\sigma}}\right)^{-1} = \frac{\hat{E}}{1-\hat{\sigma}^2}\frac{1-\hat{\sigma}}{1-2\hat{\sigma}^2} = \frac{\hat{E}}{\left(1+\hat{\sigma}\right)\left(1-2\hat{\sigma}\right)}, \quad (6.331b)$$

where (6.318a, b) were used.

The divergence of (6.325a) is (6.332a), implying that *(problem 235) for a thin plate subject only to in-plane stresses: (i) the area (volume) change satisfies (6.330a) a Poisson equation (6.332b) [(6.332c)] forced by the divergence of the surface forces:*

$$\nabla.\vec{f} = -\frac{Eh}{1-\sigma^2}\nabla\left(\nabla.\vec{u}\right) = -\frac{Eh}{1-\sigma^2}\nabla D_2 = -\frac{Eh}{\left(1+\sigma\right)\left(1-2\sigma\right)}\nabla D_3; \quad (6.332a\text{–}c)$$

*(ii) in the case of surface forces with zero divergence (6.333a), the area (6.333b) [volume (6.333c)] changes satisfy a **Laplace equation**:*

$$\nabla.\vec{f} = 0: \quad \nabla^2 D_2 = 0 = \nabla^2 D_3; \quad f = const: \quad \Theta\left(x,y\right) \in D^4\left(|R^2\right): \quad \nabla^4\Theta = 0, \quad (6.333a\text{–}f)$$

*(iii) in the case of constant surface forces (6.328a) $\equiv$ (6.333d), a four-times differentiable (6.333e) stress function satisfies a biharmonic equation (6.333f), as follows sub*stituting (6.331a) in (6.333b). Thus, both plane elasticity and in-plane stresses involve (6.333b, c) [(6.333f)] harmonic (sections I.23.1–1.23.2 and III.9.3) [biharmonic (section II.4.6)] functions. The stress function is used next (subsection 6.5.6) to specify the stresses associated with drilling a circular hole in an infinite thin elastic plate.

6.5.6 Stresses Due to the Drilling of a Screw

The methods of solution of problems of in-plane loads in thin plates are similar to plane elasticity: (i) solution (section II.4.5) of the momentum equation (6.323a, b) ≡ (6.325a–c) for the displacement vector (6.321a) to specify the stresses (6.322a–c); (ii) use a biharmonic function (sections II.4.6–II.4.7) as stress function (6.333f) to specify the stresses (6.329b–d); or (iii) use of the complex potential (section II.4.8). In the cases with radial symmetry like circular holes (subsections 6.5.6–6.5.8) or plates (subsection 6.5.9), it is convenient to use the Laplacian in polar coordinates (I.11.28b) ≡ (III.6.45a, b) to write the biharmonic equation (6.333f) satisfied by the stress function:

$$
0 = \left(\frac{1}{r} \frac{\partial}{\partial r} r \frac{\partial}{\partial r} + \frac{1}{r^2} \frac{\partial^2}{\partial \phi^2} \right)^2 \Theta(r, \phi)
$$

$$
= \left\{ \frac{1}{r} \frac{\partial}{\partial r} r \frac{\partial}{\partial r} \frac{1}{r} \frac{\partial}{\partial r} r \frac{\partial}{\partial r} + \frac{1}{r^4} \frac{\partial^4}{\partial \phi^4} + \frac{1}{r} \frac{\partial}{\partial r} r \frac{\partial}{\partial r} \frac{1}{r^2} \frac{\partial^2}{\partial \phi^2} + \frac{1}{r^3} \frac{\partial}{\partial r} r \frac{\partial^3}{\partial r \partial \phi^2} \right\} \Theta(r, \phi),
$$

$$(6.334a)$$

whose solution specifies (II.4.57b–d) ≡ (6.334b–d):

$$
\{ T_{rr}, T_{\phi\phi}, T_{r\phi} \} = \{ r^{-1} \partial_r \Theta + r^{-2} \partial_{\phi\phi} \Theta, \partial_{rr} \Theta, -\partial_r \left(r^{-1} \partial_\phi \Theta \right) \}, \qquad (6.334b\text{–}d)
$$

the polar components of the stress tensor.

A simple solution of the biharmonic equation (6.334a) is (6.335a) for which there is (6.335b, c) only one in-plane non-zero stress (6.334b–d) and strain (6.306c–e):

$$
\Theta = C\phi, \qquad T_{r\phi} = \frac{C}{r^2} = \frac{E}{1+\sigma} S_{r\phi}; \qquad Q = r 2\pi r T_{r\phi} = 2\pi C, \qquad (6.335a\text{–}d)
$$

the tangential shear stress corresponds to a constant torque or moment (6.335d). Thus *the opening of a small circular hole or screw in a thin elastic infinite plate exerts (problem 236) a torque Q that (Figure 6.11) leads to a tangential shear stress (6.335c) ≡ (6.336b) and strain (6.336c) corresponding to the stress function (6.335a, d) ≡ (6.336a):*

$$
\Theta(\phi) = \frac{Q\phi}{2\pi} : \qquad T_{r\phi} = \frac{Q}{2\pi r^2}, \qquad S_{r\phi} = \frac{1+\sigma}{E} \frac{Q}{2\pi r^2}. \qquad (6.336a\text{–}c)
$$

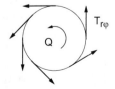

FIGURE 6.11
In contrast with a straight rod that can be subject [Figure 6.8a(b)] only to tractions (compression), the in-plane stresses on a flat plate include shear stresses, for example due to the torque applied to drill a hole.

In general, the biharmonic equation (6.333d) for the stress function is solved with boundary conditions. For example in the case of a circular hole causing a stress concentration (subsection 6.5.8) in an infinite thin elastic plate subject to in-plane stresses (subsection 6.5.7).

6.5.7 Plate with a Circular Hole Subject to In-Plane Stresses

Consider a stressed plane (Figure 6.12) with a constant stress field consisting of constant tractions or compressions along orthogonal axis and no shear at infinity:

$$\lim_{x,y\to\infty}\left\{T_{xx},T_{yy},T_{xy}\right\}=\lim_{x,y\to\infty}\left\{\partial_{yy}\Theta,\partial_{xx}\Theta,-\partial_{xy}\Theta\right\}=\left\{P,Q,0\right\};\qquad(6.337a\text{--}c)$$

a circular hole of radius (6.338a) and outer normal vector (6.338b) corresponds to the boundary conditions of zero radial (6.338c) and shear (6.338d) stresses (6.334b, d):

$$r\equiv\left|x^{2}+y^{2}\right|^{1/2}\equiv a,\ \bar{N}=-\bar{e}_{r}:\ \ 0=\left\{T_{rr},T_{r\phi}\right\}=\left\{r^{-1}\partial_{r}\Theta+r^{-2}\partial_{\phi\phi}\Theta,-\partial_{r}\left(r^{-1}\partial_{\phi}\Theta\right)\right\}.$$

$$(6.338a\text{--}d)$$

The constant normal stresses (6.339a, b) correspond (6.329b, c) to a quadratic stress function (6.339c):

$$\left\{T_{xx},T_{yy},T_{xy}\right\}=\left\{P,Q,0\right\}=constant:\qquad 2\Theta_{0}\left(x,y\right)=Py^{2}+Qx^{2}.\qquad(6.339a\text{--}c)$$

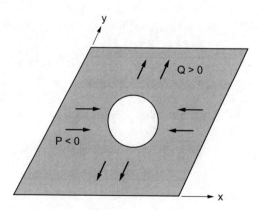

FIGURE 6.12
Changing the in-plane stresses in a flat plate from shear stresses (Figure 6.11) to normal stresses allows four combinations of compressions and tractions in orthogonal directions, for example for a stressed plate with a circular hole.

The effect of the circular hole is to create a stress concentration leading to a perturbation stress function $\Theta(x,y)$ that is of order less than (6.339c) at infinity. The perturbation stress function can be sought (section I.11.6) as the real (or imaginary) part (6.340b) of a complex differentiable or holomorphic function (6.340a):

$$f(z)\in D(|C), \quad \overline{\Theta}(x,y)=\mathrm{Re}\{f(x+iy)\}: \quad \nabla^2\overline{\Theta}=0 \;\rightarrow\; \nabla^4\overline{\Theta}=0.$$
$$(6.340a\text{-}d)$$

that satisfies a Laplace equation (6.340c) and hence also a biharmonic equation (6.340d).

The stress function is the sum of the asymptotic (6.337a–c) form (6.339a–c) plus a perturbation (6.340a–d); the choice of stress function (6.341a, b):

$$z\equiv x+iy: \qquad \Theta(x,y)=\frac{Py^2+Qx^2}{2}+\mathrm{Re}\left\{A\log z+\frac{B}{z^2}+C\frac{z^*}{z}\right\}, \qquad (6.341a, b)$$

can be justified *a priori* as follows: (i) the constant normal stresses at infinity (6.337a–c) lead to the quadratic terms (6.339a–c) first on the r.h.s. of (6.341b), and the remaining terms must be of lower order as $r\rightarrow\infty$, that is, correspond to stresses decaying at infinity; (ii–iii) the second (third) term on the r.h.s. of (6.341b) correspond [sections I.12.1–I.12.6 (I.12.7)] to a monopole (dipole) that represent the effect of the hole (6.338a, b) where two boundary conditions (6.338c, d) must be met; (iv) the first three terms correspond to an harmonic function, that is, a solution of the Laplace equations (6.342b), where general integral is (subsection II.2.4.3) of the form (II.2.152d) ≡ (6.342c):

$$f,g\in \mathcal{D}(|C): \quad \nabla^2\Theta=0 \;\Leftrightarrow\; \Theta(x,y)=\mathrm{Re}\{f(x+iy)+g(x-iy)\}, \qquad (6.342a\text{-}c)$$

involving two arbitrary functions (6.342a) analytic in the complex plane; (v) the last term is a biharmonic non-harmonic function, that is, satisfies a biharmonic equation (6.343b) but not a Laplace (6.340c) equation, because (subsection II.4.6.1) the general integral of the biharmonic equation (6.343b) is of the form (II.4.184c) ≡ (6.343c):

$$f,g,h,j\in (|C): \quad \nabla^4\Theta=0 \;\Leftrightarrow\; \Theta(x,y)=\mathrm{Re}\{f(z)+z^*h(z)+g(z^*)+zj(z^*)\},$$
$$(6.343a\text{-}c)$$

involving four arbitrary analytic functions (6.343a) in the complex plane; and (vi) the three real constants (A,B,C) are chosen so as to satisfy the biharmonic equation (6.333d) and boundary conditions (6.338a–d).

Using the Cartesian (x,y) and complex (6.341a) variables in polar coordinates:

$$\{x,y\}=r\{\cos\phi,\sin\phi\}, \quad z=x+iy=re^{i\phi}, \quad z^*=x-iy=re^{-i\phi},$$

(6.344a–d)

$$\log z=\log r+i\phi, \quad \mathrm{Re}\left(z^{-2}\right)=r^{-2}\cos(2\phi), \quad \mathrm{Re}\left(\frac{z^*}{z}\right)=\mathrm{Re}\left(e^{-i2\phi}\right)=\cos(2\phi),$$

(6.344e–h)

the stress function (6.341b) is written in polar coordinates:

$$\Theta(r,\phi)=\frac{r^2}{2}\left(P\sin^2\phi+Q\cos^2\phi\right)+A\log r+\left(\frac{B}{r^2}+C\right)\cos(2\phi)$$

(6.344i, j)

$$=\frac{r^2}{4}\left[P+Q-(P-Q)\cos(2\phi)\right]+A\log r+\left(\frac{B}{r^2}+C\right)\cos(2\phi).$$

Substitution of the stress function (6.344j) in the boundary conditions (6.338c, d) leads to (6.344a, b):

$$0=P+Q+\frac{2A}{a^2}+\left(P-Q-\frac{12B}{a^4}-\frac{8C}{a^2}\right)\cos(2\phi)=0, \quad (6.345a)$$

$$0=\left(P-Q+\frac{12B}{a^4}+\frac{4C}{a^2}\right)\sin(2\phi). \quad (6.345b)$$

Equating to zero the constant term and coefficient of $\cos(2\phi)$ in (6.345a) and the coefficient of $\sin(2\phi)$ in (6.345b) leads to a set of three equations (6.345c–e):

$$A=-\frac{P+Q}{2}a^2, 12B+8Ca^2=(P-Q)a^4=-12B-4Ca^2;$$

(6.345c–g)

$$\{C,B\}=(P-Q)\left\{\frac{a^2}{2},-\frac{a^4}{4}\right\},$$

solving (6.345d, e) for $\{B,C\}$ leads to (6.345f, g). Substitution of the three constants (6.345c, f, g) in (6.344j) determines the stress function:

$$4\Theta(r,\phi)=r^2\left[P+Q-(P-Q)\cos(2\phi)\right]-2(P+Q)a^2\log r$$

(6.346)

$$+(P-Q)a^2\left(2-\frac{a^2}{r^2}\right)\cos(2\phi),$$

that specifies the stress concentration near the circular hole (subsection 6.5.8).

6.5.8 Stress Concentration Near a Hole in a Plate

The stress function (6.346) specifies (6.334b–d) the (problem 237) polar components of the stresses at all points on the plate with a circular hole of radius a and orthogonal stresses (P,Q) at infinity:

$$2T_{rr}(r,\phi) = (P+Q)\left(1-\frac{a^2}{r^2}\right) + (P-Q)\left(1-4\frac{a^2}{r^2}+3\frac{a^4}{r^4}\right)\cos(2\phi), \qquad (6.347a)$$

$$2\,T_{\phi\phi}(r,\phi) = (P+Q)\left(1+\frac{a^2}{r^2}\right) - (P-Q)\left(1+3\frac{a^4}{r^4}\right)\cos(2\phi), \qquad (6.347b)$$

$$2T_{r\phi}(r,\phi) = -(P-Q)\left(1+2\frac{a^2}{r^2}-3\frac{a^4}{r^2}\right)\sin(2\phi). \qquad (6.347c)$$

If the stresses are equal at infinity (6.348a) there are no shear stresses anywhere on the plate (6.348b–d):

$$P=Q: \quad \{T_{rr},T_{r\phi},T_{\phi\phi}\} = P\left\{1-\frac{a^2}{r^2},1+\frac{a^2}{r^2},0\right\}, \quad T_{rr}+T_{\phi\phi}=2P, \qquad (6.348a\text{–}e)$$

and the sum of the stresses is a constant (6.348e). On the boundary of the circular hole only tangential stresses exist (6.349a–c) in agreement with the boundary conditions (6.338c, d):

$$T_{rr}(a,\phi)=0=T_{r\phi}(a,\phi): \quad T_{\phi\phi}(a,\phi)=P+Q-2(P-Q)\cos(2\phi). \qquad (6.349a\text{–}c)$$

Designating P as the larger of the two stresses at infinity (6.350a), they may be both tractions Q > 0 or both compressions P < 0 or one traction and one compression P > 0 > Q; in all cases the tangential stresses at the hole (6.349c):

$$P \geq Q: \quad \left[T_{\phi\phi}(a,\phi)\right]_{\max} = T_{\phi\phi}(a,\pm\pi/2) = 3P-Q \geq P+Q$$

$$= T_{\phi\phi}(a,\pm\pi/4) \geq 3Q-P = T_{\phi\phi}(a,0) = T_{\phi\phi}(a,\pi) \quad (6.350a\text{–}d)$$

$$= \left[T_{\phi\phi}(a,\phi)\right]_{\min},$$

are maximum (6.350b) [minimum (6.350d)] in orthogonal directions, with an intermediate value (6.350c) in the diagonal directions. The complementary domain of a plane with a circular hole (Figure 6.11) is a circular thin plate or disk (Figure 6.12) that is considered next (subsection 6.5.9).

6.5.9 Disk under Axial Compression

The preceding results (subsections 6.5.6–6.5.8) also apply in two-dimensional elasticity (chapter II.4) with the transformation (6.318a, b). Conversely, *the results in two-dimensional elasticity* $\left(\hat{\sigma}, \hat{E}\right)$ *apply to thin (section 6.5) plates* $\left(\sigma, E\right)$ *using the inverse (6.351a, b) of (6.318a, b):*

$$\hat{\sigma} = \frac{\sigma}{1+\sigma} \, , \qquad \hat{E} = E\frac{1+2\sigma}{\left(1+\sigma\right)^2} . \qquad (6.351a, b)$$

where: (i) inversion of (6.318a) proves (6.351a); and (ii) substitution of (6.318a) in (6.318b) leads to:

$$\hat{E} = E\left(1-\hat{\sigma}^2\right) = E\left[1-\left(\frac{\sigma}{1+\sigma}\right)^2\right] = E\frac{1+2\sigma}{\left(1+\sigma\right)^2} \, , \qquad (6.351c)$$

that coincides with (6.351b) ≡ (6.351c). An example is the analogy between an elastic cylinder (section II.4.5) and a disk (subsection 6.5.9). For a disk under (Figure 6.13) uniform compression p at the radius a in (6.352a) in the absence of forces (6.352b), the displacement is radial and depends on the radius only (6.352c):

$$T_{rr}\left(a, \phi\right) = -p, \vec{f} = 0: \qquad \vec{u} = \vec{e}_r u(r), \quad \nabla \wedge \vec{u} = 0, \nabla\left(\nabla.\vec{u}\right) = 0,$$
$$2C_1 = \nabla.\vec{u} = r^{-1}\left(ru\right)' = D_2, \qquad (6.352a–f)$$

leading (6.325b) by (6.352d) to (6.352e) and hence constant (6.352f) area change (6.352g). In the integral (6.353b) of (6.352g):

$$u(0) < \infty: \qquad ru = C_1 r^2 + C_2 , \qquad C_2 = 0, \qquad u(r) = C_1 r , \qquad (6.353a–d)$$

one constant is zero (6.353c) in order for the displacement to be finite at the center (6.353a), implying that the displacement is proportional to the

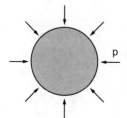

FIGURE 6.13
The case of a circular plate under radial inward pressure differs from the hole in the stressed plate (Figure 6.12) in the location of the material and direction of the normal stresses.

radius (6.353d). In linear plane elasticity, the polar components of the strain tensor and displacement vector are related by (II.4.27a, b;II.4.28) ≡ (6.354a–c):

$$S_{rr} = \partial_r u_r, \quad S_{\phi\phi} = r^{-1}\left(u_r + \partial_\phi u_\phi\right), \quad 2S_{r\phi} = \partial_r u_\phi + r^{-1}\left(\partial_\phi u_r - u_\phi\right). \qquad (6.354a\text{–}c)$$

Substituting (6.353d) in (6.354a–c), it follows that there are no shear strains (6.355a–c) and only normal in-plane (6.355d, e) and (6.313c) out-of-plane (6.355f) strains:

$$S_{r\phi} = S_{rz} = S_{\phi z} = 0, \qquad S_{rr} = C_1 = S_{\phi\phi}, \qquad S_{zz} = -\frac{2C_1\sigma}{1-\sigma}. \qquad (6.355a\text{–}f)$$

From (6.306c–e; 6.307a–c) it follows that there are no shear stresses (6.356a–c) and the normal stresses lie in the plane of the disk (6.356d–f):

$$T_{r\phi} = T_{rz} = T_{\phi z} = 0 = T_{zz}, \qquad T_{rr} = \frac{C_1 E}{1-\sigma} = T_{\phi\phi}. \qquad (6.356a\text{–}f)$$

The remaining constant of integration is determined (6.356e, f) ≡ (6.357a, b) by the pressure (6.357a, b), leading to (6.357e) and to radial displacement vector (6.353d) as linear function (6.357d) of the radius:

$$T_{rr} = -p = T_{\phi\phi}, \qquad C_1 = -\frac{1-\sigma}{E}p, \qquad \bar{u} = -\bar{e}_r\frac{1-\sigma}{E}pr. \qquad (6.357a\text{–}d)$$

The plane stresses (6.357a, b; 6.356a) ≡ (6.358a–c) correspond (6.334b–d) to the stress function (6.358d) that depends only on the radius:

$$\{T_{\phi\phi}, T_{r\phi}, T_{r\phi}\} = \{-p, -p, 0\}: \qquad \Theta = -\frac{p}{2}r^2, \qquad (6.358a\text{–}d)$$

and (6.355d–f) to (6.357c) to the non-zero strains (6.359a–c):

$$S_{rr} = S_{\phi\phi} = -\frac{1-\sigma}{E}p, \qquad S_{zz} = \frac{2\sigma}{E}p. \qquad (6.359a\text{–}c)$$

Thus, *a solid disk of radius a under an axial compression p applied (Figure 6.13) uniformly around its edge (6.352a), has (problem 238): (i) uniform radial (6.358a) and tangential (6.358b) compressions and no normal or shear stresses (6.358c; 6.356a–d); (ii) uniform radial (6.359a) and tangential (6.359b) contractions, normal (6.359c) extension, and no shear strains (6.355a–c); (iii) inward radial displacement*

*(6.357d) proportional to the radius; and (iv) stress function (6.358d) that is propor-
tional to the square of the radius and independent of the properties of the material.
The inward pressure at the rim of the circular disk of radius a reduces the radius to
(6.360a):*

$$\bar{a} = a + u(a) = a\left(1 - \frac{1-\sigma}{E}p\right), \qquad \bar{h} = h(1 + S_{zz}) = h\left(1 + \frac{2\sigma}{E}p\right), \qquad \text{(6.360a, b)}$$

and increases the thickness to (6.360b). These results can be extended to a circular hole (hollow disk), as in plane elasticity (chapter II.4), respectively subsection [(II.5.5.2 (II.4.5.3)] for a cylindrical cavity (hollow cylinder). The case of a
disk (cylinder) with [subsection(s) II.4.5.4 (II.4.5.5–II.4.5.7)] thin walls (multiple layers) is analogous to steady heat conduction (sections I.32.6–I.32.8). The
analogy extends to the deformation of a rotating disk (cylinder (subsections
II.4.5.8–II.4.5.9) due to centrifugal forces.

6.6 Deflection of a Membrane under Anisotropic Tension

Proceeding from longitudinal (in-plane) deformation of a one(two)-
dimensional elastic body, namely [section 6.4 (6.5)] a rod (plate) to transversal deflection, the simplest case that is without stiffness is the string
[chapter II.2) [membrane (section II.6.1–II.6.2). The linear (non-linear); that
is, small (large) deflection of a membrane can be considered for anisotropic stresses (subsections 6.6.1–6.6.2) including the particular case of isotropic stresses (sections II.6.1–II.6.2). The strain tensor is used to specify the
elastic energy (subsection 6.6.1) leading to the non-linear (linear) equations
specifying the large (small) deflection of a membrane by transverse loads
when subject to anisotropic stresses (subsections 6.6.1–6.6.2), including
the particular case of isotropic stresses (sections II.6.1–II.6.2). The linear
case can be reduced to a Poisson equation, thus generalizing the two-
dimensional Green function from the logarithmic potential of the Laplace
operator in the isotropic case, to the more general case of an anisotropic
second-order homogeneous partial differential operator, also linear and
with constant coefficients (subsections 6.6.3–6.6.4). The anisotropic membrane equation can be considered in a bounded (unbounded) medium
with (without) boundary conditions [subsection(s) 6.6.6 (6.6.5 and 6.6.7)].
The linear deflection of an elliptic membrane under anisotropic stresses
(subsection 6.6.6) includes as a particular case the linear deflection of a
circular membrane under isotropic stresses; the latter has also considered
in the non-linear case (sections II.6.1–II.6.2).

6.6.1 Non-Linear Strain Tensor and Elastic Energy of a Membrane

The (x_1, x_2)-plane is taken to coincide with the undeflected membrane (Figure 6.14a), leading to the arc length (6.361b) that is increased to (6.361c) when the membrane is deflected (Figure 6.14b) to the position (6.361a):

$$z = \zeta(x_1, x_2): \qquad (ds)^2 = (dx_1)^2 + (dx_2)^2, \quad (dL)^2 = (ds)^2 + (d\zeta)^2. \qquad (6.361a\text{–}c)$$

The increase in arc length due to the deflection of the membrane is given (6.362a–c) by the difference between (6.361c) and (6.361b):

$$(dL)^2 - (ds)^2 = (d\zeta)^2 = \left[(\partial_1 \zeta)\, dx_1 + (\partial_2 \zeta)\, dx_2 \right]^2$$
$$= (\partial_1 \zeta)^2 (dx_1)^2 + (\partial_2 \zeta)^2 (dx_2)^2 + 2(\partial_1 \zeta)(\partial_2 \zeta)\, dx_1\, dx_2, \qquad (6.362a\text{–}c)$$

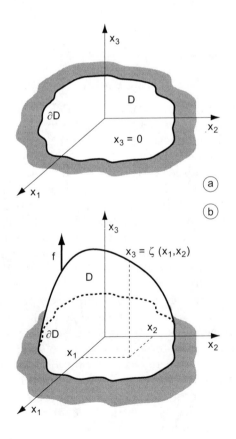

FIGURE 6.14

The deflection of an elastic membrane with flat boundary curve (a) requires the presence of transverse loads (b).

and specifies the **strain tensor** in (6.363c) where a repeated index implies summation (6.363b) over its range of values (6.363a) in the plane:

$$\alpha, \beta = 1, 2: \quad (dL)^2 - (ds)^2 = \sum_{\alpha,\beta=1}^{2} (\partial_\alpha \zeta)(\partial_\beta \zeta) \, dx_\alpha dx_\beta \equiv 2 S_{\alpha\beta} dx^\alpha dx^\beta. \quad (6.363a-c)$$

Thus, *(problem 239) the deflection (Figure 6.14b) of a flat membrane (Figure 6.14a) to a position (6.361a) increases the arc length from (6.361b) to (6.361c), and the difference (6.362a–c) ≡ (6.363a–c) specifies the exact strain tensor (6.364a) consisting of: (i) the extensions $S_{\alpha\alpha} > 0$ or contractions $S_{\alpha\alpha} < 0$ along the x_α-axis; (ii) the distortion of a segment along the x_α-axis into the positive $S_{\alpha\beta} > 0$ (negative $S_{\alpha\beta} < 0$) direction along the x_β-axis:*

$$S_{\alpha\beta} \equiv \frac{1}{2}(\partial_\alpha \zeta)(\partial_\beta \zeta) \equiv S_{\beta\alpha}; \quad 2E_c = S_{\alpha\beta} T_{\alpha\beta} = T_{\alpha\beta}(\partial_\alpha \zeta)(\partial_\beta \zeta), \quad T_{\alpha\beta} = T_{\beta\alpha},$$

$$(6.364a-e)$$

the elastic energy by (II.4.86a, b) ≡ (6.364c, d) is the double contracted product of the strain $S_{\alpha\beta}$ and stress $T_{\alpha\beta}$ tensors. The stress tensor is symmetric (6.364e) because the strain tensor (6.364a) is also symmetric (6.364b). The last statement can be proved from the quadratic form (6.364c) ≡ (6.365a) for the elastic energy:

$$2E_e = T_{\alpha\beta} S_{\alpha\beta} = T_{\beta\alpha} S_{\beta\alpha} = T_{\beta\alpha} S_{\alpha\beta} \quad \Rightarrow \quad T_{\beta\alpha} = T_{\alpha\beta}, \quad (6.365a-d)$$

where: (i) since the indices (6.363a) represent a summation (6.363b) their designations can be interchanged $(\alpha, \beta) \to (\beta, \alpha)$, leading from (6.365a) to (6.365b); (ii) the definition (6.363a–c) ≡ (6.364a) of strain tensor shows that it is symmetric (6.364b), leading from (6.365b) to (6.365c); and (iii) the identity (6.365a) ≡ (6.365c) for arbitrary strain tensor (6.364a) shows that the stress tensor is symmetric (6.365d). From the elastic energy (6.364c) can be derived the equation of non-linear deflection of a membrane and the boundary condition (subsection 6.6.2): (i) as for the non-linear deflection of strings (section III.2.2) and bars (section III.4.2); and (ii) extending the results for isotropic stresses (section II.6.1) to anisotropic stresses (subsection 6.6.2).

6.6.2 Non-Linear Deflection of a Membrane under Anisotropic Stresses

The principle of virtual work (subsections II.6.1.2, III.2.2.2, and III.4.2.4) states that the work of the downward external applied forces f per unit area in a transverse deflection $\delta\zeta$ (6.366a):

$$\int_D f \, \delta\zeta \, dA = \delta W = \delta \bar{E}_c \equiv \int_D \delta E_c \, dA = \int_D T_{\alpha\beta} (\partial_\alpha \zeta) [\partial_\beta (\delta\zeta)] dA, \quad (6.366a-e)$$

equals the variation of the total elastic energy (6.366c); that is, the elastic energy density (6.364d) integrated (6.366e) over the area (6.366d) of the undeflected membrane. The integral balance equation (6.366e) leads to a differential balance equation by integration by parts of the last term leading to:

$$T_{\alpha\beta}\left(\partial_\alpha \zeta\right)\left[\partial_\beta\left(\delta\zeta\right)\right] = \partial_\beta\left[T_{\alpha\beta}\left(\partial_\alpha \zeta\right)\delta\zeta\right] - \delta\zeta\,\partial_\beta\left[T_{\alpha\beta}\left(\partial_\alpha \zeta\right)\right]. \qquad (6.367a)$$

Substituting (6.367a) in (6.366a), yields (6.367b):

$$\int_D \left\{\partial_\beta\left[T_{\alpha\beta}\left(\partial_\alpha\zeta\right)\right] + f\right\}d\zeta\,dA = \int_D \partial_\beta\left[T_{\alpha\beta}\left(\partial_\alpha\zeta\right)\delta\zeta\right]dA$$

$$ (6.367b, c) $$

$$= \int_{\partial D} T_{\alpha\beta}\left(\partial_\alpha \zeta\right)\delta\zeta\,n_\beta\,ds = 0,$$

where the divergence theorem (III.5.163a, c) ≡ (III.9.401a–d) was used to transform the last term into an integral over the boundary (6.367c) with unit outer normal n_β and arc length ds. The surface and volume integrals can be equal for arbitrary transverse deflection $\delta\zeta$ only if (6.367c) both sides vanish.

The vanishing of the integrand on the r.h.s. of (6.367b) is the condition (6.368b) stating that the projection of the **in-plane stress vector** (6.368a) on the gradient of the transverse displacement is zero:

$$T_\beta = T_{\alpha\beta}\,n_\beta: \qquad\qquad 0 = T_{\alpha\beta}\left(\partial_\alpha\zeta\right)n_\beta = T_\beta\,\partial_\beta\zeta = \vec{T}.\nabla\zeta; \qquad (6.368a, b)$$

the boundary condition (6.369b) is met in three cases:

$$0 = T_\alpha\,\partial_\alpha\zeta = \vec{T}.\nabla\zeta \quad\left\{\begin{array}{lll} \vec{T} \perp \nabla\zeta & \text{tangential stress,} & (6.368c)\\[4pt] \zeta = \text{const} & \text{fixed,} & (6.368d)\\[4pt] \vec{T} = 0 & \text{free,} & (6.368e) \end{array}\right.$$

namely: (i) the stress vector is orthogonal to the displacement (6.368c); (ii) the displacement is zero (6.368d), that is, the membrane is fixed at the boundary; and (iii) the in-plane stress vector is zero (6.368e), that is, the boundary is free. The boundary condition (6.368d) that the membrane is fixed is used most often. The vanishing of the integrand on the l.h.s. of (6.367b) specifies the balance equation (6.369a, b) for the non-linear deflection of the membrane under a transverse force per unit area:

$$-f = \partial_\alpha\left(T_{\alpha\beta}\,\partial_\beta\zeta\right) = T_{\alpha\beta}\,\partial_{\alpha\beta}\zeta + \left(\partial_\beta\zeta\right)\partial_\alpha\left(T_{\alpha\beta}\right). \qquad (6.369a, b)$$

The non-linearity arises in (6.369b) if the stresses (6.364e) depend non-linearly on the strains (6.364a). In the case of constant stresses (6.370a), the deflection of the membrane is specified by an **anisotropic Poisson equation** (6.370b):

$$T_{\alpha\beta} = \text{const:} \qquad -f(x_\gamma) = T_{\alpha\beta}\,\partial_{\alpha\beta}\,\zeta \equiv T_{\alpha\beta}\,\partial_\alpha\,\partial_\beta\,\zeta \equiv T_{\alpha\beta}\,\frac{\partial^2\zeta}{\partial x_\alpha\,\partial x_\beta}, \qquad (6.370a,\,b)$$

forced by minus the external applied transverse per unit area.

Thus, *the non-linear deflection of a membrane (problem 240) is specified by the strain tensor (6.364a, b) and elastic energy (6.364c, d) under anisotropic in-plane stresses (6.364e), leading to the balance equation (6.369a, b) where f is the **shear stress** that is the external applied transverse force per unit area. If the stresses applied at the boundary are much larger than the internal stresses due to deflection, the latter may be taken as constant (II.6.13c) ≡ (6.370a), leading to the linear balance equation (6.370b). If the stresses are isotropic (6.371a) where δ_{αβ} is the identity matrix (6.305a–c) in two dimensions:*

$$T_{\alpha\beta} = T\,\delta_{\alpha\beta}: \quad T_{12} = 0, \quad T_{11} = T = T_{22}, \quad -\frac{f}{T} = \delta_{\alpha\beta}\,\frac{\partial^2\zeta}{\partial x_\alpha\,\partial x_\beta} = \frac{\partial^2\zeta}{\partial x_\alpha\,\partial x_\alpha} = \nabla^2\zeta,$$

$$(6.371a\text{–}e)$$

the balance equation (6.370b) reduces to the Poisson equation (II.6.13c) ≡ (6.371e) for the transverse displacement, forced by minus the ratio f/T of the transverse shear stress to the isotropic stress; note that isotropic stresses (6.371a) mean no shear stress (6.371b) and equal normal stresses (6.371c, d). The boundary condition (6.368b) of zero projection of the in-plane stress vector (6.368a) on the gradient of the transverse displacement can be met by (6.368a–e), including zero displacement (6.368d) for a membrane fixed at the boundary. Since the elastic membrane has no bending stiffness, the angle at the boundary is determined by the deflection in the interior, as for an elastic string (chapter III.2); thus, the angle at the boundary cannot be specified *a priori* as in the case of bending of a bar (chapter III.4) [plate (sections 6.7–6.9)] that have bending stiffness. The anisotropic Poisson equation (6.370b) involves the anisotropic Laplace operator; that is, (i) diagonalized (subsection 6.6.3) and (ii) re-scaled (subsection 6.6.4), leading to the isotropic Poisson equation. The same transformations (i) and (ii) in reverse extend the Green function from the isotropic to the anisotropic Laplace operator.

6.6.3 Diagonalization of the Anisotropic Laplace Operator

In the case (6.371a) of isotropic stresses, the two-dimensional Green's function for the Laplace operator (6.371b) is the deflection due to a concentrated force equal to minus the stress (6.372a) where δ is the **Dirac delta function** (chapters IIII.1,III.3,III.5):

$$\nabla^2 g(\bar{x}) = \delta(\bar{x}), \qquad\qquad 2\pi g(\bar{x}) = \log|\bar{x}|, \qquad (6.372\text{a, b})$$

and corresponds (chapter III.9) to the **logarithmic potential** (III.9.42d) $\equiv$ (6.372b). The Green's function for the **anisotropic Laplace operator** (6.370b) will be obtained next by reducing it to the isotropic Laplace operator (6.372b) in two steps: (i) a rotation to eliminate (subsection 6.6.3) the cross terms $\partial_{12} \equiv \partial x_1 \, \partial x_2$; and (ii) changes of scale along each axis (subsection 6.6.4) to make the coefficients of $(\partial_{11}, \partial_{22})$ both unity. This process (i) and (ii) applies to any second-order linear partial differential operator with constant coefficients that is homogeneous of degree two; that is, a linear combination of second-order partial derivatives. A rotation of axis by an angle ϕ in the positive, or counter-clockwise, direction (Figure 6.15a) corresponds to the coordinate transformation from (x,y) to (x_1, x_2) specified by (I.16.56a, b) $\equiv$ (III.6.51d) $\equiv$ (6.373a, b):

$$x_1 + ix_2 = (x + iy)e^{-i\phi}: \quad x + iy = (x_1 + ix_2)e^{i\phi} = (x_1 + ix_2)(\cos\phi + i\sin\phi)$$

$$= (x_1 \cos\phi - x_2 \sin\phi) + i(x_1 \sin\phi + x_2 \cos\phi),$$

$$(6.373\text{a, b})$$

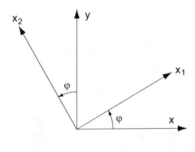

(a)

(b)

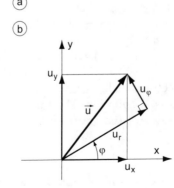

FIGURE 6.15

A plane rotation (a) corresponds to the transformation (b) between the Cartesian and polar components of a vector.

leading to (6.373b) ≡ (6.373c, d):

$$x = x_1 \cos\phi - x_2 \sin\phi, \qquad y = x_1 \sin\phi + x_2 \cos\phi, \qquad \text{(6.373c, d)}$$

that implies the partial derivatives:

$$\partial_1 \equiv \frac{\partial}{\partial x_1} = \frac{\partial x}{\partial x_1}\frac{\partial}{\partial x} + \frac{\partial y}{\partial x_1}\frac{\partial}{\partial y} = \cos\phi\frac{\partial}{\partial x} + \sin\phi\frac{\partial}{\partial y} \equiv \cos\phi\,\partial_x + \sin\phi\,\partial_y\,,$$

$$\text{(6.374a)}$$

$$\partial_2 \equiv \frac{\partial}{\partial x_2} = \frac{\partial x}{\partial x_2}\frac{\partial}{\partial x} + \frac{\partial y}{\partial x_2}\frac{\partial}{\partial y} = -\sin\phi\frac{\partial}{\partial x} + \cos\phi\frac{\partial}{\partial y} = -\sin\phi\,\partial_x + \cos\phi\,\partial_y.$$

$$\text{(6.374b)}$$

Substituting (6.374a, b) in the anisotropic Laplace operator (6.371b) yields:

$$
\begin{aligned}
-f &= T_{11}\,\partial_{11}\,\zeta + T_{22}\,\partial_{22}\,\zeta + 2T_{12}\left(\partial_1\,\zeta\right)\left(\partial_2\,\zeta\right) \\
&= T_{11}\left(\cos\phi\,\partial_x + \sin\phi\,\partial_y\right)^2\zeta \\
&\quad + T_{22}\left(-\sin\phi\,\partial_x + \cos\phi\,\partial_y\right)^2\zeta \\
&\quad + 2T_{12}\left(\cos\phi\,\partial_x + \sin\phi\,\partial_y\right)\left(-\sin\phi\,\partial_x + \cos\phi\,\partial_y\right)\zeta,
\end{aligned}
$$

$$\text{(6.375)}$$

where ϕ is constant and thus unaffected by the differentiations, leading to:

$$-f = T_{xx}\left(\phi\right)\partial_{xx}\zeta + T_{yy}\left(\phi\right)\partial_{yy}\zeta + 2T_{xy}\left(\phi\right)\partial_{xy}\zeta, \qquad \text{(6.376)}$$

involving as coefficients the stress tensor in Cartesian axis rotated by the angle ϕ:

$$T_{xx}\left(\phi\right) = T_{11}\cos^2\phi + T_{22}\sin^2\phi - T_{12}\sin\left(2\phi\right), \qquad \text{(6.377a)}$$

$$T_{yy}\left(\phi\right) = T_{11}\sin^2\phi + T_{22}\cos^2\phi + T_{12}\sin\left(2\phi\right), \qquad \text{(6.377b)}$$

$$T_{xy}\left(\phi\right) = \left(T_{11} - T_{22}\right)\sin\left(2\phi\right) + T_{12}\cos\left(2\phi\right). \qquad \text{(6.377c)}$$

The transformation of the stress tensor (6.377a–c) by (problem 241) rotation by an angle ϕ in the positive or counterclockwise direction (6.373a–d) corresponds (6.378a):

$$\left\{T_{11}, T_{22}, T_{12}\right\} \;\;\rightarrow\;\; \left\{T_{xx}, T_{yy}, T_{xy}\right\} \;\leftarrow\; \left\{T_{rr}, T_{\phi\phi}, T_{r\phi}\right\}, \qquad \text{(6.378a, b)}$$

to the transformation (6.378b) from polar to Cartesian components (6.377a–c) ≡ (II.4.253a–c) that is also a rotation by φ in the positive direction; this rotation can also be applied to the components of a vector (Figure 6.15b). The same result (6.377a–c) [≡(II.4.254a–c)] has be proved via quadratic forms [subsection 6.6.3 (II.4.7.1)]; namely, the Cartesian (6.374a, b) [polar (II.4.251a)] coordinate transformation [Figure 6.15a(b)] applied to the anisotropic Laplace operator (6.375) [invariant stress bilinear form (II.4.252)]. The rotation angle φ can be chosen to cancel the shear stress $\bar{T}_{12}$ in (6.377c), diagonalizing the anisotropic Laplace operator. The normal stresses (6.377a, b) can be reduced to unity by re-scaling the coordinates along the axis (subsection 6.6.4), leading to the isotropic Laplace operator.

6.6.4 Green's Function for the Anisotropic Laplace Operator

The choice of rotation angle (6.379b) makes the cross-term (6.377c) ≡ (6.379a) vanish in (6.375) ≡ (6.379c):

$$T_{xy}\left(\bar{\phi}\right)=0:\quad \cot\left(2\bar{\phi}\right)=\frac{T_{22}-T_{11}}{T_{12}},\quad -f=T_{xx}\left(\bar{\phi}\right)\partial_{xx}\zeta+T_{yy}\left(\bar{\zeta}\right)\partial_{yy}\zeta. \quad (6.379a–c)$$

The coefficients in (6.379c) are the **principal stresses** in a reference frame rotated by an angle $\bar{\phi}$ in (6.379b) such that (Figure 6.16) there are no shears (6.379a). In (6.379b) it is assumed that $T_{12}\neq 0$; if $T_{12}=0$ then the original axis $\left(x_1,x_2\right)$ would be already **principal axis** and no rotation would be necessary.

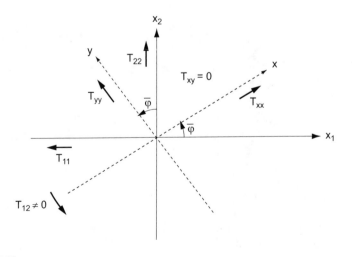

FIGURE 6.16
A plane stress state with normal stresses and shear stresses leads to the elimination of shear stresses by rotation (Figure 6.15) to the principal stress axis.

The principal stresses determine the **change of scale** along each axis (6.380a, b) that transforms (6.379c) to the Laplace operator (6.380c):

$$X \equiv x \left| T_{xx}(\bar{\phi}) \right|^{-1/2}, \quad Y \equiv y \left| T_{yy}(\bar{\phi}) \right|^{-1/2} : \qquad -f = \frac{\partial^2 \zeta}{\partial X^2} + \frac{\partial^2 \zeta}{\partial Y^2}. \qquad (6.380\text{a–c})$$

The same transformation (6.380a, b) applied to the Green function for the Laplace operator (6.372b) $\equiv$ (6.381a, b):

$$4\pi G(x_1, x_2) = 4\pi g(X,Y) = \log(X^2 + Y^2) = \log\left[\frac{x^2}{\left| T_{xx}(\bar{\phi}) \right|} + \frac{y^2}{\left| T_{yy}(\bar{\phi}) \right|} \right],$$

$$(6.381\text{a–c})$$

leads (problem 242) to the Green function (6.381c; 6.373c, d) $\equiv$ (6.382b) for the aniso-tropic Laplace operator (6.372a) $\equiv$ (6.382a):

$$\left\{ T_{11} \frac{\partial^2}{\partial x_1\, \partial x_1} + T_{22} \frac{\partial^2}{\partial x_2\, \partial x_2} + 2 T_{12} \frac{\partial^2}{\partial x_1\, \partial x_2} \right\} G(x_1, x_2) = \delta(x_1)\delta(x_2): \qquad (6.382\text{a})$$

$$2\pi G(x_1, x_2) = \log\left[\frac{\left(x_1 \cos\bar{\phi} - x_2 \sin\bar{\phi} \right)^2}{\left| T_{xx}(\bar{\phi}) \right|} + \frac{\left(x_1 \sin\bar{\phi} + x_2 \cos\bar{\phi} \right)^2}{\left| T_{yy}(\bar{\phi}) \right|} \right], \qquad (6.382\text{b})$$

*involving: (i) a rotation (6.373a–d) by (Figure 6.15a) an angle (6.379b) from the plane stress system with shear stress $T_{12} \neq 0$ to the **reference frame of principal stresses** (Figure 6.16) where there is no shear stress (6.379a); and (ii) the use of (6.377a, b), which leads to the principal stresses (6.347a, b) for re-scaling:*

$$\left\{ T_{xx}(\bar{\phi}), T_{yy}(\bar{\phi}) \right\} = T_{11}\left\{ \cos^2\bar{\phi}, \sin^2\bar{\phi} \right\} + T_{22}\left\{ \sin^2\bar{\phi}, \cos^2\bar{\phi} \right\} + T_{12} \sin(2\bar{\phi})\left\{ -1, +1 \right\}.$$

$$(6.383\text{a, b})$$

*If there are no shear strains in the original reference frame (6.384a), no rotation is needed (6.384b), simplifying the Green function to (6.384d) corresponding to the **diagonal anisotropic Laplace operator** (6.384c):*

$$T_{12} = 0; \bar{\phi} = 0: \qquad \left\{ T_{11}\, \partial_{11} + T_{22}\, \partial_{22} \right\} G\{x_1, x_2\} = \delta(x_1)\delta(x_2),$$

$$4\pi G(x_1, x_2) = \log\left(\frac{x_1^2}{T_{11}} + \frac{x_2^2}{T_{22}} \right). \qquad (6.384\text{a–d})$$

The case of isotropic stresses (6.371b, c) equal to unity T = 1 leads back to (6.372a, b). A constant λ with the dimensions of length squared divided by stress, or inverse force may be used in (6.380a, b) to make the arguments of the logarithms in (6.381c; 6.382b; 6.384d) dimensionless. A similar transformation would apply to Green's functions in dimensions higher than two (chapter III.9). The linear deflection of an elastic membrane under uniform anisotropic stresses is considered next for an infinite (finite elliptic) plane shape [subsection 6.6.5 (6.6.6)].

6.6.5 Characteristics as the Lines of Constant Deflection

Considering an unbounded membrane with no transverse forces (6.385a), the shape of the membrane is specified (6.371b) by the anisotropic Laplace operator (6.385b):

$$f_z = 0: \qquad T_{xx}\frac{\partial^2\zeta}{\partial x^2} + T_{yy}\frac{\partial^2\zeta}{\partial y} + 2T_{xy}\frac{\partial^2\zeta}{\partial x\,\partial y} = 0. \qquad \text{(6.385a, b)}$$

Since (6.385b) is a linear partial differential equation with (i) all derivatives of the same order two, (ii) constant coefficients, and (iii) without forcing, a solution is an arbitrary (6.386b) twice differentiable (6.386a) function of a linear combination (6.386c) of the independent variables:

$$f\in D^2(|R), \quad \zeta(x,y)=f(\eta), \quad \eta=x+ay; \quad \{\partial_x\zeta,\partial_y\zeta\}=\frac{df}{d\eta}\{1,a\},$$
$$\text{(6.386a–e)}$$

implying (6.386d, e). Substituting (6.386d, e) in (6.385b) leads to (6.386f):

$$0=\frac{d^2f}{d\eta^2}\left(T_{xx}+2aT_{xy}+a_2T_{yy}\right): \qquad f=A\eta+B, \qquad \text{(6.386f, g)}$$

that is satisfied by: (i) either the function *f* being linear (6.386g); or (ii) allowing an arbitrary function (6.386a–c) ≡ (6.387a) and choosing the constant *a* to be a root (6.387c) of (6.387b):

$$\zeta(x,y)=f(x+ay): \qquad a^2T_{yy}+2aT_{xy}+T_{xx}=T_{yy}(a-a_+)(a-a_-). \qquad \text{(6.387a–c)}$$

If the roots (6.388c) are distinct (6.388a, b), then (6.386b) specifies two solutions of (6.386c) and their sum is the general integral because it involves two arbitrary functions (6.388d):

$$T_{xx}T_{yy}\neq T_{xy}^2: \qquad T_{yy}\,a_\pm=-T_{xy}\pm\sqrt{T_{xy}^2-T_{xx}T_{yy}}, \qquad \text{(6.388a, b)}$$

$$a_+\neq a_-: \qquad \zeta(x,y)=h(x+a_-y)+j(x+a_+y). \qquad \text{(6.388c–d)}$$

If the roots (6.389b) of (6.387b, c) coincide (6.389a), the two particular solutions in (6.388d) reduce to one (6.387a), and another solution is obtained (section 1.3.7) by parametric differentiation with regard to a, which is equivalent to multiplying by y in the second term on the r.h.s. of (6.388d):

$$T_{xx} T_{yy} = T_{xy}^2: \qquad a_\pm = -\frac{T_{xy}}{T_{yy}}, \qquad \zeta(x,y) = h(x + ay) + y\, j(x + ay), \qquad (6.389a\text{–}c)$$

leading to (6.389c).

The lines (6.390a) are (problem 243) the **characteristics** (Figure 6.17) of the differential operator (6.385b) and appear in the solutions where:

$$\eta_\pm = x + a_\pm\, y: \qquad T_{xy}^2 - T_{xx} T_{yy} = \begin{cases} >0: & \text{two real characteristics,} \\ = 0: & \text{one characteristic,} \\ < 0: & \text{no real characteristics,} \end{cases} \qquad (6.390a\text{–}d)$$

there are three cases: (i) one real characteristic (6.390c) $\equiv$ (6.389a) for equal roots (6.389b) and solution (6.389c); and (ii/iii) two (no) real characteristics for real distinct (6.390b) [complex conjugate (6.390d)] roots (6.388b) and solution (6.388d). The characteristics (6.390a) are the lines (6.391b) of constant deflection (6.391a) that (Figure 6.17) have non-unit tangent vectors (6.391c):

$$\zeta_\pm(x,y) = f_\pm(x + ay): \qquad \eta_\pm = x + a_\pm\, y = const, \qquad \bar{m}_\pm = \{1, a_\pm\}, \qquad (6.391a\text{–}c)$$

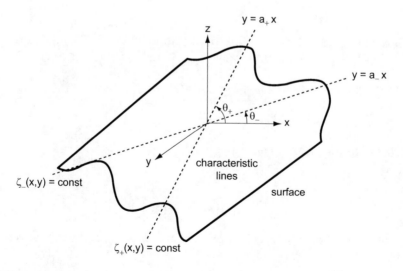

FIGURE 6.17

For an elastic membrane (Figure 6.14) under anisotropic stresses (Figure 6.16) the rotation (Figure 6.15) to the principal stress axis leads to the characteristic lines of constant deflection.

specifying: (i) the angles of the characteristics with the x-axis (6.392):

$$\cos \phi_\pm = \frac{\vec{e}_x . \vec{m}_\pm}{|\vec{m}_\pm|} = \left|1 + a_\pm^2\right|^{-1/2} ; \tag{6.392}$$

$$\phi_0 \equiv \phi_+ - \phi_- : \qquad \cos \phi_0 = \frac{(\vec{m}_+ . \vec{m}_-)}{|\vec{m}_+| \, |\vec{m}_-|} = (1 + a_+ a_-) \left|(1 + a_+^2)(1 + a_-^2)\right|^{-1/2} , \tag{6.393a, b}$$

and (ii) the angle (6.393a) between the two characteristics (6.393b) that is expressed in terms of the stresses by (6.394a) whose inverse is (6.394b):

$$\cos^2 \phi_0 = \frac{\left(T_{yy} + T_{xx}\right)^2}{\left(T_{yy} - T_{xx}\right)^2 + 4T_{xy}^2} : \qquad \sec^2 \phi_0 = 1 + 4\frac{T_{xy}^2 - T_{xx} \, T_{yy}}{\left(T_{xx} + T_{yy}\right)^2} . \tag{6.394a, b}$$

From (6.394b) can be confirmed (6.390b–d), namely: (i) in the case (6.390b) the r.h.s. of (6.394b) is larger than unity and ϕ_0 is the real angle between the two distinct characteristics; (ii) in the case (6.390c) the r.h.s. of (6.394b) is unity so $\phi_0 = 0$ and the two characteristics coincide; and (iii) in the case (6.390d) the r.h.s. of (6.394b) is less than unity and the angle ϕ_0 is imaginary so no characteristics exist.

The proof of (6.394a) can be made as follows: (i) from (6.387c) ≡ (6.395a) follows the sum (6.395b) and product (6.395c) of the roots:

$$a^2 T_{yy} + 2a T_{xy} + T_{xx} = T_{yy}\left[a^2 - (a_+ + a_-)a + a_+ a_-\right]: \quad a_+ + a_- = -2\frac{T_{xy}}{T_{yy}}, \quad a_+ a_- = \frac{T_{xx}}{T_{yy}}, \tag{6.395a–c}$$

that can be checked from (6.388b); (ii) the numerator of (6.393b) is determined by (6.395c) and the denominator by:

$$(1 + a_+^2)(1 + a_-^2) = 1 + a_+^2 + a_-^2 + a_+^2 a_-^2 = 1 + (a_+ + a_-)^2 - 2a_+ a_- + (a_+ a_-)^2$$

$$= (a_+ + a_-)^2 + (1 - a_+ a_-)^2 ; \tag{6.396}$$

(iii) substituting (6.396) in (6.393b) gives:

$$\cos^2 \phi_0 = \frac{(1 + a_+ a_-)^2}{(1 - a_+ a_-)^2 + (a_+ + a_-)^2} ; \tag{6.397a}$$

(iv) substitution of (6.395b, c) in (6.397a) proves (6.394a); and (v) the inverse of (6.394a) is:

$$\sec^2 \phi_0 = \frac{T_{xx}^2 + T_{yy}^2 - 2T_{xx} \, T_{yy} + 4T_{xy}^2}{T_{xx}^2 + T_{yy}^2 + 2T_{xx} \, T_{yy}} , \tag{6.397b}$$

that simplifies to (6.394b). The arbitrary functions (6.386a, b) that appear in the solution of the membrane equation (6.385b) are determined by the boundary condition (6.369a) in the case of a bounded region, such as an elliptic membrane (subsection 6.6.6).

6.6.6 Deflection of an Elliptic Membrane by Its Own Weight

The deflection of a membrane under isotropic stress by its own weight in the gravity field (6.398a) is specified by (6.371e) ≡ (6.398c) that may be written in polar coordinates (6.398d) for a displacement depending only on the radius (6.398b):

$$f = \rho g, \qquad \zeta = \zeta(r): \qquad -\frac{\rho g}{T} = \nabla^2 \zeta = \frac{1}{r}\frac{d}{dr}\left(r\frac{d\zeta}{dr}\right). \qquad (6.398\text{a--d})$$

The deflection is obtained integrating (6.398d) twice, with each integration introducing an arbitrary constant:

$$r\frac{d\zeta}{dr} = -\frac{\rho g}{2T}r^2 + C_1, \qquad \zeta(r) = -\frac{\rho g}{4T}r^2 + C_1 \log r + C_2. \qquad (6.399\text{a, b})$$

In the case of a circular membrane (6.400a) with radius a the condition of finite displacement at the center (6.400b) eliminates one constant (6.400c):

$$0 \le r \le a: \qquad \zeta(0) < \infty \implies C_1 = 0, \qquad 0 = u(a) = C_2 - \frac{\rho g a^2}{4T}, \qquad (6.400\text{a--e})$$

and the boundary condition (6.368d) of zero displacement (6.400d) determines the other constant (6.400e). Substituting of (6.400c, e) in (6.399b) shows that *the linear deflection (6.398d) ≡ (6.401b) of a circular elastic membrane with radius (6.401a) is given (problem 244) by (6.401c) ≡ (II.6.30a):*

$$0 \le x^2 + y^2 \le a^2: \qquad -\frac{\rho g}{T} = \frac{d^2\zeta}{dr^2} + \frac{1}{r}\frac{d\zeta}{dr}, \qquad \zeta(r) = \frac{\rho g}{4T}(a^2 - r^2). \qquad (6.401\text{a--c})$$

The maximum deflection (6.402a) of the membrane may be introduced in (6.401c), leading to (6.402b):

$$\zeta_{max} = \zeta(0) = \frac{\rho g a^2}{4T}: \qquad \zeta(x,y) = \zeta_{max}\left(1 - \frac{x^2 + y^2}{a^2}\right). \qquad (6.402\text{a, b})$$

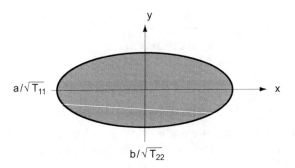

FIGURE 6.18
An example of deflection of elastic membrane (Figure 6.14) under constant anisotropic stresses (Figure 6.16) is the elliptic shape with axis along the principal stress axis or characteristics (Figure 6.17).

The transformation (6.403a, b) suggests that (6.403c) specifies the deflection of an elliptic membrane (Figure 6.18) with half-axis (A,B):

$$\frac{\{x,y\}}{a} = \left\{ \frac{x_1}{A}, \frac{x_2}{B} \right\}: \qquad \zeta(x,y) = \zeta_{max} \left[1 - \left(\frac{x_1}{A} \right)^2 - \left(\frac{x_2}{B} \right)^2 \right]. \qquad (6.403a–c)$$

It can be confirmed that the anisotropic Poisson equation (6.404a) with arbitrary stresses (6.70b) and uniform weight (6.398a):

$$-\rho g = T_{11} \partial_{11} \zeta + T_{22} \partial_{22} \zeta + 2 T_{12} \partial_{12} \zeta: \qquad \rho g = 2 \zeta_{max} \left(\frac{T_{11}}{A^2} + \frac{T_{22}}{B^2} \right), \qquad (6.404a, b)$$

is satisfied by (6.403c) with maximum amplitude given by (6.404b).

Thus, *an elliptic membrane (Figure 6.18) with half-axis (A,B) under uniform anisotropic stresses (6.404a) under its own weight has (problem 245) deflection (6.403c) with maximum (6.404b) at the center. In the case (problem 244) of a circular membrane (6.405a) with radius a and anisotropic stresses, the deflection (6.403c) simplifies to (6.402b) ≡ (6.405c) with maximum (6.405b):*

$$A = B \equiv a: \qquad \zeta_{max} = \frac{\rho g\, a^2}{2(T_{11} + T_{22})}, \qquad \zeta(r) = \frac{\rho g}{2} \frac{a^2 - r^2}{T_{11} + T_{22}}. \qquad (6.405a–c)$$

If, in addition, the stresses are isotropic (6.406a), the deflection simplifies to (6.406b) ≡ (6.401c):

$$T_{11} = T_{22} \equiv T: \qquad \zeta(r) = \frac{\rho g}{4T} \left(a^2 - r^2 \right). \qquad (6.406a, b)$$

In all cases the shear stresses T_{12} play no role because they appear in the anisotropic Poisson equation (6.404a), multiplying a mixed derivative that is zero

$\partial_{12}\zeta = 0$ for the deflection (6.402b). The transformation (6.403a, b) is similar to (6.380a, b) with a scaling factor ρg to render it dimensionless. The transformation (6.380a, b) was used (subsection 6.6.4) together with (6.379b) to determine the Green function in an unbounded membrane; the Green function can be used (Chapter III.7) to specify the deflection under arbitrary loading (subsection 6.6.7).

6.6.7 Deflection by Arbitrary Loads for an Unbounded Membrane

The linear deflection of an elastic membrane under uniform anisotropic stresses due to an arbitrary loading as a function of position (6.370b) ≡ (6.407a) is specified (problem 246) by an anisotropic Poisson equation (6.407a) involving the anisotropic Laplace operator that is: (i) linear, so the principle of superposition (subsection III.7.6.2) holds and the solution forced by an arbitrary function (III.7.77b) ≡ (6.407a) is given by the integration after multiplication by the Green function (III.7.78b) ≡ (6.407b):

$$T_{11}\,\partial_{11}\,\zeta + T_{22}\,\partial_{22} + 2T_{12}\,\partial_{12}\zeta = -f\left(x_1,x_2\right); \qquad (6.407a)$$

$$\zeta\left(x_1,x_2\right) = -\iint_D G\left(x_1 - y_1 ; x_2 - y_2\right) f\left(y_1,y_2\right) dy_1\,dy_2 ; \qquad (6.407b)$$

*and (ii) is self-adjoint (subsection III.7.8.5), so the principle of reciprocity (subsection III.7.6.3) holds and the Green function depends only on the difference of positions $\bar{x} - \bar{y}$, and (6.407b) ≡ (III.7.36) is a **convolution integral** (section III.7.4). The boundary condition is replaced by an asymptotic condition in the case of the Green function for an infinite membrane with: (i) unequal normal stress (6.384d):*

$$4\pi\zeta(x_1,x_2) = -\int_-^+ \int_\infty^\infty f\left(y_1,y_2\right)\log\left[\frac{\left(x_1 - y_1\right)^2}{T_{11}} + \frac{\left(x_2 - y_2\right)^2}{T_{22}}\right] dy_1\,dy_2 ; \qquad (6.408)$$

and (ii) arbitrary stresses including shears taken in the principal stress coordinate system (6.382b):

$$4\pi\zeta(x_1,x_2) = -\int_-^+ \int_\infty^\infty f\left(y_1,y_2\right) dy_1\,dy_2$$

$$\log\left\{\frac{\left[\left(x_1 - y_1\right)\cos\bar\phi - \left(x_2 - y_2\right)\sin\bar\phi\right]^2}{T_{11}\left(\bar\phi\right)} + \frac{\left[\left(x_1 - y_1\right)\sin\bar\phi + \left(x_2 - y_2\right)\cos\bar\phi\right]^2}{T_{22}\left(\bar\phi\right)}\right\}.$$

$$\qquad (6.409)$$

The asymptotic scaling of the deflection at large distance is determined by the evaluation of the integral (6.409), of which (6.408) is the particular case $\bar\phi = 0$ without shear: (i) the integral is finite for bounded loads in a compact region: and (ii) for loads in an unbounded region the integral (6.409) must converge for finite displacements.

6.7 Linear Bending of a Thin Plate

The consideration (Diagram 6.1) of transverse deflections of one(two)-dimensional elastic bodies: (i) starts with the cases of strings (membranes) without bending stiffness [chapter III.2 (sections II.6.1–II.6.2 and 6.6)]; (ii) proceeds with the cases of bars (plates) with bending stiffness [chapter III.4 (section 6.7)]; and (iii) combines (i) and (ii) in the case of beams (stressed plates) that can lead to elastic instability or buckling [sections 6.1–6.3 (6.8–6.9)]. The weak bending will be considered for thin (thick) plates [sections 6.7 (6.8)] in the linear case of small slopes, before proceeding to strong bending that couples non-linearly in-plane and out-of-plane deformations (section 6.9). As for strings (bars) there are [sections II.2.1–II.2.2 (II.4.1–II.4.3) two approaches to (subsection 6.7.1) weak bending of thin plates: (i) the bending moments (subsection 6.7.2) and curvatures and twist (subsection 6.7.3) lead through the stress and twist couples (subsection 6.7.4) to the elastic energy (subsection 6.7.5) and turning moments (subsection 6.7.6) and to the differential equation for the displacement; and (ii) the elastic energy of bending (subsection 6.7.5) can be obtained in an alternate way (subsection 6.7.8)

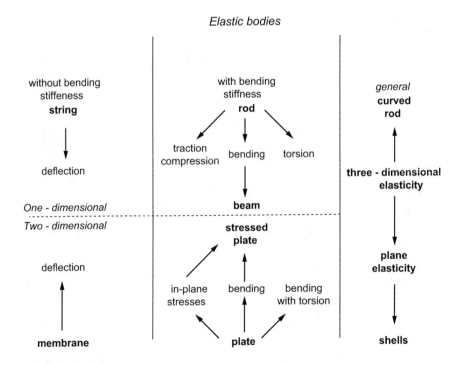

DIAGRAM 6.1
Relation between one- and two-dimensional elastic bodies (Table 6.9) with and without bending stiffness, together with some related cases and extensions.

from the displacements, strains, and stresses (subsection 6.7.7) and balanced against the virtual work of external forces (subsection 6.7.9) leads to the same differential equation for the bending of a plate (subsection 6.7.10) that can be compared with the bending of a beam (subsection 6.7.11). The boundary conditions to be satisfied at the edges of the plate (subsection 6.7.12) can be obtained for clamped, supported, pinned, or free edges (subsection 6.7.13) of plates with arbitrary shape (subsection 6.7.14), including rectangular and circular. Three examples of the weak linear bending of a circular plate are given: (i) clamped or pinned due to a concentrated force at the center (subsections 6.7.15–6.7.16); and (ii–iii) due to its own weight (subsection 6.7.17) either clamped or pinned at the boundary (subsection 6.7.18) or suspended from the center with free edge (subsection 6.7.19)

6.7.1 Linear/Non-Linear and Weak/Strong Bending of Plates

A plate is (Figure 6.19a) a two-dimensional elastic body whose thickness h is small compared (6.410a) with the transverse dimensions L. Two approximations are made (Figure 6.19b) in the theory of bending of plates: (i) the **linear (non-linear) bending** neglects (does not neglect) slopes (6.410b) implying that the deflection is negligible (may not be negligible) compared with the transverse dimensions (6.410c):

$$h^2 \ll L^2; \qquad \left(\nabla \zeta\right)^2 \ll 1: \quad \zeta^2 \ll L^2; \qquad \zeta^2 \ll h^2, \qquad (6.410a\text{–}d)$$

(ii) the linear approximation does not specify the relative scaling of the thickness h and deflection ζ, leaving two possibilities **weak (strong) bending** if the deflection is small (comparable) to the thickness (6.410d) implying that in-plane stresses can (cannot) be neglected [section(s) 6.7 (6.8–6.9)]. The linear

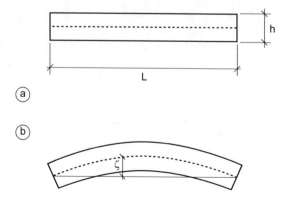

FIGURE 6.19
The bending of a plate involves a transverse deflection ζ and is : (i) linear (non-linear) if the slope is small everywhere (not small somewhere): and (ii) weak (strong) if the transverse displacement is small (not small) compared with the thickness h.

bending may be weak (strong) that is for small slope of a thick (thin) plate. The non-linear bending always causes in-plane stresses and thus is also strong bending regardless of whether the plate is thin or thick. Thus there is a hierarchy of three problems of increasing complexity: (i) weak bending with small slope (6.410b) and deflection (6.410c) of thick (6.410d) plates (section 6.7); (ii) strong bending with small slope (6.410b) and deflection of a thin plate (section 6.8); and (iii) non-linear coupling of bending an in-plane stresses for large slope or large deflection of a thin plate (section 6.9). The simplest case (i) is the starting point (subsection 6.7.2).

6.7.2 Bending Moment and Stiffness and Principal Curvatures

In the weak bending of a thin plate (Figure 6.19b), there is contraction (extension) in the inner (outer) side (Figure 6.20), so that there is in the interior an unstressed neutral surface, or **directrix,** in analogy with the **elastica** of a bar (section III.4.1 and subsection 6.6.1). The simplest theory of bars (plates) aims to specify the shape of the elastica (directrix). Choosing the axis (x_1, x_2) along the lines of principal curvature of the directrix (Figure 6.21a), the weak bending of the plate may be taken as the weak bending of two orthogonal bars (chapter III.4); namely: (i) the bending moment M_1 with x_1-axis causes a curvature (III.4.4b) ≡ (6.411a) along the x_1-axis and a cross-curvature (6.411b) along the orthogonal x_2-axis:

$$k_{11} = -\frac{M_1}{EI}, \qquad k_{21} = -\sigma k_{11} = \frac{M_1 \sigma}{EI}; \qquad \text{(6.411a, b)}$$

$$k_{22} = -\frac{M_2}{EI}, \qquad k_{12} = -\sigma k_{22} = \frac{M_2 \sigma}{EI}, \qquad \text{(6.411c, d)}$$

(ii) conversely, the bending moment M_2 with x_2-axis causes a curvature (6.411c) along the x_2-axis and a cross-curvature (6.411d) along the x_1-axis; (iii) the plate is assumed to be isotropic, since in (6.411a–d) appear the same

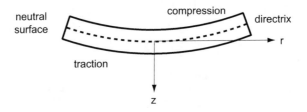

FIGURE 6.20
A beam (plate) under bending [Figure 6.1c (6.20)] is stretched (shortened) on the outer (inner) side leading to a traction (compression), with the transition along a curve (surface); namely, the elastica (characteristic) that is undeformed and subject to no stresses. For a thin bar (plate) the elastica (characteristic) specifies the bent shape.

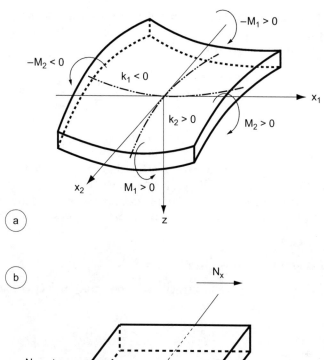

(a)

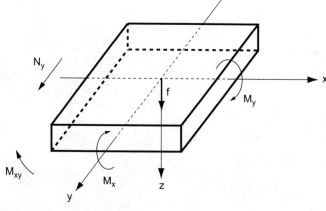

(b)

FIGURE 6.21
The bending of a plate may be considered: (a) starting with principal curvatures due to bending moments; and (b) a rotation leads to the curvatures and twist and to the stress couples. The stress couples imply the existence of turning moments that balance the transverse forces leading to the equation for the directrix.

values of the Young modulus E and Poisson ratio σ, and the moment of inertia (6.412a) of the cross-section of thickness h:

$$I \equiv \int_{-h/2}^{h/2} z^2 \, dz = \frac{h^3}{12}; \quad k_1 = k_{11} + k_{12} = \frac{M_2 \sigma - M_1}{EI}, \quad k_2 = k_{21} + k_{22} = \frac{M_1 \sigma - M_2}{EI},$$

$$(6.412a\text{–}c)$$

and (iv) the sum of (6.411a, d) [(6.411b, c)] specifies the **principal curva-tures** (6.412b) [(6.412c)] along the x_1 (x_2)-axis. Solving (6.412b, c) specifies the **bending moments** (6.413a, b):

$$\{M_1, M_2\} = -D\{k_1 + k_2\sigma, k_2 + k_1\sigma\}: \qquad D \equiv \frac{EI}{1-\sigma^2} = \frac{Eh^3}{12(1-\sigma^2)}, \qquad \text{(6.413a–d)}$$

of *(problem 247) an elastic plate: (i) with principal curvatures k_1 (k_2) along the x_1 (x_2)-axis; (ii) made of a material with Young modulus E and Poisson ratio σ; and (iii) involving the moment of inertia (6.412a) in the* **bending stiffness** *(6.413c) ≡ (6.413d).* The preceding equations are valid in a Cartesian frame with axis along the principal curvatures; they are generalized to any Cartesian reference frame with the same origin by a rotation (subsection 6.7.3).

6.7.3 Twist and Curvatures in Rotated Axis

Rotating by an angle ψ to arbitrary axis the **quadratic curvature form** is invariant:

$$K \equiv k_1(dx_1)^2 + k_2(dx_2)^2 = k_x(dx)^2 + k_y(dy)^2 + 2\tau\,dx\,dy, \qquad \text{(6.414)}$$

where τ is the **twist,** and k_x (k_y) the curvature along the $x(y)$-axis that are no longer lines of principal curvature, since they are rotated by an arbitrary angle ψ. The (x_1, x_2)-axis rotate in the positive or counterclockwise direction by an angle ψ toward the $x(y)$-axis; that is, the reverse of Figure 6.15a, so that φ is replaced (6.415a) by −ψ in (6.373b), leading to (6.415b):

$$\psi = -\phi: \qquad x + iy = (x_1 + ix_2)e^{-i\psi} = (x_1 + ix_2)(\cos\psi - i\sin\psi), \qquad \text{(6.415a, b)}$$

that implies:

$$x = x_1\cos\psi + x_2\sin\psi, \qquad y = -x_1\sin\psi + x_2\cos\psi; \qquad \text{(6.415c, d)}$$

substitution of (6.415c, d) in (6.414) leads to (6.415e):

$$
\begin{aligned}
K &\equiv k_x(dx)^2 + k_y(dx)^2 + 2\tau\,dx\,dy \\
&= k_1(\cos\psi\,dx_1 + \sin\psi\,dx_2)^2 + k_2(-\sin\psi\,dx_1 + \cos\psi\,dx_2)^2 \\
&= (k_1\cos^2\psi + k_2\sin^2\psi)(dx_1)^2 + (k_1\sin^2\psi + k_2\cos^2\psi)(dx_2)^2 \\
&\quad + 2(k_1 - k_2)\cos\psi\sin\psi\,dx_1\,dx_2.
\end{aligned}
\qquad \text{(6.415e)}
$$

Since (6.415e) must hold for arbitrary (dx_1, dx_2), *the curvatures* (k_x, k_y) *and twist* τ *for axis* (x, y) *making an angle* $\psi = -\phi$ *with (Figure 6.15a) the principal curvatures* $x_1(x_2)$ *are related (problem 248) by:*

$$k_x = k_1 \cos^2 \psi + k_2 \sin^2 \psi = \frac{k_1 + k_2}{2} + \frac{k_1 - k_2}{2} \cos(2\psi), \qquad (6.416a)$$

$$k_y = k_1 \sin^2 \psi + k_2 \cos^2 \psi = \frac{k_1 + k_2}{2} - \frac{k_1 - k_2}{2} \cos(2\psi), \qquad (6.416b)$$

$$\tau = (k_1 - k_2)\cos\psi \sin\psi = \frac{k_1 - k_2}{2} \sin(2\psi). \qquad (6.416c)$$

In the absence of rotation (6.417a) there is no twist (6.417b) and the curvatures coincide with the principal curvatures (6.417c, d):

$$\psi = 0: \qquad \tau = 0, \qquad k_x = k_1, \qquad k_y = k_2. \qquad (6.417\text{a–d})$$

For an arbitrary rotation, (6.416a–c) lead to the identities:

$$k_x + k_y = k_1 + k_2, \quad k_x - k_y \equiv (k_1 - k_2)\cos(2\psi), \quad 2\tau = (k_1 - k_2)\sin(2\psi). \qquad (6.418\text{a–c})$$

that are applied to the bending moments (6.413a, b), leading to the twist and stress couples (subsection 6.7.4).

6.7.4 Twist and Stress Couples on a Plate

The relation between the principal curvatures (subsection 6.7.2) and the curvatures and twist (subsection 6.7.3) by an arbitrary rotation also lead from the bending moments (subsection 6.7.2) to the stress and twist couples (subsection 6.7.4). From (6.413a, b) follow the sum (6.419a) and difference (6.419b) of the bending moments in principal axis of curvature:

$$M_1 + M_2 = -D(1+\sigma)(k_1 + k_2), \qquad M_1 - M_2 = -D(1-\sigma)(k_1 - k_2). \qquad (6.419\text{a, b})$$

The rotation relations (6.416a–c) also apply to the bending moments, for example: (i) the **stress couple** (6.416a; 6.419a, b) along the *x*-axis:

$$\begin{aligned} M_x &= \frac{M_1 + M_2}{2} + \frac{M_1 - M_2}{2}\cos(2\psi) \\ &= -\frac{D}{2}\left[(1+\sigma)(k_1 + k_2) + (1-\sigma)(k_1 - k_2)\cos(2\psi)\right] \\ &= -\frac{D}{2}\left[(1+\sigma)(k_x + k_y) + (1-\sigma)(k_x - k_y)\right] = -D(k_x + k_y\sigma), \end{aligned} \qquad (6.420)$$

where were used (6.418a, b); (ii) the **twist couple** (6.416c; 6.419a, b) in the (x, y)-plane:

$$M_{xy} = \frac{M_1 - M_2}{2} \sin\left(2\,\psi\right) = -\frac{D}{2}(1 - \sigma)(k_1 - k_2)\sin\left(2\,\psi\right) = -D(1 - \sigma)\tau; \quad (6.421)$$

and (iii) a relation (6.422b) similar to (6.420):

$$\left\{ M_x, M_y, M_{xy} \right\} = -D\left\{ k_x + k_y\,\sigma\, , \, k_y + k_x\,\sigma\, , \, (1 - \sigma)\tau \right\}, \quad (6.422\text{a–c})$$

$$\left\{ k_x\, , \, k_y\, , \tau \right\} = \left\{ \partial_{xx}\zeta, \partial_{yy}\zeta, \partial_{xy}\zeta \right\} = \left\{ \frac{\partial^2\zeta}{\partial x^2}, \frac{\partial^2\zeta}{\partial y^2}, \frac{\partial^2\zeta}{\partial x\,\partial y} \right\}. \quad (6.423\text{a–c})$$

Thus, *for a thin elastic plate under weak (problem 249) bending the stress (6.422a, b) [twist (3.422c)] couples are proportional to the curvatures (6.423a, b) [twist (6.423c)] through the bending stiffness (6.413c, d); the latter involves the thickness of the plate, the Young modulus, and Poisson ratio of the material, with the last also appearing in (6.422a–c).* The stress (twist) couples and curvatures (twist) specify the elastic energy of weak bending of a thin plate (subsection 6.7.5).

6.7.5 Elastic Energy of Bending

The elastic energy of bending of a bar (III.4.32b) ≡ (6.424b) is one-half of minus the product of the bending moment (III.4.4b) ≡ (6.411a) ≡ (6.424a) by the curvature (6.424c) leading to (6.424e):

$$M = -EI\,k: \quad 2\bar{E}_d = -M\zeta'' = EI\zeta''k; \quad k = \zeta'', \quad 2\bar{E}_d = -Mk, \quad (6.424\text{a–e})$$

in the case of linear bending with small slope (6.424d). The elastic energy of weak bending of a thin plate is the sum of two bars along the principal curvatures (6.425a):

$$2\bar{E}_d = -M_1k_1 - M_2\,k_2 = \frac{M_1^2 + M_2^2 - 2\sigma\,M_1M_2}{EI} = D\left(k_1^2 + k_2^2 + 2\sigma\,k_1\,k_2\right),$$
$$(6.425\text{a–c})$$

leading to (6.425b) [(6.425c)] by (6.412b, c) [(6.413a, b)]. From (6.416a–c) it follows that:

$$k_x\,k_y - \tau^2 = \left(\frac{k_1 + k_2}{2}\right)^2 - \left(\frac{k_1 - k_2}{2}\right)^2\left[\cos^2\left(2\,\psi\right) + \sin^2\left(2\,\psi\right)\right] = k_1\,k_2, \quad (6.426)$$

that may be substituted together with (6.418a) to express the elastic energy (6.425c) ≡ (6.427a) in terms of the curvatures and twist (6.427b):

$$2\bar{E}_d = D\left[(k_1+k_2)^2 - 2(1-\sigma)k_1 k_2\right] = D\left[(k_x+k_y)^2 - 2(1-\sigma)(k_x k_y - \tau^2)\right];$$

$$(6.427a, b)$$

thus derivatives of the elastic energy with regard to the curvature (6.428a, b) [twist (6.428c)] equal minus the stress (6.422a, b) [twist (6.422c)] couples:

$$\left\{\frac{\partial \bar{E}_d}{\partial k_x}, \frac{\partial \bar{E}_d}{\partial k_y}, \frac{\partial \bar{E}_d}{\partial \tau}\right\} = D\left\{k_x + k_y\,\sigma\,,\,k_y + k_x\,\sigma\,,\,2\,(1-\sigma)\tau\right\} = -\left\{M_x, M_y, 2\,M_{xy}\right\}.$$

$$(6.428a\text{--}c)$$

It has been shown that *the elastic energy (problem 250) of weak linear bending of a plate (6.425a) is specified: (i) by (6.425b) [(6.425c)] in terms of bending moments (principal curvatures); and (ii) by (6.427b) [(6.428a–c)] in terms of the curvatures and twist (stress and twist couples).*

6.7.6 Balance of Turning Moments and Transverse Forces

The stress couples $(M_x, M_{xy})\left[(M_y, M_{xy})\right]$ on the face of Figure 6.21b orthogonal to the $x(y)$-axis are (6.422a–c; 6.423a–c) balanced by the **turning moments**:

$$N_x = -\partial_x M_x - \partial_y M_{xy} = D\left[\partial_x k_x + \sigma\,\partial_x k_y + (1-\sigma)\,\partial_y\,\tau\right]$$

$$= D(\partial_{xxx}\zeta + \sigma\,\partial_{xyy}\zeta + (1-\sigma)\,\partial_{yxy}\,\zeta) = D(\partial_{xxx}\zeta + \partial_{xyy}\,\zeta) = D\partial_x(\nabla^2\zeta),$$

$$(6.429)$$

and likewise in the y-direction (6.430a, b):

$$\{N_x, N_y\} = D\{\partial_x, \partial_y\}(\nabla^2\zeta); \quad f = \partial_x N_x + \partial_y N_y, \quad (6.430a\text{--}c)$$

the balance with the transverse force per unit area (6.430c) leads to (6.431b–d):

$$D = const: \quad f(x,y) = D\{\partial_{xx} + \partial_{yy}\}\nabla^2\zeta = D\nabla^4\zeta = D(\partial_{xx} + \partial_{yy})^2\zeta, \quad (6.431a\text{--}d)$$

with the bending stiffness (6.413c, d) assumed to be constant (6.431a) in (6.429; 6.430a, b; 6.431b–d). It has been shown that *the transverse displacement of a plate under weak linear bending (6.410a–d) satisfies (problem 251) a biharmonic equation (6.431b–d) forced by the transverse force per unit area divided by the con- stant (6.431a) bending stiffness (6.413c, d), where h is the thickness of the plate, and (E,σ) the Young modulus and Poisson ratio of the material. The deflection specifies* *through its second-order derivatives: (i) the curvatures (6.423a, b) and twist (6.423c); (ii) the stress (6.422a, b) and twist (6.422c) couples; and (iii) the elastic energy (6.425a–c). All three (i–iii) are related by (6.427b). The elastic energy is specified equivalently by: (i) the principal curvatures (6.425c) ≡ (6.427a); (ii) the curvatures and twist (6.427b); (iii) the bending moments (6.425b); and (iv) specifies the stress and twist couples (6.428a–c). The third-order derivatives of the transverse displacement specify the turning moments (6.430a, b).* The preceding relations hold in a Cartesian reference frame (Figure 6.21a, b) with the vertical out-of-plane axis downward, thus: (i) (x,y,z) or (x_1, x_2, x_3) are left-handed reference frames; and (ii) a downward displacement, such as under its own weight, is positive. The same reference frame is used for elastic membranes (sections II.6.1–II.6.2 and 6.6), strings (chapter III.2), bars (Chapter III.4), beams (sections 6.1–6.3), and plates (sections 6.7–6.9). The equation (6.431b–d) specifying the transverse displacement in the weak bending of a thin plate was derived (subsections 6.7.1–6.7.6) for constant (6.431a) bending stiffness (6.413c, d) and is generalized next (subsections 6.7.7–6.7.9) to non-uniform bending stiffness using an energy method instead of balance of forces and moments.

6.7.7 Bending Displacement, Strain, and Stress

For a plate (bar) under weak bending [Figure 6.20 (6.1c)], the inner side is subject to a compression and the outer side to a traction. There is in the interior a neutral surface (line), called the **directrix** (elastica) that is not subject to change of area (length). The weak bending of the thin plate is described by the deformation of the directrix, corresponding to the displacement (6.432a):

$$\vec{u} = \vec{e}_z \, \zeta(x,y); \quad \partial_z u_x = -\partial_x u_z = -\partial_x \zeta, \quad \partial_z u_y = -\partial_y u_z = -\partial_y \zeta; \quad (6.432\text{a–e})$$

neglecting the transverse stresses (6.312a–e) compared with the longitudinal stresses leads to (6.313a, b) that (6.304c) becomes (6.432b, d) where (6.432a) is used leading to (6.432c, e). Integrating (6.432c, e) leads to (6.433c, d), where the constants of integration are zero because there is no horizontal displacement on the directrix (6.433a, b):

$$u_x(0) = 0 = u_y(0): \qquad \{u_x(z), u_y(z)\} = -z\big(\partial_x \zeta \,, \partial_y \zeta\big). \qquad (6.433\text{a–d})$$

The equation of the directrix (6.434a) leads to the unit normal vector (6.434b):

$$0 = z - \zeta(x,y) \equiv \Phi(x,y,z): \quad \vec{N} \equiv \{N_x, N_z\} = \frac{\nabla \Phi}{|\nabla \Phi|}$$

$$= \left|1 + \big(\partial_x \zeta\big)^2 + \big(\partial_y \zeta\big)^2\right|^{-1/2} \{-\partial_x \zeta, -\partial_x \zeta, 1\};$$

$$(6.434\text{a, b})$$

in the linear approximation of small slope (6.435a) the unit normal simplifies to (6.435b):

$$1 \gg |\nabla \zeta|^2 = (\partial_x \zeta)^2 + (\partial_y \zeta)^2 : \quad \vec{N} = \{-\partial_x \zeta, -\partial_y \zeta, 1\}, \{u_x(z), u_y(z)\} = z\{N_x, N_y\},$$

$$(6.435a\text{--}c)$$

and the horizontal or in-plane displacements (6.435c) are proportional to the distance from the directrix and to the corresponding components of the unit normal (6.435b).

The in-plane components of the strain tensor (6.304c) are (6.436a):

$$\{S_{xx}, S_{yy}, S_{xy}\} = \left\{ \partial_x u_x, \partial_y u_y, \frac{1}{2}(\partial_x u_y + \partial_y u_x) \right\}$$

$$(6.436a\text{--}c)$$

$$= -z\{\partial_{xx}\zeta, \partial_{yy}\zeta, \partial_{xy}\zeta\} = -z\{k_x, k_y, \tau\},$$

and are: (i) related to the displacements (6.433c, d) by the second-order derivatives (6.436b); and (ii) proportional (6.436c) to the distance from the directrix and to the curvatures (6.423a, b) [twist (6.423c)] for the normal (shear) strains. The out-of-plane shear strains are zero (6.313a, b) ≡ (6.437a, b) and the out-of-plane normal strain (6.313c; 6.436a, b) ≡ (6.437c–f):

$$S_{xz} = 0 = S_{yz}: \quad S_{zz} = -\frac{\sigma}{1-\sigma}(S_{xx} + S_{yy}) = \frac{\sigma z}{1-\sigma}(\partial_{xx}\zeta + \partial_{yy}\zeta)$$

$$(6.437a\text{--}f)$$

$$= \frac{\sigma z}{1-\sigma}(k_x + k_y) = \frac{\sigma z}{1-\sigma}\nabla^2 \zeta,$$

is proportional to the Laplacian of the transverse displacement (6.432a), which also appears in the area (6.438a–c) [volume (6.439a–c)] change:

$$D_2 \equiv S_{xx} + S_{yy} = -z(\partial_{xx}\zeta + \partial_{yy}\zeta) = -z\nabla^2\zeta, \quad (6.438a\text{--}c)$$

$$D_3 = D_2 + S_{zz} = z\left(\frac{\sigma}{1-\sigma} - 1\right)\nabla^2\zeta = -z\frac{1-2\sigma}{1-\sigma}\nabla^2\zeta. \quad (6.439a\text{--}c)$$

The direct Hooke law (6.306c–e; 6.307a–c) applied to (6.436a–b; 6.437a–f) specifies the zero (6.440a–c) and non-zero (6.440d–f) stresses:

$$0 = T_{zz} = T_{xz} = T_{yz}; \quad T_{xy} = -\frac{Ez}{1+\sigma}\partial_{xy}\zeta, \quad (6.440a\text{--}d)$$

$$\{T_{xx}, T_{yy}\} = -\frac{Ez}{1-\sigma^2}\{\partial_{xx}\zeta + \sigma\partial_{yy}\zeta, \partial_{yy}\zeta + \sigma\partial_{xx}\zeta\}. \quad (6.440e, f)$$

Thus were obtained *(problem 252) the displacement vector (6.432a; 6.433a–d:6.435a–c), strain (6.436a–c; 6.437a–f) and stress (6.440a–f) tensors for the weak linear bending of a plate.*

6.7.8 Balance of Elastic Energy and Work of the Normal Forces

The elastic energy per unit volume is given by (II.4.86b) ≡ (6.441a):

$$2E_d = \sum_{i,j=1}^{3} T_{ij}S_{ij} = \sum_{\alpha,\beta=1}^{3} T_{\alpha\beta}S_{\alpha\beta} = T_{xx}S_{xx} + T_{yy}S_{yy} + 2\,T_{xy}S_{xy}$$

$$= \frac{E}{1-\sigma^2}\Big[S_{xx}\big(S_{xx}+\sigma\,S_{yy}\big) + S_{yy}\big(S_{yy}+\sigma\,S_{yy}\big)\Big] + \frac{2\,E}{1+\sigma}\big(S_{xy}\big)^2$$

$$= \frac{E}{1-\sigma^2}\Big[\big(S_{xx}\big)^2 + \big(S_{yy}\big)^2 + 2\sigma\,S_{xx}S_{yy} + 2\,(1-\sigma)\big(S_{xy}\big)^2 \Big]$$

$$= \frac{E}{1-\sigma^2}\Big\{ \big(S_{xx}+S_{yy}\big)^2 + 2(1-\sigma)\Big[\big(S_{xy}\big)^2 - S_{xx}\,S_{yy}\Big]\Big\},$$

(6.441a–f)

where (6.440a–c) appear only the in-plane stresses and strains (6.441b, c), that are related by (6.314a–c), leading to (6.441d–f). *The elastic energy per unit volume of the weak linear bending of a bar is (problem 253) given by: (i) (6.441f) in terms of the in-plane strains; (ii) (6.442a) in terms (6.436a) of the curvatures and twist; and (iii) (6.442c) in terms (6.436b) of the second-order derivatives of the transverse displacement:*

$$2E_d = \frac{z^2 E}{1-\sigma^2}\Big[\big(k_x+k_y\big)^2 + 2\,(1-\sigma)\big(\tau^2 - k_x k_y\big)\Big]$$

$$= \frac{z^2 E}{1-\sigma^2}\Big\{ \big(\partial_{xx}\zeta + \partial_{yy}\zeta\big)^2 + 2(1-\sigma)\Big[\big(\partial_{xy}\zeta\big)^2 - \big(\partial_{xx}\zeta\big)\big(\partial_{yy}\zeta\big)\Big]\Big\}.$$

(6.442a, b)

Integrating over the thickness of the plate (6.412a) leads to the elastic energy per unit area (6.443a) ≡ (6.443b):

$$2\bar{E}_d \equiv 2\int_{-h/2}^{+h/2} E_d\, dz = \frac{h^3 E}{12\big(1-\sigma^2\big)}\Big\{ \big(\partial_{xx}\zeta + \partial_{yy}\zeta\big)^2 + 2(1-\sigma)\Big[\big(\partial_{xy}\zeta\big)^2 - \big(\partial_{xx}\zeta\big)\big(\partial_{yy}\zeta\big)\Big]\Big\}$$

$$= D\Big\{ \big(\nabla^2\zeta\big)^2 + 2(1-\sigma)\Big[\big(\partial_{xy}\zeta\big)^2 - \big(\partial_{xx}\zeta\big)\big(\partial_{yy}\zeta\big)\Big]\Big\},$$

(6.443a–c)

where was introduced (6.443c) the bending stiffness (6.413d). The expressions (6.443b) ≡ (6.427b) for the elastic energy of weak bending of a thin plate coincide in the linear approximation (6.423a–c), showing the equivalence of two methods: (i) balance of bending, coupling, turning, and twisting moments and transverse forces (subsections 6.7.1–6.7.6) from (6.411a–d) to (6.430a–c); and (ii) strains and stresses associated with the transverse deflection (subsections 6.7.7–6.7.8), leading to the elastic energy from (6.432a–e) to (6.443a–c). The method (i) takes longer to arrive at the elastic energy and leads directly (subsection 6.7.6) to the balance equation (6.431b–d) for constant (6.431a) bending stiffness (6.413c, d). The method (ii) arrives sooner at the elastic energy and through the principle of virtual work (subsection 6.7.8) leads to: (ii-1) the balance equation (subsections 6.7.9–6.7.10) valid for non-uniform bending stiffness; and (ii-2) the boundary conditions (subsections 6.7.11–6.7.12).

6.7.9 Principle of Virtual Work and Bending Vector

The **principle of virtual work** (subsections II.6.1.2–II.6.1.3; section III.2.2; subsections III.4.2.4–III.4.2.7, 6.6.2) states that the work of external applied transverse force per unit area balances the variation of the elastic energy:

$$\int_D f \, \delta\zeta \, dA = \delta W = \delta\bar{\bar{E}}_d = \delta \int_D \bar{E}_d \, dA = \delta \int_D D\left[\frac{1}{2}\left(\nabla^2\zeta\right)^2 + (1-\sigma)\nabla\cdot\vec{C}\right] dA,$$
(6.444)

where was introduced: (i) the **bending vector** (6.445a):

$$2\vec{C} = \vec{e}_x\left[(\partial_y\zeta)(\partial_{xy}\zeta) - (\partial_x\zeta)(\partial_{yy}\zeta)\right] + \vec{e}_y\left[(\partial_x\zeta)(\partial_{xy}\zeta) - (\partial_y\zeta)(\partial_{xx}\zeta)\right],$$
(6.445a)

$$\nabla\cdot\vec{C} = \left(\partial_{xy}\zeta\right)^2 - \left(\partial_{xx}\zeta\right)\left(\partial_{yy}\zeta\right),$$
(6.445b)

whose divergence (6.445b) equals the last term in square brackets in (6.443c). Thus, *an elastic plate under weak linear bending (problem 254) has: (i) elastic energy density E_d per unit volume (6.441f) ≡ (6.442a, b); (ii) elastic energy density $\bar{E}_d$ per unit area (6.443c) obtained (6.443b) integrating (i) over the thickness of the plate (6.443a); and (iii) total elastic energy $\bar{\bar{E}}_d$ for the whole plate (6.444; 6.445a) specified by integrating over its area.* The variation of the elastic energy in (6.444) will give rise to volume and surface integrals. The surface integrals specify the general boundary conditions for the bending of a plate (subsections 6.7.11–6.7.12). The volume integrals in (6.444) affect the force balance (subsections 6.7.9–6.7.10). The variation of the r.h.s. of (6.444) is:

$$\int_C f \, \delta\zeta \, dA = \int_C D(\nabla^2\zeta)\delta(\nabla^2\zeta) dA + \int_C D(1-\sigma)\left[\delta(\nabla\cdot\vec{C})\right] dA,$$
(6.447)

where only the displacement of the directrix of the plate is varied $\delta\zeta$, not the physical properties $\delta D = 0 = \delta\sigma$ of the plate.

The variation of the divergence (6.445b) of the bending vector (6.445a) appears in the second term on the r.h.s. of (6.447) and is given by (6.448a) ≡ (6.448b):

$$\delta\left(\nabla.\vec{C}\right)=2\left(\partial_{xy}\zeta\right)\delta\left(\partial_{xy}\zeta\right)-\left(\partial_{xx}\zeta\right)\delta\left(\partial_{yy}\zeta\right)-\left(\partial_{yy}\zeta\right)\delta\left(\partial_{xx}\zeta\right)$$

$$=\partial_x\left[\left(\partial_{xy}\zeta\right)\partial_y\left(\delta\zeta\right)-\left(\partial_{yy}\zeta\right)\partial_x\left(\delta\zeta\right)\right]+\partial_y\left[\left(\partial_{xy}\zeta\right)\partial_x\left(\delta\zeta\right)-\left(\partial_{xx}\zeta\right)\partial_y\left(\delta\zeta\right)\right]$$

$$=\nabla.\vec{I},$$

(6.448a–c)

that is, the divergence (6.448c) of **deformation vector** (6.448d):

$$\vec{I}\equiv\vec{e}_x\left[\left(\partial_{xy}\zeta\right)\partial_y\left(\delta\zeta\right)-\left(\partial_{yy}\zeta\right)\partial_x\left(\delta\zeta\right)\right]+\vec{e}_y\left[\left(\partial_{xy}\zeta\right)\partial_x\left(\delta\zeta\right)-\left(\partial_{xx}\zeta\right)\partial_y\left(\delta\zeta\right)\right];$$

(6.448d)

the analogy (problem 255) between the bending (6.445a) and deformation (6.448b) vector applies with the substitution of the gradient (6.448f):

$$2\vec{C}\leftrightarrow\vec{I}:\qquad\nabla\zeta=\left\{\partial_x\zeta,\partial_y\zeta\right\}\leftrightarrow\nabla\left(\delta\zeta\right)=\left\{\partial_x\left(\delta\zeta\right),\partial_y\left(\delta\zeta\right)\right\},\quad\text{(6.448e, f)}$$

leaving the second-order derivatives unchanged. Substituting (6.448c) in (6.447) leads to:

$$\int_C f\,\delta\zeta=\int_C D\left(\nabla^2\zeta\right)\delta\left(\nabla^2\zeta\right)dS+\int_C D(1-\sigma)\left(\nabla.\vec{I}\right)dS,\qquad\text{(6.449)}$$

involving the deformation vector (6.448d).

6.7.10 Deformation Vector and Balance Equation

The property (6.450a) of the divergence is equivalent to (6.450b):

$$\nabla.\left(\lambda\vec{B}\right)=\lambda\left(\nabla.\vec{B}\right)+\vec{B}.\nabla\lambda\quad\Leftrightarrow\quad\partial_i\left(\lambda\vec{B}_i\right)=\lambda\,\partial_i B_i+B_i\,\partial_i\lambda;\qquad\text{(6.450a, b)}$$

applied to (6.450c, d) it leads to (6.450e):

$$\lambda=D\left(\nabla^2\zeta\right),\quad\vec{B}=\nabla\left(\delta\zeta\right):\qquad\text{(6.450c, d)}$$

$$\nabla.\left[D\left(\nabla^2\zeta\right)\nabla\left(\delta\zeta\right)\right]=D\left(\nabla^2\zeta\right)\nabla.\left[\nabla\left(\delta\zeta\right)\right]+\nabla\left(\delta\zeta\right).\nabla\left[D\left(\nabla^2\zeta\right)\right];\quad\text{(6.450e)}$$

$$D\left(1-\sigma\right)\left(\nabla.\vec{I}\right)=\nabla.\left[D\left(1-\sigma\right)\vec{I}\right]-\vec{I}.\nabla\left[D\left(1-\sigma\right)\right], \qquad (6.450\text{f})$$

and likewise holds (6.450f). Substituting (6.450e, f) in (6.449) leads to (6.451a):

$$\int_{C}\left\{f\,\delta\zeta+\nabla\left[D\left(\nabla^{2}\zeta\right)\right].\nabla\left(\delta\zeta\right)+\vec{I}.\nabla\left[D\left(1-\sigma\right)\right]\right\}dS$$

$$=\int_{C}\left\{\nabla.\left[D\left(\nabla^{2}\zeta\right)\nabla\left(\delta\zeta\right)\right]+\nabla.\left[D\left(1-\sigma\right)\vec{I}\right]\right\}dS \qquad (6.451\text{a, b})$$

$$=\int_{\partial C}\left\{D\left(\nabla^{2}\zeta\right)\partial_{n}\left(\delta\zeta\right)+D\left(1-\sigma\right)I_{n}\right\}ds,$$

where the divergence theorem (III.5.163a–c) ≡ (6.451a, b) was applied, assuming: (i) that (Figure 6.22) the plate occupies a region C with area element dS with closed regular boundary ∂C with arc length ds and outer normal $\vec{n}$; and (ii) the normal component of a vector (normal derivative) is denoted by (6.451d) [(6.541e)] and the transverse displacement has (6.451c) continuous fourth-order derivatives in the region C:

$$\zeta\in D^{4}\left(C\right): \qquad \partial_{n}=\vec{n}.\nabla=n_{x}\partial_{x}+n_{y}\partial_{y}, \qquad I_{n}=\vec{I}.\vec{n}. \qquad (6.451\text{c–e})$$

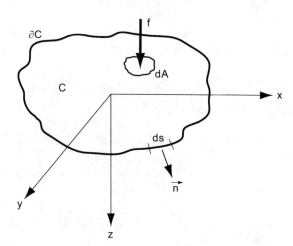

FIGURE 6.22
The equation for the directrix of a bent plate can be obtained by another method (as an alternative to that in Figure 6.21) that also supplies the boundary conditions (Figure 6.23). This method uses the principle of virtual work to balance: (i) the work of the transverse forces per unit area f in a transverse displacement $\delta\zeta$; and (ii) the variation of the elastic energy of the plate occupying the domain C with area element dS, whose boundary is a closed regular curve ∂C, with arc length ds and unit outer normal $\vec{n}$.

The second term on the l.h.s. of (6.451a) is subject to another integration by parts (6.452a) and another application of the divergence theorem (III.5.163a–c):

$$\int_C \left\{ \nabla\left[D(\nabla^2\zeta) \right].\nabla(\delta\zeta) \right\} dS = \int_C \nabla.\left\{ D\left[\nabla(\nabla^2\zeta) \right]\delta\zeta \right\} dS$$

$$- \int_C \nabla.\left\{ \nabla\left[D(\nabla^2\zeta) \right] \right\} d\zeta \, dS = \int_{\partial C} \partial_n \left[D(\nabla^2\zeta) \right] \delta\zeta \, ds \qquad (6.452a, b)$$

$$- \int_C \nabla^2 \left[D(\nabla^2\zeta) \right] \delta\zeta \, dS,$$

leading in succession to (6.452a) and (6.452b).
   Substitution of (6.452b) in (6.451b) leads to:

$$\int_C \left\{ f - \nabla^2 \left[D(\nabla^2\zeta) \right] \delta\zeta + \vec{i}.\nabla\left[D(1-\sigma) \right] \right\} dS$$

$$= \int_{\partial C} \left\{ D\left(\nabla^2\zeta \right) \partial_n(\delta\zeta) - \partial_n\left[D(\nabla^2\zeta) \right]\delta\zeta + D(1-\sigma)I_n \right\} ds = 0; \qquad (6.453a, b)$$

the equality of the boundary (surface) in the r.h.s. (l.h.s.) of (6.453a) implies that both must vanish (6.453b). The vanishing of the surface integral on the r.h.s. of (6.453b) is valid for arbitrary $\delta\zeta$ specifying *(problem 256) the* **balance equation** *for the transverse deflection of a plate under weak linear bending* (6.454b) ≡ (6.454c) *by a transverse force f per unit area:*

$$D(1-\sigma) = const: \qquad f(x,y) = \nabla^2 \left(D\nabla^2\zeta \right) = \left(\partial_{xx} + \partial_{yy} \right)\left[D\left(\partial_{xx}\zeta + \partial_{yy}\zeta \right) \right],$$
$$(6.454a–c)$$

that holds for non-uniform bending stiffness (6.413c, d) provided that (6.454a) is satisfied involving the Poisson ratio σ. If, in addition to (6.454a) ≡ (6.455a), the bending stiffness is also constant (6.431a) ≡ (6.455b) then (6.454b, c) simplifies to (6.431b–d) ≡ (6.455c):

$$\sigma, D = const: \qquad f(x,y) = D\left(\partial_{xxxx}\zeta + \partial_{yyyy}\zeta + 2\partial_{xxyy}\zeta \right). \qquad (6.455a–c)$$

   The constancy of the Poisson ratio (6.455a) ≡ (6.456a) and (6.455b) ≡ (6.456b) or (6.456c):

$$\sigma, D = const: \qquad D(1-\sigma) = \frac{E h^3}{12\left(1-\sigma^2 \right)} = const, \qquad E h^3 = const, \qquad (6.456a–d)$$

implies that the product of the Young modulus by the cube of the thickness of the plate is constant. The general boundary condition arising from the r.h.s. of (6.453b) is considered in Example 10.15. The boundary conditions in the most important cases of clamping, pinning, support, or free boundary are considered for the linear bending of a thin plate whose boundary is a closed regular curve, including the particular cases of straight and circular edges (subsections 6.7.12–6.7.14), after the comparison of bars (plates) as elastic bodies with stiffness in one (two) dimension(s) next (subsection 6.7.11).

6.7.11 Comparison of the Bending of Bars and Plates

The first method to establish the equation satisfied by the linear bending of a thin plate (6.431a–d) started from the equation for the displacement in the weak bending of a bar (6.411a, c), that in the absence of tangential tension (6.457a) and in the linear case (6.14a) is (6.14f) $\equiv$ (6.457c), allowing for non-uniform bending stiffness (6.457b):

$$T = 0: \qquad B \equiv EI, \qquad f = \left(B\zeta''\right)'', \qquad (6.457\text{a–c})$$

suggesting the comparison *(problem 257): the transverse displacement in the weak linear bending of a non-uniform bar (plate) satisfies similar equations (6.457c) [(6.454b, c)] replacing: (i) the second-order spatial derivative in one-dimension by the two-dimensional Laplacian (6.458a) and hence the fourth-order derivative by the biharmonic operator (6.458b):*

$$\frac{d^2}{dx^2} \leftrightarrow \nabla^2, \qquad \frac{d^4}{dx^4} \leftrightarrow \nabla^4; \qquad \frac{dF}{dx} \leftrightarrow \frac{dF}{dS}, \qquad (6.458\text{a–c})$$

(ii) the force (6.458c) per unit length (area) since the bar (plate) is a one (two) dimensional elastic body; and (iii) the bending stiffness of a plate (6.413d) $\equiv$ (6.459c) by that of a bar (6.459d):

$$\sigma = 0, \qquad I = \frac{h^3}{12}: \qquad D \equiv \frac{E h^3}{12\left(1-\sigma^2\right)} \quad \rightarrow \quad \frac{E h^3}{12} = EI = B, \qquad (6.459\text{a–e})$$

bearing in mind that: (iii-1) the Poisson ratio is zero (6.459a) for a bar, because the transverse displacement is neglected, leading from (6.459c) to (6.459d); (iii-2) using the moment of inertia of the cross-section (6.412a) $\equiv$ (6.459b) leads from (6.459d) to (6.459e) $\equiv$ (6.457b); that is, the bending stiffness of a bar.

The equation (6.431b–d) for the linear bending of a thin plate was obtained by two distinct methods based [subsections 6.7.2–6.7.6 (6.7.7–6.7.10)] on the balance of forces and moments (principle of virtual work). The first method: (i) starts with the weak bending equation for a beam (6.457a–c) along

(6.411a–d) the two lines of principal curvature (subsection 6.7.2); (ii) a rotation in the plane leads to a general Cartesian reference frame (subsection 6.7.3) where exist both curvatures and twist; (iii) the associated twist and stress couples (subsection 6.7.4) specify (iv) the elastic energy of bending (subsection 6.7.5); and (v) the twist and stress couples are related to the turning moments and transverse force per unit area (subsection 6.7.6) leading to the equation (6.431b–d) for the deflection of the plate with constant bending stiffness (6.431a). The second method is shorter: (a) starting from the displacements to obtain the strains and stresses (subsection 6.7.7) that lead to the elastic energy (b) [(iv)] by a different method [subsection 6.7.8 (6.7.5)]: (c) the elastic energy is balanced against the virtual work of the transverse forces (subsection 6.7.9) leading to (6.454a–c) the (c) [(v)] displacement equation [subsection 6.7.10 (6.7.6)] without the assumption of constant bending stiffness. The second method (α) extends the first to non-uniform bending stiffness, such as a homogeneous plate with variable thickness and (β) can also be used to obtain the general boundary conditions. The general boundary conditions for the linear bending of a thin plate can be obtained from the vanishing of the boundary integral in (6.453a). As for a bar (subsection III.4.2.7), the three most important cases of boundary conditions for a plate are (subsection 6.7.12) clamped (Figure 6.23a), supported (Figure 6.23b) or pinned (Figure 6.23c), and free (Figure 6.23d), that can be expressed (subsection 6.7.13) in terms of displacements, normal derivatives, stress couples, and turning moments. The boundary conditions for the weak linear bending

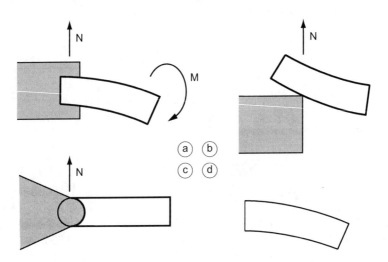

FIGURE 6.23
The four most common boundary conditions for the bending of a plate are: (a) clamped, that is, with fixed displacement and slope, leading to the existence of stress couple and turning moment; (b) supported or (c) pinned, with fixed displacement and stress couple, leading to non-zero slope and turning moment; (d) free, where at a free boundary the stress couple and turning moment vanish but not the displacement and slope.

of a thin elastic plate (subsection 6.7.14) may be considered: (i) in the general case when the boundary is a closed regular curve with arbitrary shape (Example 10.13) using the boundary integral in (6.453a); (ii–iii) simpler methods (subsection 6.7.12) can be used in the particular cases of straight or circular boundaries (subsection 6.7.13) covering also some cases of arbitrary boundaries (subsection 6.7.14).

6.7.12 Clamped, Pinned, and Free Boundaries

The three most common boundary conditions (problem 258) for the weak linear bending of an elastic plate:

$$\text{boundary} \begin{cases} \zeta = 0 = \partial_n\zeta: & \text{clamped,} & (6.460\text{a,b}) \\ \zeta = 0 = M_n: & \text{pinned or supported,} & (6.460\text{c,d}) \\ M_n = 0 = N_n: & \text{free,} & (6.460\text{e,f}) \end{cases}$$

*are: (i) **clamped** (Figure 6.23a), that is with zero displacement (6.460a) and slope (6.460b); (ii) **supported** (Figure 6.23b) or **pinned** (Figure 6.23c), with zero displacement (6.460c) and stress couple (6.460d); and (iii) **free** boundary (Figure 6.23d), with zero stress couple (6.460e) and zero turning moment (6.460f). Thus, the boundary conditions (i–iii) in (6.460a–f) involve the: (a) displacement; (b) slope; (c) stress couple; and (d) turning moment. All four (a–d) are considered next in turn at the boundary. For a plate (problem 259) occupying a domain C with arbitrary shape (Figure 6.24a) with regular boundary ∂C, the transverse deflection is a function of the Cartesian coordinates (6.461a), and the boundary curve (6.459b) is specified by the arc length s as a function of the angle θ of the normal with the x-axis, with the derivative specifying the radius of curvature (6.3b) ≡ (6.461c) that is the inverse of the curvature (6.461d):*

$$D: \quad z = \zeta(x,y); \quad \partial D: \quad s(\theta) \in C^1(\partial C), \quad R = \frac{ds}{d\theta} = \frac{1}{k}. \quad (6.461\text{a–d})$$

The unit normal (6.462a) [tangent (6.462c)] to the boundary specify the normal (6.462c) [tangential (6.462d)] derivatives:

$$\vec{n} = \{\cos\theta, \sin\theta\}: \quad \partial_n = \vec{n}.\nabla = \cos\theta\,\partial_x + \sin\theta\,\partial_y, \quad (6.462\text{a, b})$$

$$\vec{s} = \{-\sin\theta, \cos\theta\}: \quad \partial_s = \vec{s}.\nabla = -\sin\theta\,\partial_x + \cos\theta\,\partial_y, \quad (6.462\text{c, d})$$

where θ is the angle of the normal with a fixed direction like the x-axis (Figure 6.24a). The relation between the normal (6.462b) and tangential (6.462d) derivatives

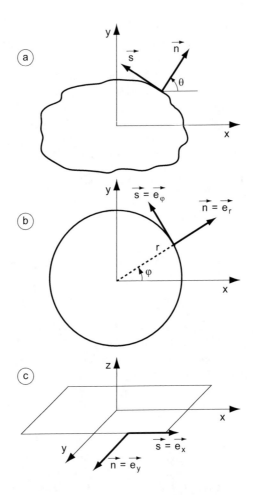

FIGURE 6.24
The balance equation specifying the shape of the directrix (Figure 6.20) of a bent plate
(Figure 6.21a, b) and the associated boundary conditions (Figures 6.23a–d) may be applied
(Figure 6.22) to the general case (a) of a plate whose boundary is a closed regular curve. The
most common particular cases are a (b) circular [(c) rectangular] plate whose boundary curve
is regular everywhere (except at the corners, that are an infinitesimal of order two, compared
with the sides that are an infinitesimal of order one, and the interior that has finite area).

and the Cartesian derivatives is inverted by (6.463b, c) using the transformation
(6.463a):

$$\{\partial_x,\partial_y,\theta\} \leftrightarrow \{\partial_n,\partial_s,-\theta\}: \quad \partial_x=\cos\theta\,\partial_n-\sin\theta\,\partial_s, \quad \partial_y=\sin\theta\partial_n+\cos\theta\,\partial_s.$$

$$(6.463\text{a--c})$$

The condition of zero displacement (6.461a) applies to a clamped (6.460a) or pinned
(6.460c) plate. The clamped condition (6.460b) of zero slope:

$$0=\partial_n\zeta=\cos\theta\partial_x\zeta+\sin\theta\partial_y\zeta \rightarrow r=a: \partial_r\zeta=0 \rightarrow y=const: \partial_y\zeta=0, \quad (6.464\text{a--e})$$

is: (i) for arbitrary shape (Figure 6.24a) given by (6.464a); (ii) in the case (6.464b) of a circular plate (Figure 6.24b) reduces to the vanishing of the radial derivative (6.464c); and (iii) for the straight y = const side (6.464d) of a rect-angular plate parallel to the x-axis (Figure 6.24c) reduces to (6.464e). Besides the displacement (6.461a–d) and slope (6.464a–c), the boundary conditions (6.460a–f) involve the stress couple and turning moment that are considered next (subsection 6.7.12).

6.7.13 Normal Stress Couple and Turning Moment

The turning moment is specified by (6.430a, b) ≡ (6.465a) involving the gradient (Laplacian) that is specified by (I.11.50) ≡ (6.465b) [(I.11.52) ≡ (6.465c)] for orthogonal curvilinear coordinates in the plane:

$$\vec{N} = D\nabla(\nabla^2\zeta): \qquad \nabla = \frac{\vec{e}_1}{h_1}\partial_1 + \frac{\vec{e}_2}{h_2}\partial_2, \qquad (6.465a, b)$$

$$\nabla^2 = \frac{1}{h_1 h_2}\left[\partial_1\left(\frac{h_2}{h_1}\partial_1\right) + \partial_2\left(\frac{h_2}{h_2}\partial_2\right)\right], \qquad (6.465c)$$

where $(\vec{e}_1, \vec{e}_2)$ are the unit base vector along the (x_1, x_2)-axis and (h_1, h_2) the corresponding scale factors. The scale factors: (i) are (III.6.10a) ≡ (6.466a, b) in Cartesian coordinates (x, y); (ii) are (III.6.14a) ≡ (6.466c, d) in polar coordinates (r, θ):

$$h_x = 1 = h_y; \qquad h_r = 1, \ h_\theta = r; \qquad h_n = 1, \ h_s = R = \frac{ds}{d\theta}, \ \partial_n R = 1, \qquad (6.466a–g)$$

and (iii) are equal to unity (6.466e) [the radius of curvature (6.461c) ≡ (6.466f)] for orthogonal curvilinear coordinates normal and tangent to an arbitrary regular curve, that satisfy (6.466g). *Considering (problem 260) respectively a straight (Figure 6.24c) / circular (Figure 6.24b) / arbitrary regular (Figure 6.24a) boundary to which the plate is fixed (6.467a/c/e), the turning moment (6.465a–c) is given: (i) by (6.467b) for (6.466a, b) the y-component orthogonal to the straight boundary along the x-axis (6.467a); (ii) by (6.467d) for the radial component (6.466c, d) orthogonal to (6.467c) the circle of radius a; and (iii) by (6.467f) for the normal component (6.466e, f) to an arbitrary regular boundary curve (6.467e):*

$$y = const: \qquad N_y = D\,\partial_y\big(\partial_{xx}\zeta + \partial_{yy}\zeta\big), \qquad (6.467a, b)$$

$$r = a: \qquad N_r = D\partial_r\left(\partial_{rr}\zeta + \frac{1}{r}\partial_r\zeta\right); \qquad (6.467c, d)$$

$$s(\theta) \in C^1(\partial C): \qquad N_n = D\partial_n\left(\partial_{nn}\zeta + \frac{d\theta}{ds}\partial_n\zeta\right). \qquad\qquad (6.467e, f)$$

In (6.467d) [(6.467f)] were used (6.468a) [(6.468b)]:

$$\frac{1}{r}\partial_r\left(r\partial_r\zeta\right) = \partial_{rr}\zeta + \frac{1}{r}\partial_r\zeta, \qquad\qquad (6.468a)$$

$$\frac{1}{R}\partial_n\left(R\partial_n\zeta\right) = \partial_{nn}\zeta + \frac{1}{R}\partial_n\zeta = \partial_{rr}\zeta + \frac{d\theta}{ds}\partial_r\zeta, \qquad (6.468b\text{--}d)$$

where the passage from (6.468b) to (6.468c) [(6.468d)] uses (6.466g) [(6.461d)].

The boundary conditions (6.460a–f) involve, besides the displacement (6.461a–d), slope (6.464a–e), turning moment (6.467a–f), and also the stress couple, for which can be used the following transformation implied by (6.467a–f): *the passage (problem 261) from orthogonal curvilinear coordinates normal and tangent to an arbitrary regular curve (6.467e) ≡ (6.469a) to radial coordinates orthogonal to a circle (6.467c) ≡ (6.469b) involves: (i) exchanging normal (6.469c) by radial (6.469d) derivatives; and (ii) replacing the radius of curvature (6.469e) ≡ (6.461d) by the distance from the origin (6.469f):*

$$s(\theta) \in C^1(\partial C) \quad\leftrightarrow\quad r = a: \qquad \partial_n \leftrightarrow \partial_r, \qquad R = \frac{ds}{d\theta} \leftrightarrow r; \qquad (6.469a\text{--}f)$$

$$r = a \quad\leftrightarrow\quad y = 0: \qquad \partial_{rr} \leftrightarrow \partial_{yy}, \qquad \frac{1}{r}\partial_r \leftrightarrow \partial_{xx}, \qquad (6.470a\text{--}f)$$

the passage (problem 262) from polar coordinates in the radial direction orthogonal to a circle (6.467c) ≡ (6.470a) to Cartesian coordinates along the y-axis orthogonal to the x-axis (6.467a) ≡ (6.470b) replaces the radial derivatives according to (6.470c, d) and (6.470e, f). The stress couple (6.422b; 6.423a, b) ≡ (6.471b) orthogonal to the x-axis (6.471a):

$$y = const: \qquad -\frac{M_y}{D} = \partial_{yy}\zeta + \sigma\partial_{xx}\zeta, \qquad\qquad (6.471a, b)$$

$$r = a: \qquad -\frac{M_r}{D} = \partial_{rr}\zeta + \frac{\sigma}{r}\partial_r\zeta, \qquad\qquad (6.471c, d)$$

$$s(\theta) \in C^1(\partial C): \qquad -\frac{M_n}{D} = \partial_{nn}\zeta + \sigma\frac{d\theta}{ds}\partial_n\zeta, \qquad\qquad (6.471e, f)$$

becomes (6.471d) [(6.471f)] in the radial (normal) direction; that is, orthogonal to a circle (6.471c) [arbitrary regular curve (6.471e)], using the transformations

(6.470a–f) [(6.469a–f)]. Thus, *(problem 263) respectively for an arbitrary regular bound-ary curve (Figure 6.24a) / the radial direction orthogonal to a circle (Figure 6.24b) / the y-direction orthogonal to a straight (line parallel to the x-axis (Figure 6.24c) correspond-ing to a plate with arbitrary/circular/ rectangular shape with fixed boundary: (i) the dis-placement is given by (6.461a) in the interior with boundary (6.461b) with curvature (6.461c) and radius of curvature (6.461d); (ii) the slope is given by (6.464a/b, c/d, e); and (iii–iv) the normal/radial/orthogonal stress couple (turning moment) by (6.471a, b/c, d/e, f) [(6.467a, b/c, d/e, f)].* Applying the preceding statements (i) to (iv) to (6.460a–f) leads to the boundary conditions for the linear bending of thin plate with rectangular, circular or arbitrary shapes (subsection 6.7.13).

6.7.14 Rectangular, Circular, and Arbitrarily Shaped Plates

The three most common cases of boundary conditions (6.460a–f) are indicated in Table 6.7, and may be applied (problem 264) respectively to a straight/circular/arbi-trary regular curved boundary as follows: (i) for (6.460a, b) a clamped (Figure 6.23a) plate (6.472a, b/6.473a, b/6.474a, b) the stress couples (6.472c/6.473c/6.474c) and turning moments (6.472d/6.473d/6.474d) are non-zero:

$$\zeta(x,0)=0=\partial_y\zeta: \qquad M_y=-D\partial_{yy}\zeta, \qquad N_y=D\partial_{yyy}\zeta, \qquad (6.472a\text{–}d)$$

$$\zeta(a,\phi)=0=\partial_r\zeta: \qquad -\frac{M_r}{D}=\partial_{rr}\zeta+\frac{\sigma}{r}\partial_r\zeta, \qquad \frac{N_r}{D}=\partial_r\left(\partial_{rr}\zeta+\frac{1}{r}\partial_r\zeta\right),$$
$$(6.473a\text{–}d)$$

$$\zeta=0=\partial_n\zeta: \qquad -\frac{M_n}{D}=\partial_{nn}\zeta+\sigma\frac{d\theta}{ds}\partial_n\zeta, \qquad \frac{N_n}{D}=\partial_n\left(\partial_{nn}\zeta+\frac{d\theta}{ds}\partial_n\zeta\right);$$
$$(6.474a\text{–}d)$$

(ii) for a supported (Figure 6.23b) or pinned (Figure 6.23c) plate (6.460c, d) the dis-placement (6.475a/6.476a/6.477a) [slope (6.475b/6.476b/6.477b)] is zero (not-zero), implying a non-zero turning moment (6.477d/6.476d/6.477d) [a zero stress couple specifying the second boundary condition (6.475c/6.476c/6.477c)]:

$$\zeta(x,0)=0\neq\partial_y\zeta: \qquad \partial_{yy}\zeta=0, \qquad N_y=D\,\partial_{yyy}\zeta, \qquad (6.475a\text{–}d)$$

$$\zeta(a,\phi)=0\neq\partial_r\zeta: \qquad \partial_{rr}\zeta+\frac{\sigma}{r}\partial_r\zeta=0, \qquad \frac{N_r}{D}=\partial_r\left(\partial_{rr}\zeta+\frac{1}{r}\partial_r\zeta\right), \qquad (6.476a\text{–}d)$$

$$\zeta=0\neq\partial_n\zeta: \qquad \partial_{nn}\zeta+\sigma\frac{d\theta}{ds}\partial_n\zeta=0, \qquad \frac{N_n}{D}=\partial_n\left(\partial_{nn}\zeta+\frac{d\theta}{ds}\partial_n\zeta\right); \qquad (6.477a\text{–}d)$$

and (iii) for a (Figure 6.24d) free boundary (6.460e, f) the displacement (6.478a/6.479a/6.480a) [slope (6.478b/6.479b/6.480b)] are both non-zero, and the vanishing of the stress couple (6.478c/6.479c/6.480c) [turning moment (6.478d/6.479d/6.480d)] specifies the first (second) boundary condition:

$$\zeta(x,0) \neq 0 \neq \partial_y \zeta: \qquad \partial_{yy}\zeta + \sigma\partial_{xx}\zeta = 0 = \partial_y\left(\partial_{xx}\zeta + \partial_{yy}\zeta\right), \qquad (6.478a\text{–}d)$$

$$\zeta(a,\phi) \neq 0 \neq \partial_r \zeta: \qquad \partial_{rr}\zeta + \frac{\sigma}{r}\partial_r\zeta = 0 = \partial_r\left(\partial_{rr}\zeta + \frac{1}{r}\partial_r\zeta\right), \qquad (6.479a\text{–}d)$$

$$\zeta \neq 0 \neq \partial_n\zeta: \quad \left(\partial_{nn}\zeta + \frac{d\theta}{ds}\partial_n\zeta\right) + (1-\sigma)\left[\sin(2\theta)\partial_{xy}\zeta - \sin^2\theta\,\partial_{xx}\zeta - \cos^2\theta\,\partial_{yy}\zeta\right] = 0,$$

$$\partial_{nnn}\zeta + \frac{d\theta}{ds}\partial_{nn}\zeta - (1-\sigma)\left[\sin\theta\cos\theta\left(\partial_{xx}\zeta - \partial_{yy}\zeta\right) - \cos(2\theta)\partial_{xy}\zeta\right] = 0.$$
$$(6.480a\text{–}d)$$

The free boundary conditions (6.480c) [(6.480d)] for the linear bending of a thin plate whose boundary is an arbitrary closed regular curve are less simple than (6.471a–f) [(6.467a–f)], that can be obtained as particular cases of the general method (Example 10.15) based on the boundary integral (6.453a).

The simpler methods used before (subsections 6.7.12–6.7.14) can be used to derive the radial stress couple (6.471d) without using the transformation (6.470a–f) as shown next. The consideration of pinned and free boundary conditions for circular plates (6.473c) and hence for arbitrary (6.474c) [rectangular (6.472c)] shapes, was based on the vanishing of the stress couple (6.422a–c; 6.423a–c) that is next shown to be specified in the radial direction by (6.481c):

$$k_r = \partial_{rr}\zeta, \quad k_\phi = \frac{1}{r}\partial_r\zeta: \quad M_r = -D\left(k_r + \sigma k_\phi\right) = -D\left(\partial_{rr}\zeta + \frac{\sigma}{r}\partial_r\zeta\right), \qquad (6.481a\text{–}d)$$

where (6.481a) [(6.481b)] is the curvature along the normal (tangent) to the circle; from (6.481a–c) follows (6.481d) and the condition $M_r = 0$ leads to the boundary condition (6.479c). The curvatures (6.481a, b) that appear in the stress couple (6.481c) can be calculated in polar coordinates (6.482a, b) using (6.482c):

$$\{x,y\} = r\{\cos\phi, \sin\phi\}: \quad \frac{\partial}{\partial x} = \frac{\partial r}{\partial x}\frac{\partial}{\partial r} + \frac{\partial\phi}{\partial x}\frac{\partial}{\partial\phi} = \cos\phi\,\frac{\partial}{\partial r} - \frac{\sin\phi}{r}\frac{\partial}{\partial\phi}, \qquad (6.482a\text{–}c)$$

where one coefficient was evaluated by (II.7.123a):

$$\frac{\partial\phi}{\partial x} = \frac{\partial}{\partial x}\left[\arg\cos\left(\frac{x}{r}\right)\right] = -\left(1 - \frac{x^2}{r^2}\right)^{-1/2}\frac{\partial}{\partial x}\left(\frac{x}{r}\right) = -\frac{r}{y}\left(\frac{1}{r} - \frac{x^2}{r^3}\right) = -\frac{y}{r^2} = -\frac{\sin\phi}{r},$$
$$(6.483)$$

using (6.484b):

$$r^2 = x^2 + y^2: \qquad \frac{\partial r}{\partial x} = \frac{\partial}{\partial x}\left[\left(x^2 + y^2\right)^{-1/2}\right] = -x\left(r^2 + y^2\right)^{-3/2} = -\frac{x}{r^3}, \qquad \text{(6.484a, b)}$$

that follows from (6.484a). The curvature (6.423a) is thus given by:

$$k_x = \partial_{xx}\zeta = \left(\cos\phi\,\partial_r - \frac{\sin\phi}{r}\partial_\phi\right)\left(\cos\phi\,\partial_r - \frac{\sin\phi}{r}\partial_\phi\right)\zeta$$

$$= \cos^2\phi\,\partial_{rr}\zeta + \frac{\sin^2\phi}{r^2}\partial_{\phi\phi}\zeta - \frac{\sin(2\phi)}{r}\partial_{r\phi}\zeta + \frac{\sin(2\phi)}{2r^2}\partial_\phi\zeta + \frac{\sin^2\phi}{r}\partial_r\zeta.$$

$$\text{(6.485)}$$

The curvature normal (6.486a) [tangent (6.486b)] to the circle corresponds to constant $\phi = 0(\phi = \pi/2)$ in (6.485):

$$k_r = k_x(\phi = 0) = \partial_{rr}\zeta; \qquad \partial_\phi = 0: \qquad k_\phi = k_x\left(\phi = \frac{\pi}{2}\right) = \frac{1}{r}\partial_r\zeta, \qquad \text{(6.486a–c)}$$

in agreement with (6.481a) ≡ (6.486a) and (6.481b) ≡ (6.486b, c).

It has been shown that *(problem 265): (i) the curvature in polar coordinates (6.482a, b) is given by (6.485); (ii) in the particular case of a circle (6.486b) the radial (azimuthal) curvature is (6.486a) [(6.486c)], that specify the radial stress couple (6.481c, d) involving the bending stiffness (6.413c, d); (iii) the vanishing of the stress couple applies (6.460d, e) to a supported or pinned (Figure 6.23b, d) or free (Figure 6.23d) boundary, for arbitrary (Figure 6.24a), circular (Figure 6.24b) or rectangular (Figure 6.24c) shape; (iv) at a free boundary the turning moment vanishes (6.460f); (v) at a clamped boundary the slope (6.460b) vanishes; (vi) at a clamped or pinned or supported boundary the displacement vanishes (6.460a, c); (vii) at each boundary there is a pair of boundary conditions (6.460a–f) indicated in Table 6.7; (viii) the transformation of boundary conditions from a plate with arbitrary shape to circular (6.469a–f) [rectangular (6.470a–f)] shape is indicated in Table 6.6.* The three types of boundary conditions are applied to circular plates: (i) clamped or pinned (subsection 6.7.16) with a concentrated force at the center (subsection 6.7.15); (ii) clamped or pinned under a uniform load (subsection 6.7.16) such as its own weight (subsection 6.7.18); and (iii) held by the center and bent by its own weight with a free boundary (subsection 6.7.19).

6.7.15 Bending Due to a Concentrated Force at the Center

The weak linear bending of a plate with constant (6.431a) ≡ (6.487a) bending stiffness (6.413c, d) by a concentrated force F is specified (6.431b) by (6.487b):

$$D \equiv \text{const}: \qquad DV^4\zeta = f = F\delta(x)\delta(y) = \frac{F}{2\pi r}\delta(r), \qquad \text{(6.487a–d)}$$

TABLE 6.6

Boundary Conditions for the Bending of a Plate

Case	I	II	III
Type	clamped	supported or pinned	free
First boundary condition	$\zeta = 0$	$\zeta = 0$	$M_n = 0$
Second boundary condition	$\partial_n \zeta = 0$	$M_n = 0$	$N_n = 0$
*Displacement**		(6.461a–d)/(6.467c)/(6.467a)	
*Slope**		(6.464a, b/c, d/e)	
*Stress couple**	(6.480c/6.479c/6.478c)	(6.477c/6.476c/6.475c)	(6.474c/6.473c/6.472c)
*Turning moment**	(6.480d/6.479d/6.478d)	(6.477d/6.476c/6.475d)	(6.674d/6.473d/6.472d)

* for rectangular/circular/shape in Figure 6.24c/b/a

Note: The most common boundary conditions for the bending of a plate are clamped (Figure 6.23a), supported (Figure 6.23b) or pinned (Figure 6.23c), and free (6.23d) that may involve the displacement, slope, stress couple, and/or turning moment.

TABLE 6.7

Bending of General, Circular, and Rectangular Plates

Plate	Arbitrary Domain	Circular	Rectangular
Boundary	regular curve	circle	straight line
Figure	6.24a	6.24b	6.24c
Equation	$\zeta(\theta) \in C^1(\partial C)$	$r = \text{const} \equiv a$	$y = 0$
Radius of curvature	$R = \dfrac{ds}{d\theta}$	$R = r$	$R = \infty$
Transverse displacement	$z = \zeta(s, \theta)$	$z = \zeta(r, \phi)$	$z = \zeta(x, y)$
Zero displacement	$\zeta(s, \theta) = 0$	$\zeta(a, \phi) = 0$	$\zeta(x, 0) = 0$
Zero slope	$\partial_n \zeta = 0$	$\partial_r \zeta = 0$	$\partial_y \zeta = 0$
Stress couple	(6.474c)*	(6.473c)	(6.472c)
Turning moment	(6.474d)**	(6.473d)	(6.472d)
Clamped (Figure 6.23a)	(6.474a–d)	(6.473a–d)	(6.472a–d)
Supported (Figure 6.23b) or pinned (Figure 6.23c)	(6.477a–d)	(6.476a–d)	(6.475a–d)
Free boundary (Figure 6.23d)	(6.480a–d)	(6.479a–d)	(6.478a–d)

* assuming zero displacement; in general (10.126).

** assuming zero displacement; in general (10.127).

Note: The boundary conditions for the bending of plate (Table 6.6) are indicated in general for a plate whose boundary is an arbitrary closed regular curve (Figure 6.24a) and in particular for a circular plate (Figure 6.24b) and the straight edge along the *x*-axis of a rectangular plate (Figure 6.24c).

where: (i) a concentrated force F corresponds to a force per unit area involving (6.487c) the product of two Dirac delta functions (section III.1.3; subsection III.3.1.2) of the Cartesian coordinates (x,y) in the plane; (ii) this product is equivalent (III.5.60a, b) $\equiv$ (6.487d) to a Dirac delta function of the radius r divided by the perimeter of the circle of radius r. The radial symmetry (6.488a) in (6.487c) simplifies the biharmonic or double Laplace operator in polar coordinates (6.334a) to (6.488b) $\equiv$ (6.488c):

$$\partial_\phi = 0: \qquad \frac{F}{2\pi r}\delta(r) = D\left[\frac{1}{r}\frac{d}{dr}\left(r\frac{d}{dr}\right)\right]^2 \zeta = \frac{D}{r}\left\{r\left[\frac{1}{r}(r\zeta')'\right]'\right\}'. \qquad (6.488a\text{–}c)$$

The Green function corresponds to $F = 1$ in (6.487c, d) with the singularity of the delta function at an arbitrary position, in general not restricted to the center of the circular plate. The first integral of (6.488c) is (6.489c):

$$r > 0: \qquad \frac{F}{2\pi D} = \frac{F}{2\pi D}H(r) = r\left[\frac{1}{r}(r\zeta')'\right]' = r\zeta''' + \zeta'' - \frac{1}{r}\zeta', \qquad (6.489a\text{–}d)$$

where the Heaviside unit function (III.1.28c) is unity (6.489b) outside the origin (6.489a). The displacement is obtained by three successive integrations of (6.489c):

$$\frac{F}{2\pi D}\log r + 4C_1 = \frac{1}{r}(r\zeta')' = \nabla^2\zeta, \qquad (6.490a)$$

$$r\zeta' = \frac{F}{4\pi D}r^2\left(\log r - \frac{1}{2}\right) + 2C_1 r^2 + C_2, \qquad (6.490b)$$

$$\zeta = \frac{F}{8\pi D}r^2(\log r - 1) + C_1 r^2 + C_2\log r + C_3, \qquad (6.490c)$$

each introducing a constant of integration; the primitive:

$$\int r\log r\,dr = \int \log r\,d\left(\frac{r^2}{2}\right) = \frac{r^2}{2}\log r - \int \frac{r^2}{2}d(\log r)$$

$$= \frac{r^2}{2}\log r - \int \frac{r}{2}dr = \frac{r^2}{2}\left(\log r - \frac{1}{2}\right), \qquad (6.491)$$

was used in the passage from (6.490a) to (6.490b) and to (6.490c). The transverse displacement of the directrix of the plate is specified by the solution

(6.490c) of the differential equation (6.431a–d) forced (6.487a–d) ≡ (6.488a–c) by a unit impulse (subsection 6.7.15) at the center together with boundary conditions to determine the constants of integration.

One of the three constants of integration in (6.490c) is zero (6.492b) for a disk in order for the displacement to be finite at the center (6.492a):

$$\zeta(0) < \infty: \qquad C_2 = 0; \quad 0 = \zeta(a) = \frac{F a^2}{8\pi D}(\log a - 1) + C_1 a^2 + C_3, \qquad (6.492\text{a–c})$$

the remaining two constants of integration are determined by boundary conditions, namely for a plate clamped (supported) on a circle [Figure 6.25a(b)] of radius a: (i) the displacement is zero (6.460a) [(6.460c)] in both cases (6.492c); and (ii) in the clamped (pinned) case the slope (6.473b) [radial stress couple (6.479c)] is zero (6.493a) [(6.493b)]:

$$0 = \frac{\zeta_1'(a)}{a} = \frac{F}{4\pi D}\left(\log a - \frac{1}{2}\right) + 2C_1, \qquad (6.493\text{a})$$

$$0 = \zeta_2''(a) + \frac{\sigma}{a}\zeta_2'(a) = \frac{F}{4\pi D}\left[(1+\sigma)\left(\log a - \frac{1}{2}\right) + 1\right] + 2C_1(1+\sigma). \qquad (6.493\text{b})$$

Substituting (6.492c) in (6.490c) leads to the transverse displacement:

$$\zeta(r) = \frac{F}{8\pi D}\left[r^2 \log r - a^2 \log a + a^2 - r^2\right] + C_1\left(r^2 - a^2\right), \qquad (6.494)$$

that applies both to the clamped (pinned) case with (subsection 6.7.15) different values (6.493a) [(6.493b)] of the constant C_1.

6.7.16 Bending of a Clamped/Supported Circular Plate

Substituting (6.493a) [(6.493b)] in (6.494) leads to:

$$\{\zeta_1(r), \zeta_2(r)\} = \frac{F}{16\pi D}\left[2r^2 \log\left(\frac{r}{a}\right) + (a^2 - r^2)\left\{1, \frac{3+\sigma}{1+\sigma}\right\}\right], \qquad (6.495\text{a, b})$$

showing *that the weak linear bending of a circular plate of radius a, with a concentrated force F at the center, clamped (pinned) the edge in Figure 6.25a(b) leads [problem 266 (267)] to: (i) the displacement (6.495a) [(6.495b)] that is maximum (6.496b) [(6.496c)] at the center (6.496a):*

$$r = 0: \qquad \zeta_{1\max} = \frac{1+\sigma}{3+\sigma}\zeta_{2\max} = \frac{F a^2}{16\pi D} = \frac{3\left(1-\sigma^2\right) F a^2}{4\pi E h^3}, \qquad (6.496\text{a–d})$$

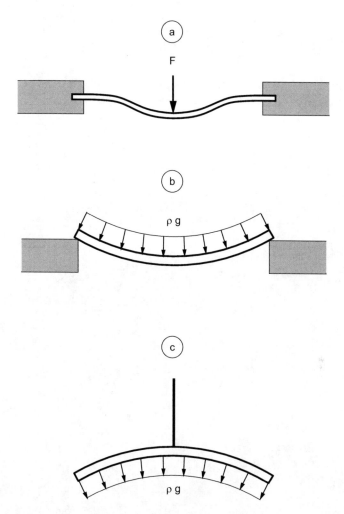

FIGURE 6.25
Three examples of the bending of an elastic plate (Figures 6.19–6.22) is the effect on a circular plate (Figure 6.24b) of a concentrated force (Figure 6.25a) or its own weight (Figures 6.25b, c) in the cases when the circular edge is: (a) clamped (Figure 6.23a); (b) supported (Figure 6.23b) or pinned (Figure 6.23a); or (c) free (Figure 6.23d) with the plate suspended from the center.

where was used (6.496d) the bending stiffness (6.413d); (ii) the slope (6.497a) [(6.497b)] that vanishes (6.497c) [does not vanish (6.497d)] at the boundary in the clamped (supported) case:

$$\left\{ \zeta_1'(r),\ \zeta_2'(r) \right\} = \frac{Fr}{4\pi D}\left[\log\!\left(\frac{r}{a}\right) + \left\{0,-\frac{1}{1+\sigma}\right\} \right], \qquad \text{(6.497a, b)}$$

$$\zeta_1'(a) = 0, \qquad \zeta_2'(a) = -\frac{Fa}{4\pi D(1+\sigma)} = -\frac{3Fa(1-\sigma)}{\pi E h^3}; \qquad (6.497\text{c, d})$$

(iii) the radial (6.481d) ≡ (6.498a) [(6.498b)] stress couple does not (does) vanish in the boundary in the clamped (6.498c) [supported (6.498d)] case:

$$M_{r1,2} = -D\left[\zeta_{1,2}''(r) + \frac{\sigma}{r}\zeta_{1,2}'(r)\right] = -\frac{F}{4\pi}\left[(1+\sigma)\log\left(\frac{r}{a}\right) + \{1,0\}\right], \quad (6.498\text{a–d})$$

$$M_{r1}(a) = -\frac{F}{4\pi}, \qquad\qquad M_{r2}(a) = 0; \qquad (6.498\text{c, d})$$

(iv) the turning moments (6.430a, b):

$$N_r = \frac{F}{2\pi r}: \qquad \{N_x(r), N_y(r)\} = D\{\partial_x, \partial_y\}\left(\zeta'' + \frac{\zeta'}{r}\right)$$

$$= \frac{F}{4\pi}\{\partial_x, \partial_y\}\left[2\log\left(\frac{r}{a}\right) + \left\{1, -\frac{1-\sigma}{1+\sigma}\right\}\right]$$

$$= \frac{F}{4\pi}\{\partial_x, \partial_y\}2\log r = \frac{F}{2\pi r^2}\{x, y\} \qquad\qquad (6.499\text{a–g})$$

$$= \frac{F}{2\pi r}\{\cos\phi, \sin\phi\} = N_r\{\cos\phi, \sin\phi\},$$

that are: (iv–1) independent of material properties and boundary conditions (6.499b–g); (iv–2) uniform along the boundary and with radial component equal to the force divided the perimeter (6.499a); and (v) the area (6.438c) ≡ (6.500a)[volume (6.439c) ≡ (6.500b)] changes are given (6.500c) ≡ (6.500d) by (6.500e) [(6.500f)]:

$$D_2 = \frac{1-\sigma}{1-2\sigma}D_3 = -z\nabla^2\zeta = -z\left(\zeta'' + \frac{\zeta}{r}\right) = -\frac{zF}{4\pi}\left[2\log\left(\frac{r}{a}\right) + \left\{1, -\frac{1-\sigma}{1+\sigma}\right\}\right].$$

$$(6.500\text{a–f})$$

Two opposite extremes are a concentrated (uniform) load [subsection 6.7.14 (6.7.16)] that can be applied to a clamped or pinned plate [subsection 6.7.15 (6.7.17)].

6.7.17 Constant Forcing of a Biharmonic Equation with Radial Symmetry

The solution of the biharmonic equation with radial symmetry and constant forcing, like the weight (6.501a):

$$f = \rho g: \quad \frac{\rho g}{D} = \nabla^4 \zeta = r^{-1}\left\{r\left[r^{-1}\left(r\zeta'\right)'\right]'\right\}' = \zeta'''' + 2r^{-1}\zeta''' - r^{-2}\zeta'' + r^{-3}\zeta'.$$

$$(6.501a\text{–}c)$$

can be obtained (6.501b, c) by two methods. The first, like (6.490a–c), is four successive integrations of (6.501b), each introducing a constant of integration:

$$r\left[r^{-1}\left(r\zeta'\right)'\right]' = \frac{\rho g r^2}{2D} + 4C_4, \qquad (6.502a)$$

$$r^{-1}\left(r\zeta'\right)' = \frac{\rho g r^2}{4D} + 4C_4\log r + 4C_3 \equiv \nabla^2\zeta, \qquad (6.502b, c)$$

$$r\zeta' = \frac{\rho g r^4}{16D} + 2C_4 r^2\left(\log r - \frac{1}{2}\right) + 2C_3 r^2 + C_2, \qquad (4.502d)$$

$$\zeta(r) = \frac{\rho g r^4}{64D} + C_4 r^2\left(\log r - 1\right) + C_3 r^2 + C_2\log r + C_1; \qquad (6.502e)$$

in the passage from (6.502b) to (6.502d) and (6.502e) was used (6.491). *The first (last four) term(s) on the r.h.s. of (6.502e) is (problem 268) the particular (general) integral (6.503d) [(6.503e)] of the forced (6.503a) [unforced (6.503b)] biharmonic equation:*

$$\nabla^2\zeta_* = \frac{\rho g}{D}, \qquad \nabla^4\overline{\zeta} = 0, \qquad \zeta(r) = \zeta_* + \overline{\zeta}(r): \qquad (6.503a\text{–}c)$$

$$\zeta_*(r) = \frac{\rho g r^4}{64D}, \qquad \overline{\zeta}(r) = C_4 r^2\left(\log r - 1\right) + C_2\log r + C_3 r^2 + C_1. \qquad (6.503d, e)$$

whose sum is the complete integral (6.503c).

The complete integral of (6.503c) can also be obtained by separately calculating the two contributions. The particular integral of (6.503a) may be sought in the form (6.504a), leading on substitution in (6.501c) to (6.504b):

$$\zeta_* = Cr^4: \quad \frac{\rho g}{D} = \nabla^4\left(Cr^4\right) = C(24 + 48 - 12 + 4) = 64C; \quad \zeta_* = \frac{\rho g r^4}{64D}; \quad (6.504a\text{–}c)$$

substituting (6.504b) in (6.504a) yields (6.504c) ≡ (6.503d), which is the particular integral of (6.503a), in agreement with the first term on the r.h.s. of (6.502e).

The general integral of (6.503b), using (6.501c), leads to a linear fourth-order ordinary differential equation (6.505b) with homogeneous power coefficients of Euler (1.291a) type:

$$\bar{\zeta} = Br^n: \qquad\qquad r^4\,\bar{\zeta}'''' + 2r^3\bar{\zeta}''' - r^2\,\bar{\zeta}'' + r\bar{\zeta}' = 0, \qquad\qquad (6.505a, b)$$

in which each derivative of order $m = 1,2,3,4$ is multiplied by a power with the same exponent $r^m\,\zeta^{(m)}$; thus the solution may be sought (6.505a) as a power with exponent n to be determined by substitution in (6.505b), leading to (6.506a–c):

$$0 = Br^n\Big[n(n-1)(n-2)(n-3) + 2n(n-1)(n-2) - n(n-1) + n\Big]$$

$$= Br^n\,n(n-2)\Big[(n-1)(n-3) + 2(n-1) - 1\Big] \qquad\qquad (6.506a–d)$$

$$= Br^n\,n(n-2)\Big[(n-1)^2 - 1\Big] = Br^n n^2\,(n-2)^2 \equiv Br^n P_4\,(n);$$

in (6.506d) the characteristic polynomial has double roots $n = 0,2$ in (6.507a), corresponding (1.296a, b) to the particular integrals (6.507b):

$$n_{1-2} = \{0,0,2,2\}, \quad \bar{\zeta}_{1-4} = \{1, \log r, r^2, r^2 \log r\}:$$

$$\bar{\zeta} = C_1\,\bar{\zeta}_1 + C_2\,\bar{\zeta}_2 + (C_3 - C_4)\,\bar{\zeta}_3 + C_4\,\bar{\zeta}_4; \qquad\qquad (6.507a–c)$$

their linear combination (6.507c) specifies the general integral of (6.504b), in agreement with the last four terms (6.504e) on the r.h.s. of (6.502e). The two equivalent (6.503a–e; 6.506a–d; 6.507a–c) ≡ (6.502a–e) methods of solution of the biharmonic equation (6.501a–c) with radial symmetry and uniform forcing are applied next to the linear bending of thin circular elastic plate by its own weight (subsection 6.7.18).

6.7.18 Bending of a Circular Plate by Its Own Weight

The condition of finite displacement at the center (6.508a) eliminates a constant of integration (6.508b) from the complete integral (6.502e):

$$\zeta(0) < \infty: \qquad C_2 = 0; \qquad F(0) = \lim_{r\to 0} D\nabla^2\zeta = 0: \quad C_4 = 0, \qquad (6.508a–d)$$

the condition that there is no concentrated force at the center, as in the first term on the r.h.s. of (6.490b), eliminates (6.508c) the corresponding coefficient

(6.502d) in (6.508d). The remaining two constants of integration (C_1, C_3) in the complete integral (6.502e) ≡ (6.509a) are determined by the two boundary conditions:

$$\zeta(r) = \frac{\rho g \, r^4}{64 D} + C_3 \, r^2 + C_1: \qquad 0 = \zeta(a) = \frac{\rho g \, a^4}{64 D} + C_3 \, a^2 + C_1, \qquad \text{(6.509a, b)}$$

namely: (i) that the boundary of the circular plate is level (6.509b) ≡ (6.460a) ≡ (6.460c); and (ii) the condition that the plate is clamped (6.460b) ≡ (6.473b) ≡ (6.510a) [supported (6.460d) ≡ (6.476c) ≡ (6.510b)] at the edge:

$$0 = \frac{\zeta'(a)}{2a} = \frac{\rho g \, a^2}{32 D} + C_3, \quad 0 = \zeta''(a) + \frac{\sigma}{a} \zeta'(a) = \frac{\rho g \, a^2}{16 D}(3+\sigma) + 2C_3(1+\sigma).$$

$$\text{(6.510a, b)}$$

Substituting (6.509b) in (6.509a) leads to:

$$\zeta(r) = \frac{\rho g}{64 D}(r^4 - a^4) + C_3(r^2 - a^2) = (r^2 - a^2)\left[\frac{\rho g}{64 D}(r^2 + a^2) + C_3\right],$$

$$\text{(6.511a, b)}$$

that specifies the linear bending of the thin circular plate by its own weight with the constant C_3 specified by (6.510a) [(6.510b)] in the case of clamped (supported) edge.

Substitution of (6.510a) [(6.510b)] in (6.511b) leads to:

$$\{\zeta_1(r), \zeta_2(r)\} = \frac{\rho g}{64 D}(a^2 - r^2)\left\{a^2 - r^2, \frac{5+\sigma}{1+\sigma}a^2 - r^2\right\}, \qquad \text{(6.512a, b)}$$

showing that *the weak linear bending of a circular bar by its own weight (Figure 6.25b) clamped (6.460a, b) [supported or pinned (6.460c, d)] at its edge of radius a [in Figure 6.23a(b, c)], has [problem 269 (270)]: (i) the transverse deflection (6.512a) [(6.512b)] that is maximum (6.513b) [(6.513c)] at the center (6.513a) and involves (6.513d) the bending stiffness (6.413d):*

$$r = 0: \qquad \zeta_{1max} = \frac{1+\sigma}{5+\sigma}\zeta_{2max} = \frac{\rho g \, a^4}{64 D} = \frac{3\rho g \, a^4 (1-\sigma^2)}{16 E h^3}; \qquad \text{(6.513a–d)}$$

(ii) the maximum deflection for a clamped (supported or pinned) plate [Figure 6.25a (b, c)] is the same under its own weight (6.513a) [(6.513b)] or by a concentrated force (6.496a) [(6.496b)] if the condition (6.514a) [(6.514b)] is met:

clamped:
$$\frac{Fa^2}{16\pi D} = \zeta_{1\max} = \frac{\rho g a^4}{64 D},$$
(6.514a)

supported:
$$\frac{Fa^2}{16\pi D}\frac{3+\sigma}{1+\sigma} = \zeta_{2\max} = \frac{\rho g a^4}{64 D}\frac{5+\sigma}{1+\sigma};$$
(6.514b)

(iii) introducing the weight of the uniform plate (6.515a), the same maximum deflection is obtained for a concentrated force at the center equal to one quarter of the weight (6.515b) [multiplied by an additional factor depending on the Poisson ratio (6.515c) and larger than unity] for a clamped (supported) plate:

$$w = \pi\rho g\, a^2: \qquad F = \pi\rho g\, a^2\left\{\frac{1}{4}, \frac{5+\sigma}{3+\sigma}\right\} = \frac{w}{4}\left\{1, \frac{5+\sigma}{3+\sigma}\right\};$$
(6.515a–c)

(iv) conversely, a concentrated force at the center equal to the weight (6.516a) would multiply the displacement by a factor of four (6.516b) [larger than four (6.516c)] for a clamped (supported) beam:

$$F = w = \pi\rho g\, a^2: \qquad \left(\zeta_{1\max}, \zeta_{2\max}\right) \;\rightarrow\; \times\; 4\left\{1, \frac{3+\sigma}{5+\sigma}\right\},$$
(6.516a–c)

because the same load applied close to the center causes a larger deflection than applied close to the boundary; (v) the slope (6.517a) [(6.517b)] does (6.517c) [does not (6.517d)] vanish at the boundary in the clamped (supported) case:

$$\left\{\zeta_1'(r),\, \zeta_2'(r)\right\} = \frac{\rho g r}{16 D}\left\{r^2 - a^2,\; r^2 - \frac{3+\sigma}{1+\sigma}a^2\right\},$$
(6.517a, d)

$$\zeta_1'(a) = 0, \qquad \zeta_2'(a) = -\frac{\rho g a^3}{8 D(1+\sigma)} = -\frac{3\rho g a^3(1-\sigma)}{2 E h^3};$$
(6.517c, d)

(vi) the stress couples (6.481d) ≡ (6.581a) [(6.518b)] do not (do) vanish on the clamped (6.518c) [supported (6.518d)] boundary:

$$M_{r1,2}(r) = -D\left[\zeta_{1,2}''(r) + \frac{\sigma}{r}\zeta_{1,2}'(r)\right] = -\frac{\rho g}{16}\left[(3+\sigma)r^2 - a^2\left\{1+\sigma, 3+\sigma\right\}\right],$$
(6.518a, b)

$$M_{r1}(a) = -\frac{\rho g a^2}{8}, \qquad\qquad M_{r2}(a) = 0;$$
(6.518c, d)

and (vii) the Cartesian turning moments (6.430a, b) are specified by (6.519a–f):

$$\left\{N_x, N_y\right\} = D\{\partial_x, \partial_y\}\left(\zeta_{1,2}'' + \frac{\zeta_{1,2}'}{r}\right) = \frac{\rho g}{8}\{\partial_x, \partial_y\}\left[2r^2 - a^2\left\{1, \frac{2+\sigma}{1+\sigma}\right\}\right]$$

$$= \frac{\rho g}{4}\{\partial_x, \partial_y\}\left(x^2 + y^2\right) = \frac{\rho g}{2}\{x, y\} \qquad (6.519a\text{–}f)$$

$$= \frac{\rho g r}{2}\{\cos\phi, \sin\phi\} = N_r\{\cos\phi, \sin\phi\},$$

and correspond to a radial turning moment (6.520b) that equals the weight of the circular plate (6.520a) of radius r divided by the perimeter (6.520c):

$$w = \pi \rho g r^2: \qquad\qquad N_r = \frac{\rho g r}{2} = \frac{w}{2\pi r}. \qquad (6.520a\text{–}c)$$

The bending of a circular plate by its own weight can be considered [subsection 6.7.17 (6.7.18)] for [Figure 6.25a, b(c)] clamping or pinning at the edge (hanging from the center with a free edge).

6.7.19 Bending of a Heavy Suspended Circular Plate

In the transverse displacement of a heavy circular plate (6.502e) suspend from the center (Figure 6.25c) two constants vanish (6.521b, c) because the displacement vanishes at the center (6.521a):

$$\zeta(0) = 0: \quad C_1 = 0 = C_2; \quad \bar{C}_3 \equiv C_3 - C_4: \quad \zeta(r) = \frac{\rho g r^4}{64D} + C_4 r^2 \log r + \bar{C}_3 r^2;$$

$$(6.521a\text{–}e)$$

substitution of (6.521b, c) in (6.502e) leads to the transverse displacement (6.521d, e) and hence (6.471d) [(6.467d)] to the stress couple (6.522a) [turning moment (6.522b)]:

$$M_r(r) = -D\left(\zeta'' + \frac{\sigma}{r}\zeta'\right) = -(3+\sigma)\left(C_4 D + \frac{\rho g r^2}{16}\right) - 2(1+\sigma)D\left(\bar{C}_3 + C_4 \log r\right),$$

$$(6.522a, b)$$

$$N_r(r) = D\left(\zeta'' + \frac{\zeta'}{r}\right)' = \frac{\rho g r}{2} + \frac{4C_4 D}{r}. \qquad (6.522b)$$

The vanishing of the turning moment (6.522b) [stress couple (6.522a)] at the free edge (6.523a) [(6.523c)] specifies the two constants of integration (6.523b) [(6.5235d)]:

$$0 = N_r(a): \quad C_4 = -\frac{\rho g a^2}{8D}; \quad 0 = M_r(a): \quad \bar{C}_3 = -C_4 \log a + \frac{3+\sigma}{1+\sigma}\frac{\rho g a^2}{32D}.$$

$$(6.523a\text{–}d)$$

Substitution of (6.523b, d) in (6.521e) specifies *(problem 271) the transverse displacement (6.524b) in the weak linear bending of a heavy circular plate suspended from the center (Figure 6.25c):*

$$0 = \zeta(0) = \zeta_{\min} \leq \zeta(r) = \frac{\rho g r^2}{64D}\left[r^2 + 8a^2 \log\left(\frac{a}{r}\right) + 2a^2 \frac{3+\sigma}{1+\sigma} \right]$$

$$(6.524a\text{–}c)$$

$$\leq \zeta_{\max} = \zeta(a) = \frac{\rho g a^4}{64D}\frac{7+3\sigma}{1+\sigma} = \frac{3\rho g a^4(1-\sigma)(7+3\sigma)}{16Eh^3},$$

that is minimum (maximum) at the center (6.524a) [free edge (6.524c)]. The slope (6.525b):

$$0 = \zeta'(0) = \zeta'_{\min} \leq \zeta'(r) = \frac{\rho g r}{16D}\left\{ r^2 + a^2\left[4\log\left(\frac{a}{r}\right) + \frac{1-\sigma}{1+\sigma} \right] \right\}$$

$$(6.525a\text{–}c)$$

$$\leq \zeta'_{\max} = \zeta'(a) = \frac{\rho g a^3}{8D(1+\sigma)} = \frac{3\rho g a^3(1-\sigma)}{2Eh^3},$$

is also minimum (6.525a) [maximum (6.525c)] at the center (free boundary). The stress couple (6.522a; 6.523b, d) ≡ (6.526b):

$$0 = M_r(a) < M_r(r) = \frac{\rho g}{16}(3+\sigma)(a^2 - r^2) + \frac{\rho g a^2}{4}(1+\sigma)\log\left(\frac{r}{a}\right) < M_r(0) = -\infty,$$

$$(6.526a\text{–}c)$$

vanishes at the free edge (6.526c) ≡ (6.523a) and is minus infinity (6526c) at the suspension point. The turning moment (6.522b; 6.523b) ≡ (6.527b):

$$0 = N_r(a) = N_{r\max} \geq N_r(r) = \frac{\rho g}{2}\left(r - \frac{a^2}{r} \right) > N_{r\min} = N_r(0) = -\infty, \quad (6.527a\text{–}c)$$

has a zero maximum (6.527a) at the free edge and a negative infinity (6.527c) at the center. The case of a circular plate with a circular concentric hole (Problem 272) is considered in Example 10.11.

6.8 Elastic Stability of a Stressed Orthotropic Plate

The buckling of a beam (plate) arises [sections 6.1–6.3 (6.7)] from the super-position at linear or non-linear level of: (i) the transverse deflection of a plate (section 6.7) [bar (chapter III.4)]; and (ii) in-plane stresses (section 6.5) [axial tension (section 6.4)]. The combination (i–ii) specifies (subsections 6.8.1–6.8.2) the linear transverse deflection of a (i) plate made of an isotropic material (section 6.7) under (ii) in-plane anisotropic stresses (sections 6.5). This may be extended (i) to a plate made of an anisotropic material, such as an ortho-tropic plate whose stiffness depends on direction. The consideration of aniso-tropic materials starts with the momentum equation balancing the inertia, volume, and surface forces (subsection 6.8.3) and their moments (subsection 6.8.4) leading to the work of deformation of the stresses upon the strains (sub-section 6.8.5). This specifies the thermodynamic internal energy (subsection 5.5.8) and thus the constitutive relation between the strains and residual, elas-tic and inelastic stresses (subsection 6.8.6). The strains are related to the elas-tic stresses through a stiffness matrix (subsection 6.8.7) with: (i) a maximum of 21 distinct elastic moduli for an anisotropic material without symmetries; (ii) a minimum of 2 elastic moduli, namely the Young modulus and Poisson ratio, for an isotropic material (subsection 6.8.8) for which all directions are equivalent; and (iii) an intermediate case of an orthotropic material that has 3 orthogonal planes of symmetry, leading to 9 distinct elastic moduli (subsec-tion 6.8.9). The constitutive relation between stresses and strains is specified by the stiffness and compliance matrices (subsection 6.8.10), for example for an orthotropic material (subsection 6.8.11); this leads to the elastic energy of defor-mation of an orthotropic plate (subsection 6.8.1.12) that in the pseudo-isotropic case (subsection 6.8.13) is similar to that of an isotropic plate with different bending stiffness; this implies similar equations for the bending (buckling) of unstressed (stressed) plates (subsection 6.8.14) and related boundary condi-tions (subsection 6.8.15). The elastic stability or buckling of isotropic plates is considered for a rectangular shape with biaxial (uniaxial) loads [subsection 6.8.17 (6.8.18–6.8.20)]. As for a beam, the most common boundary conditions are clamped, pinned, and free (subsection 6.8.18) and buckling can be consid-ered also for mixed boundary conditions (subsections 6.8.18–6.8.20).

6.8.1 Linear Buckling of a Plate under Tension

In the case of (i) bending of a plate (ii) subject to in-plane stresses there are two contributions to the transverse force per unit area: (i) the linear bending of thin plate (6.454a–c) makes the first contribution (6.528a) to the transverse force per unit area:

$$f_1 = \nabla^2 \left(D \, \nabla^2 \zeta \right); \qquad \frac{f_2}{h} = -\partial_\alpha \left(T_{\alpha\beta} \, \partial_\beta \zeta \right). \qquad (6.528a, b)$$

(ii) the second contribution (6.528b) due to the in-plane stresses that are generally non-uniform is similar to an elastic membrane (6.369a). In (6.528a) appears the force per unit area (6.528a):

$$f_1 = \frac{dF_1}{dS}, \qquad\qquad \frac{dF_2}{dV} = \frac{dF_2}{h\,dS} = \frac{f_2}{h}, \qquad (6.528\text{c, d})$$

and in (6.528b) the force per unit volume (6.528d) equals the force per unit area divided by the thickness. The total transverse force per unit area (6.529a) leads (6.528a, b) to (6.529b):

$$f = f_1 + f_2: \qquad\qquad f = \nabla^2\left(D\nabla^2\zeta\right) - h\,\partial_\alpha\left(T_{\alpha\beta}\,\partial_\beta\zeta\right), \qquad (6.529\text{a, b})$$

that is, *(problem 273)* **the balance equation** *satisfied by the transverse displacement in the strong linear bending of a plate of stiffness D subject to in-plane stresses* $T_{\alpha\beta}$ *across its thickness. For example, in Cartesian coordinates:*

$$f(x,y) = \left(\partial_{xx} + \partial_{yy}\right)\left[D\left(\partial_{xx}\zeta + \partial_{yy}\zeta\right)\right]$$
$$- h\left[\partial_x\left(T_{xx}\,\partial_x\zeta\right) + \partial_y\left(T_{yy}\,\partial_y\zeta\right) + \partial_x\left(T_{xy}\,\partial_y\zeta\right) + \partial_y\left(T_{yx}\,\partial_x\zeta\right)\right], \qquad (6.530)$$

where: (i) the thickness h of the plate multiplies the in-plane stresses, because f is the transverse force per unit area; (ii) appears the bending stiffness (6.413d) involving the Young modulus E and Poisson ratio σ. *The one (problem 274) dimensional case (6.531a–e) with zero Poisson ratio (6.511f) corresponds to the bending of a beam (6.531h)* ≡ *(6.15d) with I as the moment of inertia of the cross-section (6.9b)* ≡ *(6.412a) in the bending stiffness (6.413c, d)* ≡ *(6.9a)* ≡ *(6.531g):*

$$\partial_y\zeta = 0, \quad \zeta' \equiv \frac{d\zeta}{dx}, \quad T_{xx} = \frac{T}{h}, \quad T_{yy} = 0 = T_{xy}, \quad \sigma = 0,$$

$$ (6.531\text{a–h})$$

$$D = \frac{h^3 E}{12} = EI = B: \quad f = \left(B\zeta''\right)'' - \left(T\zeta'\right)'.$$

The linear equation (6.529b) [(6.531a–h)] applies to a plate (beam) with the restriction that the slope is small $\zeta'^2 \ll 1 \left(|\nabla\zeta|^2 \ll 1\right)$. *The axial T/h (in plane* $T_{\alpha\beta}$) *stresses*

may be non-uniform, and if (a) applied at the boundary and much larger than internal stresses, can be taken as constant; and (iii) the plate (beam) need not be uniform, that is, the bending stiffness may vary with position, for example, if the material is inhomogeneous and the cross-section variable. In the case (problem 275) of uniform tension (6.532b) [in-plane stresses (6.533b)] and homogeneous material (6.532a)

*[(6.533a)], the transverse displacement in the linear bending of a **uniform beam** (plate) is (6.531f) ≡ (6.532a) [(6.530) ≡ (6.533c)]:*

$$B,T = const: \qquad EI\zeta'''' - T\zeta'' = f = \frac{dF}{dx}, \qquad (6.532a\text{--}d)$$

$$D,T_{\alpha\beta} = const: \qquad D\nabla^4\zeta - hT_{\alpha\beta}\,\partial_{\alpha\beta}\zeta = f = \frac{dF}{dS}, \qquad (6.533a\text{--}d)$$

and the forcing (6.532d) [(6.533d)] is by the transverse per unit length (area). The restriction of small slope for linear bending is lifted in connection with strong bending (section 6.9).

6.8.2 Membranes and Weak/Strong Bending of Plates

The order of magnitude of the two terms on the r.h.s. of (6.529b) is: (i) for the transverse force per unit area (6.528d) due to in-plane anisotropic stresses (6.534b), the strain tensor (6.364a) ≡ (6.534a) leads to (6.534a) where L is the linear dimension of the plate, implying (6.534b) for the in-plane stresses and hence (6.534c):

$$S_{\alpha\beta} = \frac{1}{2}(\partial_\alpha\zeta)(\partial_\beta\zeta) \sim \left(\frac{\zeta}{L}\right)^2: \quad T_{\alpha\beta} \sim ES_{\alpha\beta} \sim \frac{E\zeta^2}{L^2}, \quad -f_2 \equiv hT_{\alpha\beta}\,\partial_{\alpha\beta}\zeta \sim \frac{hE\zeta^3}{L^4};$$

$$(6.534a\text{--}c)$$

(ii) for the transverse force per unit area (6.528c) due to the bending, the bending stiffness (6.413d) ≡ (6.534d) appears in (6.534e):

$$D \equiv \frac{Eh^3}{12(1-\sigma^2)} \sim Eh^3, \qquad f_1 \equiv D\nabla^4\zeta \sim \frac{Eh^3\zeta}{L^4}; \qquad -\frac{f_1}{f_2} \sim \left(\frac{h}{\zeta}\right)^2, \qquad (6.534d\text{--}f)$$

(iii) the ratio of the two terms on the r.h.s. of (6.529b) scales (6.534f) on the square of the ratio of the thickness of the plate h to the deflection ζ of the directrix. Thus, *(problem 276) two extreme cases and one intermediate case arise: (i/ii) the linear deflection of a membrane (6.535a) [weak linear bending of a plate (6.535c)] for which the transverse deflection is large (small) compared with the thickness, minus the (the) transverse force per unit area is specified by the anisotropic Laplace (6.535b) [biharmonic (6.535d)] operator:*

$$\zeta^2 \gg h^2: \quad f_2 = -h\partial_\alpha(T_{\alpha\beta}\,\partial_\beta\zeta); \qquad h^2 \gg \zeta^2: \quad f_1 = \nabla^2(D\nabla^4\zeta); \quad (6.535a\text{--}d)$$

(iii) the coefficient in the in-plane stresses (bending stiffness) may be non-uniform; and (iv) the transverse force per unit area appears with minus (plus) sign in (6.535b) [(6.535d)] because the derivation of the balance equation for the transverse displacement of a membrane by the principle of virtual work [subsection 6.6.2 (6.7.9)]

involves one (two) integrations by parts, hence one (two) minus sign(s), that is, equivalent to one minus (plus) sign. In the intermediate case of thickness of the plate comparable to the transverse deflection $\zeta \sim h$, the strong linear bending is specified (6.529b) by the combination (6.529a) of: (i) anisotropic in-plane stresses (6.528b); and (ii) weak linear bending of an isotropic plate (6.528a). The extension of (ii) from isotropic to anisotropic and orthotropic plates (subsections 6.8.3–6.8.16) is made before proceeding to consider (subsections 6.8.17–6.8.20) buckling or elastic instability of plates. The extension is important because: (i) an isotropic plate corresponds for example to an homogeneous plate of constant thickness without reinforcements (Figure 6.26a); (ii) the plate may have reinforcements in one direction (Figure 6.26b) like

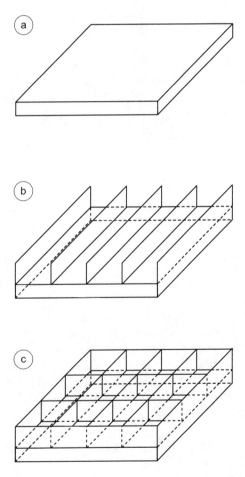

FIGURE 6.26
Taking as example a rectangular plate (Figure 6.24c) it can be: (a) isotropic if it has the same properties in all directions; the existence of (b) equal [(c) unequal] orthogonal reinforcements creates a particular type of anisotropy, called orthotropic because there are orthogonal planes of symmetry, as for an orthorhombic crystal.

the circumferential **frames** in a cylinder; (iii) more often there are also orthogonal reinforcements (Figure 6.26c) like **longerons** besides frames in a fuselage; and (iv) a **wing skin** like a fuselage skin may also have orthogonal reinforcements in the form of longerons and **ribs**. All these lead to anisotropic plates; another case is a **composite** plate consisting of several layers of fibers in distinct directions bonded together. The consideration of anisotropic elastic materials (subsections 6.8.7–6.8.16) starts with the fundamental equations of continuous deformable media (subsections 6.8.2–6.8.6).

6.8.3 Inertia, Volume, and Surface Forces

Consider (Figure 6.27) a three-dimensional region L in which: (i) the **mass** element dm has **velocity** (6.535a) equal to the time derivative of the displacement vector; (ii) the interior $L - \partial L$ is subject to a **force** with density $\vec{F}$ per unit volume dV; and (iii) the boundary ∂L is also subject forces with density or **stress vector** $\vec{T}$ per unit area dA. The balance of (i) inertia, (ii) volume, and (iii) surface force is specified by (6.535b):

$$\vec{v} \equiv \frac{d\vec{u}}{dt}: \qquad \frac{d}{dt}\left(\int_L \vec{v}\, dm\right) = \int_{L-\partial L} \vec{f}\, dV + \int_{\partial L} \vec{T}\, dA. \qquad (6.535a, b)$$

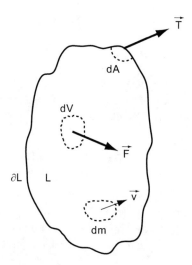

FIGURE 6.27
The beams (Figures 6.1–6.7) and rods (Figures 6.8–6.10) [membranes (Figures 6.11–6.18) and plates (Figures 6.19–6.26)] are particular cases of one(two)-dimensional elastic bodies whose properties can be considered in three dimensions for a domain L with volume element dV and a closed regular boundary ∂L with unit outer normal $\vec{N}$ and area element $d\vec{S} = \vec{N}\, dS$. Both for solid and fluid bodies the volume forces $\vec{F}$ and surface forces or stresses $\vec{T}$ are balanced by the inertia force associated with the motion of a mass element dm with velocity $\vec{v}$.

The **balance of forces** in integral form (6.535b) can re-stated in differential form by transforming the surface integral, last on the r.h.s. of (6.535b), to a volume integral; changing to index notation (notes III.9.1–III.9.50), the stress vector is related to the unit outer normal by (6.536a) the **stress tensor**, so that the last term on the r.h.s. of (6.535b) becomes (6.536b):

$$T_i = T_{ij} N_j: \qquad \int_{\partial L} T_i \, dA = \int_{\partial L} T_{ij} N_j \, dA = \int_{\partial L} T_{ij} \, dA_j = \int_L \left(\partial_j T_{ij} \right) dV, \qquad \text{(6.536a–d)}$$

where was introduced the surface element (6.536c) and applied the divergence theorem (III.9.401a–d) ≡ (6.536d). Substituting (6.536d) in (6.535) leads to a volume integral (6.537b):

$$\rho \equiv \frac{dm}{dV}: \qquad \int_L \left[\frac{d}{dt}(\rho v_i) - f_i - \partial_j T_{ij} \right] dV = 0, \qquad \text{(6.537a, b)}$$

where was introduced the mass density (6.537a) or mass per unit volume. Since (6.537b) must hold for an arbitrary volume follows *(problem 277) the* **momentum equation** *(6.538) stating the balance between: (i) the* **inertia force** *equal to the time derivative of the* **linear momentum** *that equals the velocity times mass density; (ii) the force per unit volume; and (iii) the divergence of the stress tensor:*

$$\frac{d}{dt}(\rho v_i) = f_i + \partial_j T_{ij}. \qquad \text{(6.538)}$$

If the mass density is independent of time (6.539a), the inertia force balancing the volume forces and surface stresses is (6.539b) equal to the product of the **mass density** *by the* **acceleration** *(6.539c):*

$$\frac{d\rho}{dt} = 0: \qquad f_i + \partial_j T_{ij} = \rho \frac{dv_i}{dt} = \rho a_i, \qquad a_i \equiv \frac{dv_i}{dt}, \qquad \text{(6.539a–d)}$$

defined (6.539d) as the derivative of the velocity with regard to time. In particular, (problem 278) in the absence of stresses (6.540a) and for mass density independent of time (6.540b) follows the **Newton (1686) law** *stating that the force per unit volume (6.540c) balances the product of mass density by acceleration:*

$$T_{ij} = 0 = \frac{d\rho}{dt}: \qquad f_i = \rho a_i. \qquad \text{(6.540a–c)}$$

The general case (6.538) of mass density dependent on time, also including surface stresses in addition to volume forces, is retained in the sequel, for example next when considering the balance of moments (subsection 6.8.4).

6.8.4 Balance of Moments and Symmetry of the Stresses

The **moment** $\vec{M}$ of a force $\vec{F}$ is defined (6.541a) as the outer product by the position vector:

$$\vec{M} = \vec{x} \wedge \vec{f} \quad \Leftrightarrow \quad M_i = e_{ijk}\, x_j\, f_k \,, \tag{6.541a, b}$$

or equivalently by (6.541b) in index notation involving the three-dimensional or three-index **permutation symbol** (III.5.182a–c) $\equiv$ (6.542a–c):

$$e_{ijk} = \begin{cases} +1 & \text{if } (i,j,k) \text{ is an even permutation of } (1,2,3), \\ -1 & \text{if } (i,j,k) \text{ is an odd permutation of } (1,2,3), \\ 0 & \text{if any pair of indices } i,j,k = 1,2,3 \text{ is repeated.} \end{cases} \tag{6.542a–c}$$

Applying (6.541b) to (6.538) leads to the **balance of moments** (6.543) in integral form:

$$\int_L e_{ijk}\, x_j \left[\frac{d}{dt}(\rho v_k) - f_k \right] dV = \int_{\partial L} e_{ijk}\, x_j\, T_k\, dA; \tag{6.543}$$

the balance of moments in differential form is obtained applying the divergence theorem (III.9.401a–d) to the r.h.s. of (6.543) after using (6.536a) leading to:

$$\int_{\partial L} e_{ijk}\, x_j\, T_k\, dA = \int_{\partial L} e_{ijk}\, x_j\, T_{k\ell}\, N_\ell\, dA = \int_{\partial L} e_{ijk}\, x_j\, T_{k\ell}\, dA_\ell = \int_L \partial_\ell \left(e_{ijk}\, x_j\, T_{k\ell} \right) dV. \tag{6.544}$$

Substituting (6.544) in (6.543) leads to a volume integral:

$$0 = \int_D e_{ijk} \left\{ x_j \left[\frac{\partial}{\partial t}(\rho v_k) - f_k \right] - \partial_\ell \left(x_j\, T_{k\ell} \right) \right\} dV, \tag{6.545}$$

where the permutation symbol (6.542a–c) is not differentiated because its components are constant. Since (6.545) is valid for an arbitrary volume the integrand must be zero, leading to (6.546a):

$$e_{ijk}\, T_{k\ell}(\partial_\ell x_j) = e_{ijk}\, x_j \left[\frac{\partial}{\partial t}(\rho v_k) - f_k - \partial_\ell\, T_{k\ell} \right] = 0, \tag{6.546a, b}$$

where the r.h.s. is zero (6.546b) by the balance of forces (6.538). The cross-derivatives of the position vector equal (6.547a, b) to the identity matrix (6.305a, b):

$$\partial_k x_j \equiv \frac{\partial x_k}{\partial x_j} = \delta_{k\ell} = \begin{cases} 1 & \text{if} \quad k = j, \\ 0 & \text{if} \quad k \neq j; \end{cases} \qquad (6.547\text{a, b})$$

thus (6.546a) ≡ (6.548a):

$$0 = e_{ijk} T_{k\ell} \left(\partial_\ell x_j \right) = e_{ijk} T_{k\ell} \, \delta_{\ell j} = e_{ijk} T_{kj} \Rightarrow T_{jk} = T_{kj}, \qquad (6.548\text{a, b})$$

proves that the stress tensor is symmetric (6.548b) because the permutation symbol (6.542a–c) is skew-symmetric. A formal proof is:

$$0 = 2 e_{ijk} T_{kj} = \left(e_{ijk} - e_{ikj} \right) T_{kj} = e_{ijk} \left(T_{kj} - T_{jk} \right), \qquad (6.549\text{a–e})$$

where: (i) the skew-symmetry of the permutation symbol (6.542a–c) was used in (6.549a); (ii) the dummy indices (j, k) that represent a sum over $i, j = 1, 2, 3$ can be interchanged in the second term of (6.549b); and (iii) from (6.549c) follows (6.548b). It has been shown that *(problem 279) the **balance of the moments** (6.543; 6.541b) of the inertia and volume forces and surface stresses (6.538) implies that the stress tensor is symmetric (6.548b),* in agreement with the particular case two dimensions (subsection II.4.2.1 and Figure II.4.5). The balance of the forces (subsection 6.8.3) and moments (subsection 6.8.4) is followed by the work performed in a displacement (subsection 6.8.5).

6.8.5 Kinetic Energy and Work of Deformation

A **displacement** δu_i of the body in Figure 6.27 corresponds to the work (6.550) of (6.538) the volume and surface forces:

$$\delta W = \int_L f_i \, \delta u_i \, dV + \int_{\partial L} T_i \, \delta u_i \, dA. \qquad (6.550)$$

Substituting the stress vector by the stress tensor (6.536a) in the second term on the r.h.s. of (6.550) leads to (6.551a):

$$\int_{\partial D} T_i \, \delta u_i \, dA = \int_{\partial D} T_{ij} \, \delta u_i \, N_j \, dA = \int_{\partial D} T_{ij} \, \delta u_i \, dA_j = \int_L \partial_j \left(T_{ij} \, \delta u_i \right) dV, \qquad (6.551\text{a, b})$$

where the divergence theorem (III.9.402a–d) ≡ (6.551b) was used. Substitution of (6.551b) in (6.550) leads to:

$$\delta W = \int_L \left(f_i + \partial_j T_{ij} \right) \delta u_i \, dV + \int_L T_{ij} \, \delta\left(\partial_j u_i\right) dV \equiv \delta W_v + \delta W_d, \qquad (6.552)$$

consisting of two terms. Using (6.538) in the first term (6.553a) expressed in terms of the velocity (6.535a) leads to (6.553b, c):

$$\delta W_c = \int_L \frac{d}{dt}\left(\rho v_i\right) \delta u_i \, dV = \int_L d\left(\rho v_i\right) \frac{\delta u_i}{dt} \, dV = \int_L v_i \, d\left(\rho v_i\right) dV; \qquad (6.553a\text{–}c)$$

for mass density independent of time (6.553d) to (6.553c) corresponds the **kinetic energy** per unit volume (6.553e):

$$\frac{d\rho}{dt} = 0: \qquad \frac{\delta W_c}{dV} = v_i \, d\left(\rho v_i\right) = d\left(\frac{1}{2}\rho v_i \, v_i\right) = d\left(\frac{1}{2}\rho v^2\right) \equiv dE_c. \qquad (6.553d, e)$$

Adding the second term in (6.552), it follows that *(problem 280) the work of the volume and surface forces in a displacement (6.550) consists (6.552) of: (i) the kinetic energy (6.553a–e); and (ii) the **work of deformation** that equals the double contracted product of the stress tensor by (6.554b, c) the **displacement tensor** (6.554a):*

$$D_{ji} \equiv \partial_j u_i: \qquad \delta W_b = \int_L T_{ij} \, \delta\left(\partial_j u_i\right) dV = \int_D T_{ij} \, \delta D_{ji} \, dV. \qquad (6.554a\text{–}c)$$

*The balance of moments (6.543) implies that the stress tensor is symmetric (6.548b) and thus the work of deformation (6.554c) equals the double contracted product of (6.555b, c) the stress tensor by the **strain tensor** (6.555a, b); that is, the symmetric part of the displacement tensor (6.554a):*

$$2 S_{ij} \equiv D_{ij} + D_{ji} = \partial_i u_j + \partial_j u_i = 2 S_{ji}:$$

$$\delta W_b = \frac{1}{2} \int_D T_{ij} \, \delta\left(\partial_i u_j + \partial_j u_i\right) dV = \int_D T_{ij} \, \delta S_{ij} \, dV. \qquad (6.555a\text{–}d)$$

*The skew-symmetric part of the displacement tensor (6.556a) ≡ (II.4.9a–c); that is, the local **rotation bivector** (6.556b) and performs no work (6.556c):*

$$2 \Omega_{ij} \equiv D_{ij} - D_{ji} = \partial_i u_j - \partial_j u_i, \quad \Omega_i = e_{ijk} \Omega_{ik}: \qquad \int_D T_{ij} \, \delta\Omega_{ij} \, dV = 0. \qquad (6.556a\text{–}c)$$

Thus only the strain tensor (6.555a, b) or symmetric part of the displacement tensor (6.554a) does work (6.555c, d) with the stress tensor (6.536a). The formal proof for (6.554a–c) the work of deformation uses: (i) (6.557a) the symmetry of the stress tensor (6.548b) due to the moment balance; and (ii) the interchange of dummy indices (6.557b) to show that only the symmetric part of the displacement tensor (6.554a) appears in (6.557c); that is, the strain tensor (6.555a):

$$\frac{dW_d}{dV} = \frac{1}{2}\left(T_{ij} + T_{ji}\right)dD_{ij} = T_{ji}\,d\left[\frac{1}{2}\left(D_{ij} + D_{ji}\right)\right] = T_{ij}\,dS_{ij}\,; \quad (6.557a\text{–}c)$$

$$2T_{ij}\,d\Omega_{ij} = T_{ij}\,dD_{ij} - T_{ij}\,dD_{ji} = \left(T_{ij} - T_{ji}\right)dD_{ij} = 0, \quad (6.557d, e)$$

in a similar way (6.557d, e) it is proved that the stresses perform no work in a rotation. The work together with the heat specifies the internal energy (subsections 5.5.16–5.5.17), leading to the constitutive relation between stresses and strains (subsection 6.8.6).

6.8.6 Residual, Elastic, and Inelastic Stresses

The internal energy (5.85c) ≡ (6.558a) per unit volume is (problem 281) the sum of the work (6.552) and the heat (5.85b) leading to (6.558b):

$$d\bar{U} = dW + dQ = dW_v + T_{ij}\,dS_{ij} + T\,dS, \quad (6.558a, b)$$

where T_{ij} (T) is the stress tensor (temperature) and S_{ij} (S) the strain tensor (entropy), and the kinetic energy (6.553a–e) is part of the augmented internal energy $\bar{U}$. In the case of isotropic stresses specified by the pressure (6.559a), the work of deformation (6.559c) is minus the product by the volume change (6.559b) ≡ (6.304c–g):

$$T_{ij} = -p\,\delta_{ij},\, dV = dS_{ii} = dD_{ii}: \qquad dW_d = -p\,\delta_{ij}\,dS_{ij} = -p\,dS_{ii} = -p\,dV;$$
$$(6.559a\text{–}c)$$

the corresponding internal energy is:

$$d\bar{U} - dW_v = dU = -p\,dV + T\,dS, \quad (6.559d, e)$$

in agreement with (5.85d) ≡ (6.559d) for a body at rest, for which the kinetic energy (6.553a–e) is zero. Since the internal energy is an exact differential (6.558b): (i) it depends only on the strain tensor and entropy (6.560a); (ii) the stress tensor is the derivative of the internal energy with regard to the strain tensor at constant entropy (6.560b):

$$U = U(S_{ij}, S): \qquad T_{ij} = \left(\frac{\partial U}{\partial S_{ij}}\right)_S ; \qquad T_{ij} = T_{ij} = (S_{k\ell}; S), \qquad (6.560\text{a–c})$$

and (iii) from (6.560a, b) follows that the stress tensor is a function of the strain tensor and entropy (6.560c). At constant entropy (6.561a) the stress tensor can (problem 282) be expanded in power series of the strain tensor leading to the **constitutive relation** (6.561b):

$$S = \text{const}: \qquad T_{ij}(S_{k\ell}) = \overset{0}{T}_{ij} + C_{ijk\ell}S_{k\ell} + O(S_{ij}\,S_{k\ell}), \qquad (6.561\text{a, b})$$

where: (i) the constant term is the **residual stresses** (6.562a); that is, the stresses in the absence of strain:

$$\overset{0}{T}_{ij} \equiv T_{ij}(0); \qquad C_{ijk\ell} = \frac{\partial T_{ij}}{\partial S_{k\ell}} = \frac{\partial^2 U}{\partial S_{ij}\,\partial S_{k\ell}}, \qquad (6.562\text{a, b})$$

(ii) the second term is the linear relation between the stress and strain tensor for an **elastic material** specified by the **stiffness tensor** (6.562b) with four indices; and (iii) the **inelastic stresses** correspond to higher order terms involving the products of strain tensors in (6.561b) and leading to **constitutive tensors** with 6, 8, ..., 2n indices. The linear homogeneous relation between stresses and strains for an elastic material is considered in more detail next (subsection 6.8.7).

6.8.7 Components and Symmetries of the Stiffness Tensor

The second term on the r.h.s. of (6.561b) specifies the linear relation (6.563a) between the stresses and strains in an elastic material:

$$T_{ij} = C_{ijk\ell}S_{k\ell}: \qquad C_{ijk\ell} = C_{jik\ell} = C_{ij\ell k} = C_{k\ell ij}. \qquad (6.563\text{a–d})$$

where the stiffness tensor (6.563b–d) is: (i/ii) symmetric in the first (6.563b) [second (6.563c)] pair of indices because the stress (6.548b) [strain (6.555b)] tensor is symmetric; and (iii) symmetric in the two pairs of indices (6.563d) because of the equality (6.564b) of second-order cross-derivatives of the internal energy with regard to the strain tensor (6.562b), assuming that the internal energy is twice continuously differentiable (6.564a):

$$U(S_{ij}) \in C^2(|R^6): \qquad C_{ijk\ell} = \frac{\partial^2 U}{\partial S_{ij}\,\partial S_{k\ell}} = \frac{\partial^2 U}{\partial S_{k\ell}\,\partial S_{ij}} = C_{k\ell ij}. \qquad (6.564\text{a, b})$$

The total number of components of the stiffness tensor is (6.565a) because each of the four indices can take three values:

$$\# C_{ijk\ell} = 3^4 = 81 > \#^* C_{ijk\ell} = \frac{6 \times 7}{2} = 21, \qquad (6.565a, b)$$

but the number of independent components is smaller (6.565b), as is shown next.

A pair of three-dimensional symmetric indices (6.566a) can be replaced by one six-dimensional index (6.566b):

$$i, j, k, \ell = x, y, z = 1, 2, 3 \quad \leftrightarrow \quad a, b = xx, yy, zz, xy, xz, yz = 1, 2, 3, 4, 5, 6,$$
$$(6.566a, b)$$

so that the stiffness tensor (6.562b) reduces to a 6×6 **stiffness matrix** (6.567a):

$$C_{ab} = \begin{vmatrix} C_{11} & C_{12} & C_{13} & C_{14} & C_{15} & C_{16} \\ C_{12} & C_{22} & C_{23} & C_{24} & C_{25} & C_{26} \\ C_{13} & C_{23} & C_{33} & C_{34} & C_{35} & C_{36} \\ C_{14} & C_{24} & C_{34} & C_{44} & C_{45} & C_{46} \\ C_{15} & C_{25} & C_{35} & C_{45} & C_{55} & C_{56} \\ C_{16} & C_{26} & C_{36} & C_{46} & C_{56} & C_{66} \end{vmatrix} \qquad (6.567a)$$

$$= \begin{bmatrix} C_{xxxx} & C_{xxyy} & C_{xxzz} & C_{xxxy} & C_{xxxz} & C_{xxyz} \\ C_{xxyy} & C_{yyyy} & C_{yyzz} & C_{yyxy} & C_{yyxz} & C_{yyyz} \\ C_{xxzz} & C_{yyzz} & C_{zzzz} & C_{zzxy} & C_{zzxz} & C_{zzyz} \\ C_{xxxy} & C_{yyxy} & C_{zzxy} & C_{xyxy} & C_{xyxz} & C_{xyyz} \\ C_{xxxz} & C_{yyxz} & C_{zzxz} & C_{xyxz} & C_{xzxz} & C_{xzyz} \\ C_{xxyz} & C_{yyyz} & C_{zzyz} & C_{xyyz} & C_{xzyz} & C_{yzyz} \end{bmatrix} \qquad (6.567b)$$

that is symmetric and hence has (6.565b) independent components. Thus, *(problem 283) for an elastic material the linear relation (6.563a)≡(6.586e) between* the stress *(6.568a)* and strain *(6.568b)* in tensor (vector) form:

$$T_a \quad \leftrightarrow \quad T_{ij}, \quad S_a \leftrightarrow S_{ij}, \quad C_{ab} \quad \leftrightarrow \quad C_{ijk\ell}, \quad C_{ab} = C_{ba}: \quad T_a = C_{ab} S_b, \qquad (6.568a-e)$$

involves the stiffness tensor (6.562b) [matrix (6.567a, b)] that is symmetric (6.568d) and holds in the general case of absence of any material symmetry. The symmetries of the stiffness tensor (6.562b) with four indices are taken into account: (i–ii) for the first (i, j) [second (k, ℓ)] pair (6.563b) [(6.563c)] of three-dimensional index (6.566b); and (iii) between the two pairs (i, j) and (k, ℓ) of indices (6.563d) by the symmetry (6.568d) of the stiffness matrix (6.568c) in the indices (a, b). Material symmetries between fully anisotropic (subsection 6.8.7) and fully isotropic (subsection 6.8.8) such as orthotropic (subsection 6.8.9) are considered next.

6.8.8 Isotropy as the Maximum Material Symmetry

A body has **material symmetry** if it is unchanged by a coordinate transformation, in which case: (i) every constitutive tensor, such as the stiffness tensor (6.567b) or matrix (6.567a), must have the same symmetry; and (ii) the resulting relations between the components of the constitutive tensor reduce the number of independent components, for example to less than (6.565b) for the stiffness tensor. For example, an *(problem 284)* **isotropic material** *has properties independent of direction, and hence: (i) the stiffness tensor in (6.563a) can be formed only with scalars and the identity matrix; and (ii) the symmetries (6.563b, c, d) imply that it must be of the form (6.569a):*

$$C_{ijk\ell} = \lambda\, \delta_{ij}\, \delta_{k\ell} + 2\mu\, \delta_{ik}\, \delta_{j\ell} : \qquad T_{ij} = \lambda\, \delta_{ij}\, \delta_{k\ell}\, S_{k\ell} + 2\mu\, \delta_{ik}\, \delta_{j\ell}\, S_{k\ell} = \lambda\, S_{kk}\, \delta_{ij} + 2\mu\, S_{ij}\,,$$

$$(6.569\text{a–c})$$

that leads to the direct Hooke law (6.569b, c) ≡ (6.304b), showing that an *(problem 285) elastic isotropic material has two* **elastic moduli**, *alternatively: (a) the* **Lamé moduli** (λ, μ) *that are the simplest coefficients in the elastic stress-strain relations (6.569c); or (b) the Young modulus E and Poisson ratio σ that are readily measured in an uniaxial traction or compression test (subsection II.4.3.5) and are related (6.304b)≡(6.569c) by (II.4.75b, c) ≡ (6.570a, b):*

$$2\mu = \frac{E}{1+\sigma}, \qquad\qquad \lambda = \frac{2\mu\sigma}{1-2\sigma} = \frac{E}{1+\sigma}\frac{\sigma}{1-2\sigma}. \qquad (6.570\text{a, b})$$

Thus, (problem 286) the direct Hooke law can be written in terms of: (i) the Lamé moduli (6.569c) ≡ (6.571):

$$
\begin{bmatrix} T_{xx} \\ T_{yy} \\ T_{zz} \\ T_{xy} \\ T_{xz} \\ T_{xz} \end{bmatrix}
=
\begin{bmatrix}
2\mu+\lambda & 2\mu & 2\mu & 0 & 0 & 0 \\
2\mu & 2\mu+\lambda & 2\mu & 0 & 0 & 0 \\
2\mu & 2\mu & 2\mu+\lambda & 0 & 0 & 0 \\
0 & 0 & 0 & 2\mu & 0 & 0 \\
0 & 0 & 0 & 0 & 2\mu & 0 \\
0 & 0 & 0 & 0 & 0 & 2\mu
\end{bmatrix}
\begin{bmatrix} S_{xx} \\ S_{yy} \\ S_{zz} \\ S_{xy} \\ S_{xz} \\ S_{xz} \end{bmatrix}
; \qquad (6.571)
$$

(ii) the Young modulus and Poisson ratio (6.306c–e; 6.307a–c) ≡ (6.572):

$$
\begin{bmatrix} T_{xx} \\ T_{yy} \\ T_{zz} \\ T_{xy} \\ T_{xz} \\ T_{yz} \end{bmatrix} \equiv \frac{E}{1+\sigma} \begin{bmatrix} \dfrac{1-\sigma}{1-2\sigma} & \dfrac{\sigma}{1-2\sigma} & \dfrac{\sigma}{1-2\sigma} & 0 & 0 & 0 \\[2ex] \dfrac{\sigma}{1-2\sigma} & \dfrac{1-\sigma}{1-2\sigma} & \dfrac{\sigma}{1-2\sigma} & 0 & 0 & 0 \\[2ex] \dfrac{\sigma}{1-2\sigma} & \dfrac{\sigma}{1-2\sigma} & \dfrac{1-\sigma}{1-2\sigma} & 0 & 0 & 0 \\[2ex] 0 & 0 & 0 & 1 & 0 & 0 \\ 0 & 0 & 0 & 0 & 1 & 0 \\ 0 & 0 & 0 & 0 & 0 & 1 \end{bmatrix} \begin{bmatrix} S_{xx} \\ S_{yy} \\ S_{zz} \\ S_{xy} \\ S_{xz} \\ S_{yz} \end{bmatrix}; \quad (6.572)
$$

or (iii) in an equivalent (6.571) ≡ (6.572) ≡ (6.573a) more condensed form:

$$
\begin{bmatrix} T_{xx} \\ T_{yy} \\ T_{zz} \\ T_{xy} \\ T_{xz} \\ T_{xz} \end{bmatrix} = \begin{bmatrix} C_1(1-\sigma) & C_1\sigma & C_1\sigma & 0 & 0 & 0 \\ C_1\sigma & C_1(1-\sigma) & C_1\sigma & 0 & 0 & 0 \\ C_1\sigma & C_1\sigma & C_1(1-\sigma) & 0 & 0 & 0 \\ 0 & 0 & 0 & C_2 & 0 & 0 \\ 0 & 0 & 0 & 0 & C_2 & 0 \\ 0 & 0 & 0 & 0 & 0 & C_2 \end{bmatrix} \begin{bmatrix} S_{xx} \\ S_{yy} \\ S_{zz} \\ S_{xy} \\ S_{xz} \\ S_{xz} \end{bmatrix} \quad (6.573a)
$$

in terms of:

$$
C_2 \equiv \frac{E}{1+\sigma}, \qquad C_1 = \frac{C_2}{1-2\sigma} = \frac{E}{(1+\sigma)(1-2\sigma)}. \quad (6.573b\text{–}d)
$$

Between the minimum (maximum) material symmetry, that is fully anisotropic (isotropic) with 21 (2) elastic moduli [subsection 6.8.8 (6.8.9)] there are intermediate cases such as homoclinic and orthotropic (subsection 6.8.9).

6.8.9 Homoclinic and Orthotropic Elastic Materials

A **homoclinic material** has one plane of symmetry that may taken as the (y, z)-plane (Figure 6.28a) implying that a **reflection** in the (y, z)-plane changes only the sign of x in (6.574a):

$$
x^i \equiv (x, y, z) \quad \rightarrow x^{i'} \equiv (-x, y, z): \qquad X_i^{i'} \equiv \frac{\partial x^{i'}}{\partial x^i} = \begin{bmatrix} -1 & 0 & 0 \\ 0 & 1 & 0 \\ 0 & 0 & 1 \end{bmatrix}, \quad (6.574a, b)
$$

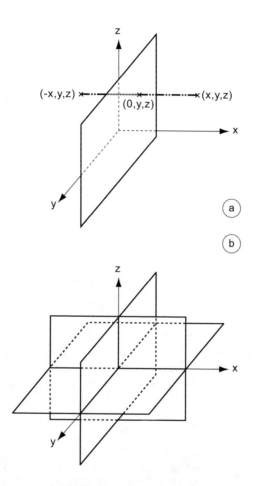

FIGURE 6.28

A homoclinic (orthotropic) elastic material has one (three orthogonal) planes of symmetry [Figure 6.28a (b)], reducing the number of independent elastic moduli to 13 (9) compared with 21 for a general anisotropic material.

leading to the **direct transformation matrix** (III.9.305b) ≡ (6.574b). The **transformation law** of a fourth-order tensor like the stiffness tensor between two coordinate system is (III.9.320) ≡ (6.575):

$$C^{i'j'k'\ell'} = X_i^{i'} X_j^{j'} X_k^{k'} X_\ell^{\ell'} C^{ijk\ell}. \tag{6.575}$$

In the case (6.574b) of reflection on the (y, z)-plane (6.574a), the transformation law (6.575) changes the sign of the components of the stiffness tensor where: (i) the x index appears an odd number of times in (6.567b); (ii) equivalently the index a in (6.566b) takes once the values 4 or 5. The **principle of material invariance** states that if the material maps onto itself by a coordinate transformation, the corresponding constitutive properties cannot change under the same transformation. In the present case, the components of the stiffness tensor that change sign in a reflection in the (y, z)-plane (6.574a, b) must vanish for a homoclinic material:

$$C_{14} = C_{15} = C_{24} = C_{25} = C_{34} = C_{35} = C_{46} = C_{56} = 0. \qquad (6.576\text{a--h})$$

Substitution of (6.576a–h) simplifies the stiffness matrix (6.567a) to:

$$
\begin{bmatrix} T_{xx} \\ T_{yy} \\ T_{zz} \\ T_{xy} \\ T_{xz} \\ T_{yz} \end{bmatrix} =
\begin{bmatrix}
C_{11} & C_{12} & C_{13} & 0 & 0 & C_{16} \\
C_{12} & C_{22} & C_{23} & 0 & 0 & C_{26} \\
C_{13} & C_{23} & C_{33} & 0 & 0 & C_{36} \\
0 & 0 & 0 & C_{44} & C_{45} & 0 \\
0 & 0 & 0 & C_{45} & C_{55} & 0 \\
C_{16} & C_{26} & C_{36} & 0 & 0 & C_{66}
\end{bmatrix}
\begin{bmatrix} S_{xx} \\ S_{yy} \\ S_{zz} \\ S_{xy} \\ S_{xz} \\ S_{yz} \end{bmatrix}, \qquad (6.577)
$$

showing that a homoclinic material has $21 - 8 = 13$ distinct elastic moduli.

An **orthotropic material** has three orthogonal planes of symmetry (Figure 6.28b), implying that: (i) the stiffness tensor in (6.567a) must be invariant with regard to reflections (6.578a–c) in the (y, z), (x, z) and (x, y) planes:

$$(x, y, z) \rightarrow (-x, y, z), (x, -y, z), (x, y, -z); \qquad (6.578\text{a--c})$$

(ii) the components of the stiffness tensor (6.567b) in which any index x or y or z appears an odd number of times must vanish; (iii) the components of the stiffness matrix where $a = 4, 5, 6$ appears once must vanish; (iv) thus, in addition to (6.576a–h) for a homoclinic material, for an orthotropic material also vanish:

$$C_{16} = C_{26} = C_{36} = C_{45} = 0, \qquad (6.579\text{a--d})$$

(iv) thus the stiffness matrix (6.567a) simplifies further to (6.580):

$$
\begin{bmatrix} T_{xx} \\ T_{yy} \\ T_{zz} \\ T_{xy} \\ T_{xz} \\ T_{yz} \end{bmatrix} =
\begin{bmatrix}
C_{11} & C_{12} & C_{13} & 0 & 0 & 0 \\
C_{12} & C_{22} & C_{23} & 0 & 0 & 0 \\
C_{13} & C_{23} & C_{33} & 0 & 0 & 0 \\
0 & 0 & 0 & C_{44} & 0 & 0 \\
0 & 0 & 0 & 0 & C_{55} & 0 \\
0 & 0 & 0 & 0 & 0 & C_{66}
\end{bmatrix}
\begin{bmatrix} S_{xx} \\ S_{yy} \\ S_{zz} \\ S_{xy} \\ S_{xz} \\ S_{yz} \end{bmatrix}, \qquad (6.580)
$$

and consists of a symmetric 3×3 matrix plus a diagonal; and (v) the number of independent elastic moduli of an orthotropic material is (6.565b) minus (6.576a–h; 6.579a–d); that is, $21 - 8 - 4 = 9$. It has been shown that *the stiffness tensor (6.563b–d) relating (6.563a) the elastic stresses to strains corresponds (6.567a, b) to a stiffness matrix that: (i/ii) has a maximum (minimum) of 21 (2) distinct elastic moduli for [problem 284 (285–286)] an anisotropic (6.567a, b) [isotropic (6.569a–c; 6.570a, b) ≡ (6.571) ≡ (6.572) ≡ (6.573a–d)] material; (iii–iv) the intermediate cases include a homoclinic (orthotropic) material [problem 287 (288)] that has one plane (three orthogonal planes) of symmetry [Figure 6.28a(b)] corresponding to a stiffness matrix (6.577) [(6.580)] with 13 (9) distinct elastic moduli.* The orthotropic elastic material is considered in more detail next (subsection 6.8.10).

6.8.10 Stiffness and Compliance Matrices as Inverses

The stiffness **(compliance) matrix** specifies (6.568d) [(6.581a)] the stresses in terms of the strains (vice-versa) and thus the two matrices must be inverse (6.581b, c):

$$S_a = A_{ab} \, T_b: \qquad\qquad C_{ab} \, A_{bc} = \delta_{ac} = A_{ab} \, C_{bc}. \qquad\qquad (6.581a\text{–}c)$$

In the case of an isotropic material, the inverse Hooke law (6.306c–e; 6.311a–c) specifies the compliance matrix (6.582):

$$
\begin{bmatrix} S_{xx} \\ S_{yy} \\ S_{zz} \\ S_{xy} \\ S_{xz} \\ S_{yz} \end{bmatrix}
=
\begin{bmatrix}
\dfrac{1}{E} & -\dfrac{\sigma}{E} & -\dfrac{\sigma}{E} & 0 & 0 & 0 \\[2mm]
-\dfrac{\sigma}{E} & \dfrac{1}{E} & -\dfrac{\sigma}{E} & 0 & 0 & 0 \\[2mm]
-\dfrac{\sigma}{E} & -\dfrac{\sigma}{E} & \dfrac{1}{E} & 0 & 0 & 0 \\[2mm]
0 & 0 & 0 & \dfrac{1+\sigma}{E} & 0 & 0 \\[2mm]
0 & 0 & 0 & 0 & \dfrac{1+\sigma}{E} & 0 \\[2mm]
0 & 0 & 0 & 0 & 0 & \dfrac{1+\sigma}{E}
\end{bmatrix}
\begin{bmatrix} T_{xx} \\ T_{yy} \\ T_{zz} \\ T_{xy} \\ T_{xz} \\ T_{yz} \end{bmatrix}
,
$$

$$(6.582)$$

in terms of two elastic moduli, namely the Young modulus E and Poisson ratio σ.

In the case of an orthotropic material, the compliance matrix that is the inverse of (6.580) may be written by analogy in a similar form (6.583) with: (i) zero top-right and bottom-left 3×3 submatrices; (ii) diagonal bottom-right 3×3 matrix with distinct diagonal elements; and (iii) symmetric top-left 3×3 matrix with 6 distinct components:

$$
\begin{bmatrix} S_{xx} \\ S_{yy} \\ S_{zz} \\ S_{xy} \\ S_{xz} \\ S_{yz} \end{bmatrix} =
\begin{bmatrix}
\frac{1}{E_x} & -\frac{\sigma_{yx}}{E_y} & -\frac{\sigma_{zx}}{E_z} & 0 & 0 & 0 \\
-\frac{\sigma_{xy}}{E_x} & \frac{1}{E_y} & -\frac{\sigma_{zy}}{E_z} & 0 & 0 & 0 \\
-\frac{\sigma_{xz}}{E_x} & -\frac{\sigma_{yz}}{E_y} & \frac{1}{E_z} & 0 & 0 & 0 \\
0 & 0 & 0 & \frac{1}{2G_{yz}} & 0 & 0 \\
0 & 0 & 0 & 0 & \frac{1}{2G_{zx}} & 0 \\
0 & 0 & 0 & 0 & 0 & \frac{1}{2G_{xy}}
\end{bmatrix}
\begin{bmatrix} T_{xx} \\ T_{yy} \\ T_{zz} \\ T_{xy} \\ T_{xz} \\ T_{yz} \end{bmatrix},
$$

$$(6.583)$$

that is symmetric (6.584b):

$$
\frac{1}{E} \to \left\{ \frac{1}{E_x}, \frac{1}{E_y}, \frac{1}{E_z} \right\}, \quad \frac{\sigma_{ij}}{E_i} = \frac{\sigma_{ji}}{E_j}; \quad \frac{1+\sigma}{E} = \frac{1}{2\mu} \to \left\{ \frac{1}{2G_{yz}}, \frac{1}{2G_{zx}}, \frac{1}{2G_{xy}} \right\}, \quad (6.584a\text{–}d)
$$

and involves: (i) three Young moduli E_i in (6.584a); (ii) six Poisson ratios σ_{ij} of which only three are independent by the symmetry conditions (6.584b); and (iii) three **shear moduli** (6.584d) replacing the isotropic shear modulus (6.584c) $\equiv$ (6.570a). Thus (i, ii, iii) imply that an orthotropic elastic material has 12 elastic moduli (6.583) subject to 3 symmetry relations (6.584b), implying 9 independent elastic moduli in agreement with (6.580).

6.8.11 Elastic Moduli of Orthotropic Materials

The upper-right 3×3 compliance sub-matrix (6.583) for an orthotropic elastic material has determinant (6.585a, b) given by (6.585c) for the 3×3 part:

$$
i,j = 1,2,3: \quad C_0 = Det(C_{ij}): \quad E_x E_y E_z C_0 = 1 - \sigma_{xy}\sigma_{yx} - \sigma_{xz}\sigma_{zx} - \sigma_{yz}\sigma_{zy} - 2\sigma_{xy}\sigma_{yz}\sigma_{zx}.
$$

$$(6.585a\text{–}c)$$

Thus the inverse of the compliance matrix (6.583) is the stiffness matrix as given by (6.586):

$$
\begin{bmatrix} T_{xx} \\ T_{yy} \\ T_{zz} \\ T_{xy} \\ T_{xz} \\ T_{yz} \end{bmatrix} = \begin{bmatrix} \dfrac{1-\sigma_{yz}\sigma_{zy}}{C_0 E_y E_z} & \dfrac{\sigma_{yx}+\sigma_{yz}\sigma_{zx}}{C_0 E_y E_z} & \dfrac{\sigma_{zx}+\sigma_{zy}\sigma_{yx}}{C_0 E_y E_z} & 0 & 0 & 0 \\[3mm] \dfrac{\sigma_{xy}+\sigma_{xz}\sigma_{zy}}{C_0 E_x E_z} & \dfrac{1-\sigma_{xz}\sigma_{zx}}{C_0 E_x E_z} & \dfrac{\sigma_{zy}+\sigma_{zx}\sigma_{xy}}{C_0 E_x E_z} & 0 & 0 & 0 \\[3mm] \dfrac{\sigma_{xz}+\sigma_{xy}\sigma_{yz}}{C_0 E_x E_y} & \dfrac{\sigma_{yz}+\sigma_{yx}\sigma_{xz}}{C_0 E_x E_y} & \dfrac{1-\sigma_{xy}\sigma_{yx}}{C_0 E_x E_y} & 0 & 0 & 0 \\[3mm] 0 & 0 & 0 & 2G_{yz} & 0 & 0 \\[2mm] 0 & 0 & 0 & 0 & 2G_{zx} & 0 \\[2mm] 0 & 0 & 0 & 0 & 0 & 2G_{xy} \end{bmatrix} \begin{bmatrix} S_{xx} \\ S_{yy} \\ S_{zz} \\ S_{xy} \\ S_{xz} \\ S_{yz} \end{bmatrix}
$$

(6.586)

that is symmetric:

$$
i,j,k=1,2,3\,;\, i\neq j\neq k\neq i: \quad \left(\sigma_{ij}+\sigma_{ik}\,\sigma_{kj}\right)E_j = E_i\left(\sigma_{ji}+\sigma_{jk}\,\sigma_{ki}\right). \tag{6.587a–c}
$$

It has been shown that *(problem 289) the elastic strains specify the stresses (vice-versa) for an elastic material by the stiffness (compliance) matrix specified: (i) by (6.572) ≡ (6.573a–d) [(6.582)] for an isotropic material with one Young modulus and one Poisson ratio σ, thus two independent elastic moduli, that specify the shear modulus (6.584c); (ii) by (6.586; 6.585c) [(6.583)] for (problem 290) an orthotropic material (problem 291) with three Young moduli E_i, six Poisson ratios σ_{ik} and three shear moduli G_{ij} with three symmetry relations (6.584b) [(6.587a–c)], hence nine independent elastic moduli (6.580). The (i) isotropic [(iii) orthotropic] elastic materials have (problem 292) the following three properties: (a) the shear stresses are specified by the shear strains in both cases (i, ii); (b) the normal stresses are specified by the normal (normal and shear) strains; and (c) the normal strains are specified by the normal (normal and shear) stresses.* The constitutive relation for an orthotropic elastic material (subsection 6.8.10–6.8.11) is applied next to the energy of deformation of an orthotropic plate (subsection 6.8.12).

6.8.12 Elastic Energy of Bending of an Orthotropic Plate

The work of the stresses on the strains (6.555a, b) per unit volume (6.555c, d) for an anisotropic elastic material (6.563a) is given by (6.588a):

$$
\frac{dW_d}{dV} = T_{ij}\,dS_{ij}\,; \quad C_{ijkl} = \text{const}: \quad \frac{dW_d}{dV} = C_{ijkl} S_{kl}\,dS_{ij} = d\left(\frac{1}{2}C_{ijkl}\,S_{kl}\,S_{ij}\right) = dE_c,
$$

(6.588a–c)

for an homogeneous material the stiffness tensor is constant (6.588b), leading to (6.588c), that coincides (6.588c) $\equiv$ (6.589a) with the **elastic energy**:

$$2E_e = C_{ijk\ell} S_{ij} S_{k\ell} = T_{ij} S_{ij} = T_a S_a = C_{ab} S_a S_b = A_{ab} T_a T_b , \qquad \text{(6.589a–e)}$$

that is specified (problem 293) for a homogeneous (6.588b) material equivalently: (i) by (6.589a) in terms of the stiffness (6.562b) and strain (6.555a–c) tensors; (ii) by (6.589b) $\equiv$ (6.441a) in terms of the stress and strain tensors; (iii) by (6.589c) in terms of the stresses (6.568a) and strains (6.568b); (iv) by (6.589d) in terms of the stiffness matrix (6.567a) $\equiv$ (6.568c) and strains (6.568b); and (v) by (6.589e) in terms of the compliance matrix (6.581a) and stresses (6.568a). In the case of a plate, the elastic energy (6.589b) $\equiv$ (6.441a) simplifies to (6.441b) due to the absence of out-of-plane stresses (6.440a–c) with (6.440a) in (6.580) implying (6.590a):

$$0 = T_{zz} = C_{13} S_{xx} + C_{23} S_{yy} + C_{33} S_{zz} ; \qquad T_{xy} = C_{44} S_{xy} , \qquad \text{(6.590a, b)}$$

the in-plane shear stresses are given by (6.590b), and the in-plane normal stresses by (6.591a, c):

$$T_{xx} = C_{11} S_{xx} + C_{12} S_{yy} + C_{13} S_{zz} = \left(C_{11} - C_{13} \frac{C_{13}}{C_{33}} \right) S_{xx} + \left(C_{12} - C_{23} \frac{C_{13}}{C_{33}} \right) S_{yy} ,$$
$$\text{(6.591a, b)}$$

$$T_{yy} = C_{12} S_{xx} + C_{22} S_{yy} + C_{23} S_{zz} = \left(C_{12} - C_{13} \frac{C_{23}}{C_{33}} \right) S_{xx} + \left(C_{22} - C_{23} \frac{C_{23}}{C_{33}} \right) S_{yy} ,$$
$$\text{(6.591c, b)}$$

where S_{zz} was substituted from (6.590a) leading to (6.591b, d). Substituting (6.590b) and (6.591b, d) in (6.441b) leads to:

$$2E_d = \left(C_{11} - C_{13} \frac{C_{13}}{C_{33}} \right) (S_{xx})^2 + \left(C_{22} - C_{23} \frac{C_{23}}{C_{33}} \right) (S_{yy})^2$$
$$\text{(6.592)}$$
$$+ 2C_{44} (S_{xy})^2 + 2 \left(C_{12} - \frac{C_{23} C_{13}}{C_{33}} \right) S_{xx} S_{yy} ,$$

(problem 294) as the elastic energy (6.592) for the weak linear deformation of an orthotropic plate. If the elastic energy (6.592) can be simplified to the form (6.443c) with more general coefficients, the transverse displacement due to bending (buckling) will be specified by (6.454a–c) [(6.530)] with the corresponding coefficients; this case leads to a pseudo-isotropic orthotropic elastic material (subsection 6.8.13).

6.8.13 Plate Made of a Pseudo-Isotropic Orthotropic Material

The elastic energy (6.592) of an orthotropic plate takes the isotropic form (6.443c) with more general coefficients if two assumptions are made. The first assumption (6.593a) simplifies the elastic energy of an orthotropic plate (6.592) to (6.593b) ≡ (6.593c):

$$\bar{D} \equiv C_{11} - C_{13} \frac{C_{13}}{C_{33}} = C_{22} - C_{23} \frac{C_{23}}{C_{33}}:$$

$$2E_d = \bar{D}\left[\left(S_{xx}\right)^2 + \left(S_{yy}\right)^2 \right] + 2C_{44}\left(S_{xy}\right)^2 + 2\left(C_{12} - \frac{C_{13}\,C_{23}}{C_{33}} \right)S_{xx}\,S_{yy}$$

$$= \bar{D}\left(S_{xx} + S_{yy}\right)^2 + 2C_{44}\left(S_{xy}\right)^3 - 2\left(\bar{D} - C_{12} + \frac{C_{13}\,C_{23}}{C_{33}} \right)S_{xx}\,S_{yy}.$$

$$(6.593\text{a–c})$$

The second assumption (6.594a) simplifies further the elastic energy of linear bending from (6.593c) to (6.594b):

$$C_{44} = \bar{D} - C_{12} + \frac{C_{13}\,C_{23}}{C_{33}}: \quad 2E_d = \bar{D}\left(S_{xx} + S_{yy}\right)^2 + 2C_{44}\left[\left(S_{xy}\right)^2 - S_{xx}S_{yy} \right]$$

$$= z^2\left\{ \bar{D}\left(\partial_{xx}\zeta + \partial_{yy}\zeta\right)^2 + 2C_{44}\left[\left(\partial_{xy}\zeta\right)^2 - \left(\partial_{xx}\zeta\right)\left(\partial_{yy}\zeta\right) \right] \right\} \qquad (6.594\text{a–d})$$

$$= z^2\left\{ \bar{D}\left(\nabla^2\zeta\right)^2 + C_{44}\left(\nabla.\vec{C}\right) \right\},$$

where substitution of (6.436b) [(6.445a, b)] leads to (6.594c) [(6.594d)]. Integrating (6.594d) over the thickness of the plate (6.412a) leads to (6.595c):

$$\left\{D, \bar{C}_{44}\right\} = I\left\{\bar{D}, C_{44}\right\} = \frac{h^3}{12}\left\{\bar{D}, C_{44}\right\}: \qquad \bar{E}_d = D\left(\nabla^2\zeta\right)^2 + \bar{C}_{44}\left(\nabla.\vec{C}\right), \qquad (6.595\text{a–c})$$

where (6.595a) [(6.595b)] is the **first (second) bending stiffness**. The principle of virtual work (6.444) applied to (6.595c) leads, as for an isotropic plate [(6.445a, b) up to (6.454a–c)] to the same balance equation for the transverse deflection with a more general bending stiffness (6.595a; 6.593a, b). Thus a **pseudo-isotropic orthotropic material** *(problem 295) satisfies the relations (6.593a, b) [(6.594a)] between elastic moduli that imply (6.596a) [(6.596b, c)]:*

$$C_{22} = C_{11} + \frac{\left(C_{23}\right)^2 - \left(C_{13}\right)^2}{C_{33}}, \qquad (6.596\text{a})$$

$$C_{44} \equiv C_{11} - C_{12} + \frac{C_{13}}{C_{33}}\left(C_{23} - C_{13}\right) = C_{22} - C_{12} - \frac{C_{23}}{C_{33}}\left(C_{23} - C_{13}\right). \qquad (6.596\text{b, c})$$

The stiffness matrix (6.567a) for an orthotropic material (6.580) simplifies further for a pseudo-isotropic orthotropic material (6.596a–c), reducing the number of independent elastic moduli from nine to seven.

6.8.14 Comparison of Isotropic and Pseudo-Isotropic Orthotropic Plates

It has been shown that *(problem 296) the weak linear bending of an elastic plate due to a transverse force per unit area is specified by (6.454a–c) for two cases: (I) an isotropic material with bending stiffness (6.413c, d); and (II) a pseudo-isotropic orthotropic material (6.580; 6.596a–c)* with **generalized bending stiffness** *(6.595a; 6.593a, b)* ≡ *(6.597a, b):*

$$D = \frac{h^3}{12}\left[C_{11} - \frac{(C_{13})^2}{C_{33}}\right] = \frac{h^3}{12}\left[C_{22} - \frac{(C_{23})^2}{C_{33}}\right] > 0, \qquad (6.597a, b)$$

that is positive because the condition of positive (6.598b) elastic energy (6.589b) for non-zero deformation (6.598a) requires that the 2 × 2 determinants (6.598c, d) along the diagonal of the stiffness matrix (6.567a) be positive:

$$S_a \neq 0, \qquad E_e > 0: \qquad \begin{vmatrix} C_{11} & C_{13} \\ C_{13} & C_{33} \end{vmatrix} > 0 < \begin{vmatrix} C_{22} & C_{23} \\ C_{23} & C_{33} \end{vmatrix}, \qquad (6.598a–d)$$

so that (6.598c, d) proves (6.597a, b).

In the particular case (a) of an isotropic material (6.306c–e; 6.307a–c) ≡ (6.572) ≡ (6.573a–d):

$$\left\{C_{11} = C_{22} = C_{33}, \quad C_{12} = C_{13} = C_{23}, C_{44} = C_{55} \equiv C_{66}\right\} = \frac{E}{1+\sigma}\left\{\frac{1-\sigma}{1-2\sigma}, \frac{\sigma}{1-2\sigma}, 1\right\},$$
$$(6.599a–c)$$

the: (i) bending stiffness (6.597a, b) simplifies to (6.600a):

$$D = \frac{h^3}{12 C_{11}}\left[(C_{11})^2 - (C_{12})^2\right] = \frac{E h^3}{12(1+\sigma)(1-2\sigma)}\left(1 - \sigma - \frac{\sigma^2}{1-\sigma}\right) = \frac{E h^3}{12(1-\sigma^2)},$$
$$(6.600a–c)$$

in agreement with (6.600c) ≡ (6.413d); (ii) the conditions (6.596a) [(6.596b, c)] simplify to (6.601a) [(6.601b, c)]:

$$C_{11} = C_{22} = \frac{E}{1-2\sigma}\frac{1-\sigma}{1+\sigma}, \quad C_{44} = C_{11} - C_{12} = \frac{E}{1+\sigma}\frac{1-\sigma-\sigma}{1-2\sigma} = \frac{E}{1+\sigma}, \qquad (6.601a, b)$$

in agreement with $(6.601a) \equiv (6.307a, b)$ $[(6.601b) \equiv (6.306c)]$. The pseudo-isotropic orthotropic plate in case II satisfies the same balance equation for the transverse displacement in linear bending, replacing the bending stiffness $(6.413c, d) \equiv (6.600a–c)$ by the generalized bending stiffness $(6.597a, b)$ as discussed next (subsection 6.8.15).

6.8.15 Generalized Bending Stiffness for Pseudo-Isotropic Orthotropic Plates

Starting (problem 297) with (i) the general anisotropic elastic material (6.563a) with 21 independent (6.567a, b) elastic moduli, there is the following hierarchy with three more levels: (ii) the orthotropic material with three orthogonal planes of symmetry (Figure 6.26c) has nine independent moduli of elasticity (6.580) of which seven appear in the energy of deformation of a plate (6.592); (iii) the two assumptions (6.593a; 6.594a) reduce the number of independent elastic moduli to seven for a pseudo-isotropic orthotropic material (6.580; 6.596a–c) of which four affect the bending of a plate (6.595a–c; 6.597a, b); and (iv) the isotropic material (6.572) $\equiv$ (6.571; 6.570a, b) $\equiv$ (6.573a–d) has two independent elastic moduli and both affect the bending of a plate (6.443a–c). In spite of these differences: (v) the transverse deflection in the weak linear bending of plate by a force per unit area is specified by (6.454a–c) that applies both to an isotropic (6.572) $\equiv$ (6.571; 6.570a, b) $\equiv$ (6.573a–d) [pseudo-isotropic orthotropic (6.580; 6.596a, b)] elastic material with different bending stiffness (6.413c, d) [(6.597a, b)]; (vi) in the presence of in-plane stresses the transverse displacement satisfies (6.530), that applies to the buckling of a plate.

The stiffness matrix (6.580) of case I, an orthotropic material, shows that: (I-i) the normal stiffness is distinct in the x, y and z directions; (I-ii) the coupling of the normal stiffness is distinct in the (x, y), (x, z), and (y, z) planes; (I-iii) there is no coupling of normal and shear strains. In case II, pseudo-isotropic orthotropic material: (II-i) relates the difference of the normal stiffnesses in the x and y directions to all shear (x, z) and (y, z) and normal (z, z) stiffness in the z-direction by (6.596a); (II-ii) also relates the shear stiffnesses in the (x, y) plane to the preceding (I-i) through (6.596b, c). In the case III, an isotropic $(6.572) \equiv (6.571; 6.570a, b) \equiv (6.573a–d)$ elastic material: (III-i) the normal stiffness is the same in the x, y, and z directions; (III-ii) the coupling of normal stiffness is the same in the (x, y), (x, z), and (y, z) planes; (III-iii) shear stiffness is the same in the three planes, and is not independent but rather determined by (III-i) and (III-ii); (III-iv) there is no coupling of the normal and shear stresses or strains.

When applied to an elastic plate the three cases (I, II, III) lead to an hierarchy with three levels as shown by the elastic energy that depends: (I) on the two moduli of elasticity for an elastic plate (6.443a–c); (II) on seven elastic moduli for an orthotropic plate (6.592); (III) on four elastic moduli for a pseudo-isotropic orthotropic plate (6.595a–c; 6.597a, b). The isotropic material (III) corresponds to a plate without reinforcements (Figure 6.26a); and pseudo-isotropic orthotropic (general orthotropic) material corresponds to a plate with equal (unequal) orthogonal reinforcements [Figure 6.26b(c)]. Using the generalized (6.597a, b) [original (6.413c, d)] bending stiffness the same balance equation (6.530) specifies the transverse displacement of (II) pseudo-isotropic [(III) isotropic] plates that specifies the buckling of plates, that is considered for rectangular plates with biaxial (uniaxial) stresses [subsections 6.8.17 (6.8.18–6.8.20)]. The buckling is also affected by boundary conditions considered next (subsection 6.8.16).

6.8.16 Boundary Conditions for Bending of a Plate

The general boundary condition (problem 298) for the bending of an isotropic (pseudo-isotropic) orthotropic plate is (6.602) [(6.603)]:

$$D(1-\sigma)I_n + \partial_n\left[D(\nabla^2\zeta)\right]\delta\zeta - D\left(\nabla^2\zeta\right)\delta(\partial_n\zeta) = 0, \tag{6.602}$$

$$\bar{C}_{44}I_n + \left\{\partial_n\left[D(\nabla^2\zeta)\right]\right\}\delta\zeta - D\left(\nabla^2\zeta\right)\delta(\partial_n\zeta) = 0; \tag{6.603}$$

where I_n is the normal component (6.451d, e) of the deformation vector (6.448d). In the case (problem 299) of constant first bending stiffness (6.604a) [and also constant second bending stiffness (6.605a, b)], the general boundary condition (6.602) [(6.603)] simplifies to (6.604b) [(6.605c)]:

$$D = \text{const:} \qquad (1-\sigma)I_n + \left[\partial_n\left(\nabla^2\zeta\right)\right]\delta\zeta - \left(\nabla^2\zeta\right)\delta(\partial_n\zeta) = 0, \tag{6.604a, b}$$

$$D, \bar{C}_{44} = \text{const:} \qquad \chi I_n + \left[\partial_n\left(\nabla^2\zeta\right)\right]\delta\zeta - \left(\nabla^2\zeta\right)\delta(\partial_n\zeta) = 0; \tag{6.605a–c}$$

*the latter (6.605c) involves the **stiffness ratio parameter** (6.600a–c):*

$$\frac{1}{\chi} \equiv \frac{D}{\bar{C}_{44}} = \frac{\bar{D}}{C_{44}} = 1 + \frac{C_{12}}{C_{44}} - \frac{C_{13}}{C_{33}}\frac{C_{23}}{C_{44}}, \tag{6.606a–c}$$

$$\frac{1}{\chi} = 1 + \frac{\sigma}{1-2\sigma}\left(1 - \frac{\sigma}{1-\sigma}\right) = 1 + \frac{\sigma}{1-\sigma} = \frac{1}{1-\sigma}, \tag{6.607a–c}$$

that in the isotropic case (6.599a–c) simplifies to (6.607a–c) in agreement with (6.604b).

The preceding results are proved (Example 10.15) as follows: (i) the vanishing of the integrand of the surface (boundary) integral on l.h.s. (r.h.s.) of (6.453a) specifies the balance equation for the transverse displacement (6.454a–c) [the general boundary condition (6.602)] for an isotropic plate; (ii) for a pseudo-isotropic orthotropic plate the same balance equation (boundary condition) applies using (6.608a) the generalized bending stiffness (6.597a) instead of (6.413d) [and making the substitution (6.608b)]:

$$\frac{E}{1-\sigma^2} \to \bar{D} \equiv C_{11} - \frac{(C_{13})^2}{C_{33}}, \qquad 2D(1-\sigma) \to \bar{C}_{44}, \qquad (6.608a, b)$$

as follows from the comparison of the elastic energy density per unit area of an isotropic (6.443c) and pseudo-isotropic orthotropic (6.595c) plate; (iii) in the case of constant first bending stiffness (6.604a) it is a common factor in (6.602) that drops out in (6.604b) for an isotropic plate; and (iv) for an pseudo-isotropic orthotropic plate (6.603) simplifies to (6.605c) with the additional condition of constant second bending stiffness (6.605b) that introduces the stiffness ratio factor (6.606a–c), generalizing (6.607a–c) in the isotropic case (6.604b). Performing integrations by parts in the boundary integral on the r.h.s. of (6.453b) leads to differences at a point that vanish by continuity (Example 10.15). Thus the integrand that specifies *(problem 300) the elastic energy per unit length of boundary is a linear combination (6.609a) of the displacement and slope:*

$$0 = \tilde{E}_d = \frac{\delta \hat{E}_d}{ds} = -N_n\,\delta\zeta - M_n\,\delta(\partial_n\zeta)\text{:}\quad M_n = -\frac{\partial \hat{E}_e}{\partial\big[\delta(\partial_n\zeta)\big]}, \quad N_n = -\frac{\delta \hat{E}_e}{\partial(\delta\zeta)},$$

$$(6.609a\text{–}c)$$

with coefficients; that is, the derivatives of the elastic energy per unit area and per unit length of the boundary with regard to the deflection (6.609b) [slope (6.609c)] that specify minus the component normal to the boundary of the stress couple (turning moment). The **general boundary condition** *(6.609a) for the bending of a plate is satisfied in the particular cases of a boundary that is: (i) clamped (6.460a, b); (ii) pinned or supported (6.460c, d); or (iii) free (6.460e, f). The* general boundary condition (6.609a) including the expressions for the stress couple (6.609b) and stress couple (6.609c) are obtained (Problems 301–306) in the Example 10.15 where non-uniform pseudo-isotropic orthotropic plates are considered.

6.8.17 Rectangular Plate Supported on All Four Sides

Consider a rectangular plate (Figure 6.29a) with sides a (b) subject to stresses P (Q), that are only (6.610c) tractions > 0 or compressions < 0; that is, there are no shears (6.610b) in (6.530) $\equiv$ (6.610d) in the absence of external forces (6.610a):

$$f = 0 = T_{xy}, \quad \{T_{xx}\,T_{yy}\} = \{P, Q\}\text{:}\quad P\,\partial_{xx}\zeta + Q\,\partial_{xx}\zeta = \frac{D}{h}\big(\partial_{xx}+\partial_{yy}\big)^2\zeta.$$

$$(6.610a\text{–}d)$$

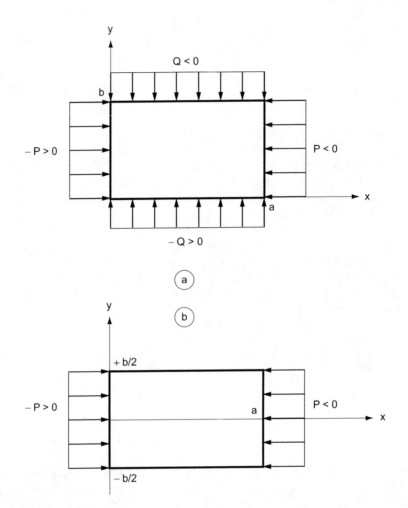

FIGURE 6.29
Buckling can occur for a bar (plate) under [Figures 6.1–6.6 (6.19–6.24)] axial compression (in-plane stresses). In the case of a stressed plate (Figure 6.26) buckling can occur under uniaxial compression (b) or biaxial stresses with dominant compression (a).

The plate is supported (6.460c, d) at all edges (6.611a, b, e, f); namely, (6.475a, c): (i) the displacement is zero at all edges (6.611c, g):

$$x = 0, a: \quad \zeta = 0 = \partial_{yy}\zeta = -\frac{M_y}{D}; \quad y = 0, b: \quad \zeta = 0 = \partial_{xx}\zeta = -\frac{M_x}{D}; \qquad (6.611a–h)$$

(ii–iii) the stress couples (6.422a–c; 6.423a–c) ≡ (6.612a–c):

$$\{M_x, M_y, M_{xy}\} = -D\{\partial_{xx}\zeta + \sigma\partial_{yy}\zeta, \partial_{yy}\zeta + \sigma\partial_{xx}\zeta, (1-\sigma)\partial_{xy}\zeta\}, \qquad (6.612a–c)$$

normal (6.612a, b) to the sides vanish (6.611d, h) in agreement with (6.471a, b) ≡ (6.611d, h); (iii) the boundary conditions (6.611a–c) ≡ (6.613a–c) [(6.611e–g) ≡ (6.614a–c)]:

$x = 0, a:$ $\qquad \zeta = 0 \Rightarrow \partial_x \zeta = 0 \Rightarrow 0 = M_y = -D \partial_{yy} \zeta,$ $\qquad$ (6.613a–f)

$y = 0, b:$ $\qquad \zeta = 0 \Rightarrow \partial_y \zeta = 0 \Rightarrow 0 = M_x = -D \partial_{xz} \zeta,$ $\qquad$ (6.614a–f)

imply (6.613d) [(6.614d)], simplifying the zero (6.613e) [(6.614e)] stress couples (6.612b) [(6.612a)] to (6.613f) ≡ (6.611d)[(6.614f) ≡ (6.611h)]; (iv) the stress couples (6.612a, b) apply to an isotropic plate and in the case of a pseudo-isotropic orthotropic plate (6.607c) the Poisson ratio $\sigma = 1 - \chi$ is replaced by the stiffness ratio; (v) since σ does not appear in the boundary conditions (6.611a–h), χ also does not appear, and the same boundary conditions apply to an isotropic and to a pseudo-isotropic orthotropic plate; and (vi) the balance equation (6.610d) is also the same for pseudo-isotropic orthotropic (isotropic plates with different bending stiffness (6.597a, b) [(6.413c, d)] so the analysis that follows applies to both cases using $1 - \chi(\sigma)$.

The displacement (6.615a) where (m, n) are arbitrary positive integers (6.615a, b):

$m, n \in | N:$ $\qquad \zeta_{m,n}(x, y) = A_{m,n} \sin\left(\dfrac{m \pi x}{a}\right) \sin\left(\dfrac{n \pi y}{b}\right);$

$$\{\partial_{xx} \zeta, \partial_{yy} \zeta\} = -\pi^2 \left\{\frac{m^2}{a^2} + \frac{n^2}{b^2}\right\} \zeta(x, y),$$ $\qquad$ (6.615a–e)

leads to (6.615d, e), that imply that: (i) the boundary conditions (6.611a–h) are satisfied; and (ii) the balance equation (6.610d) leads to the algebraic **buckling condition** (6.616a):

$$\left(P \frac{m^2}{a^2} + Q \frac{n^2}{b^2}\right) = -\frac{D}{h} \pi^2 \left(\frac{m^2}{a^2} + \frac{n^2}{b^2}\right)^2 = -\frac{\pi^2 E h^2}{12(1 - \sigma^2)} \left(\frac{m^2}{a^2} + \frac{n^2}{b^2}\right)^2,$$ $\quad$ (6.616a, b)

where: (i) was substituted the bending stiffness (6.413d) of an isotropic plate yielding (6.616b), for the mode (m, n) in the (x, y)-direction; and (ii) for a pseudo-isotropic orthotropic plate the Poisson ratio σ is replaced (6.607c) by $1 - \chi$ where χ is the stiffness ratio parameter (6.606a–c). For the fundamental mode (6.617a, b), the buckling occurs for (6.617c):

$$m = 1 = n: \qquad \frac{P}{a^2} + \frac{Q}{b^2} = -\frac{\pi^2 E h^2}{12(1 - \sigma^2)} \left(\frac{1}{a^2} + \frac{1}{b^2}\right)^2, \qquad \frac{\zeta_{1,1}(x, y)}{A_{11}} > 0, \quad (6.617a–d)$$

and the whole plate deflects (6.615c) in the same direction (6.617d) specified by the sign of A_{11}. Thus, *(problem 307) an isotropic or pseudo-isotropic orthotropic rectangular plate of sides (a, b) under stresses $P(Q)$ in the x(y)-direction has a displacement (6.618) consisting of a superposition of* **normal modes** *(6.615a–c) with amplitudes $A_{m,n}$:*

$$\zeta(x,y)= \sum_{m,n=1}^{\infty} A_{m,n}\,\zeta_{m,n}(x,y)= \sum_{m,n=1}^{\infty} A_{mn}\,\sin\left(\frac{m\pi x}{a}\right)\sin\left(\frac{n\pi y}{b}\right). \quad (6.618)$$

The mode (m, n) buckles (problem 308) if the condition (6.616a) is met, implying that: (i) there can be no buckling under tractions $P > 0 < Q$, because the r.h.s. and l.h.s. of (6.616) have opposite signs, and the equality is impossible; (ii) buckling is possible only if the r.h.s. of (6.616a) is negative, implying a predominance of compressions $P < 0$ and/or $Q < 0$. The condition (6.616b) is met for example (6.619c) [(6.620c)] for equal biaxial (6.619a, b) [a uniaxial (6.620a, b)] compression:

$$Q = P_2 < 0: \qquad\qquad -P_2 = \frac{\pi^2 E h^2}{12(1-\sigma^2)}\left(\frac{m^2}{a^2}+\frac{n^2}{b^2}\right), \qquad\qquad (6.619a–c)$$

$$Q = 0 > P_1: \qquad -P_1 = \frac{\pi^2 E h^2 a^2}{12(1-\sigma^2) m^2}\left(\frac{m^2}{a^2}+\frac{n^2}{b^2}\right)^2 = -P_2\left(1+\frac{a^2 n^2}{b^2 m^2}\right)\geq -P_2,$$

$$(6.620a–e)$$

leading (6.619d) to a larger buckling load in the latter case (6.620e). In the case of one compression (6.621a) and one traction (6.621b) buckling is possible if (6.621c) the former predominates:

$$P < 0 < Q: \ \ -P > Q\frac{n^2 a^2}{m^2 b^2}; \ \ \{F_x, F_y\}=\{bP, aQ\}: \ \ F_x > -F_y\frac{n^2 a}{m^2 b}, \qquad (6.621a–e)$$

thus the forces on the two sides, that equal (6.621d) the stresses times the length of the sides, must satisfy (6.621e). This option is not available for (problem 309) a beam (6.622a, b) of length (6.622c) whose m-th mode satisfies (6.616b) the buckling condition (6.622d):

$$n = 0 = \sigma, a = L: \qquad -P = \frac{\pi^2 E h^2 m^2}{12 a^2} = \frac{\pi^2 E I m^2}{L^2} = -T_{3,m}, \qquad (6.622a–g)$$

where: (i) in (6.622e) was used the moment of inertia of the cross-section (6.412a); (ii) the critical buckling tension (6.622f) simplifies to (6.39d) for the fundamental mode m = 1 of a pinned beam; and (iii) the stress P for a plate is multiplied by the thickness h leading to P h for the tangential tension along a beam.

6.8.18 Mixed Supported and Free Boundary Conditions

The plate (Figure 6.29a) of sides $a(b)$ can be used (Figure 6.29b) as a strut by: (i) applying uniaxial loads in the x-direction, so that (6.610d) is replaced by (6.623):

$$P\, \partial_{xx}\zeta = \frac{E h^2}{12\left(1-\sigma^2\right)}\left(\partial_{xxxx}\zeta + 2\,\partial_{xxyy}\zeta + \partial_{yyyy}\zeta\right);\qquad (6.623)$$

(ii) the boundary conditions are unchanged (6.611a–d) along the sides $x = 0, a$, whereas along the sides (6.624a) the plate is free so the stress couple (6.422b; 6.423a, b) ≡ (6.624b) ≡ (6.478c) and turning moment (6.430b) ≡ (6.624c) ≡ (6.478d) vanish:

$$y=\pm\frac{b}{2}: \qquad -\frac{M_y}{D}=\partial_{yy}\zeta+\sigma\,\partial_{xx}\zeta=0=\partial_y\left(\partial_{xx}\zeta+\partial_{yy}\zeta\right)=\frac{N_y}{D};\qquad (6.624a\text{–}c)$$

in (6.624b) the Poisson ratio σ from (6.478d) for an isotropic plate can be replaced (6.607c) by $\sigma = 1-\chi$ to apply also to a pseudo-isotropic orthotropic plate with stiffness ratio χ. The boundary conditions (6.611a–d) at the supported edge are satisfied by the displacement (6.625b):

$$\Phi_m \in \mathcal{D}^4\left(-\frac{b}{2},+\frac{b}{2}\right): \qquad \zeta_m(x,y)=\Phi_m(y)\sin\left(\frac{m\pi x}{a}\right),\qquad (6.625a, b)$$

where the function (6.625a) is four times differentiable and (6.623) implies that it satisfies for each mode (6.626a):

$$m\in|N: \quad \Phi_m'''' - \frac{2m^2\pi^2}{a^2}\Phi_m'' + \frac{m^2\pi^2}{a^2}\left[\frac{m^2\pi^2}{a^2}+\frac{12\left(1-\sigma^2\right)P}{Eh^2}\right]\Phi_m = 0,\qquad (6.626a, b)$$

the linear fourth-order differential equation with constant coefficients (6.626b).

The differential equation (6.626b) has exponential solutions (1.56a) ≡ (6.627a) with coefficients specified by the roots of the characteristic polynomial (6.627b):

$$\Phi_m(y)=e^{\vartheta y}: \quad P_4(\vartheta)=\left(\vartheta^2-\frac{m^2\pi^2}{a^2}\right)^2-\frac{m^2\pi^2 k^4}{a^2}=0,\quad k^4\equiv-\frac{12\left(1-\sigma^2\right)P}{Eh^2},$$

$$(6.627a\text{–}c)$$

where was introduced the factor (6.627c) that is positive for a compression $P < 0$, when buckling is possible. The roots of the characteristic polynomial (6.627b) are (6.628a–c):

$$\left(\vartheta_\pm\right)^2 = \frac{m^2\pi^2}{a^2} \pm \frac{m\pi k^2}{a}, \qquad \vartheta_{\pm\pm} = \pm\sqrt{\vartheta_\pm} = \pm\frac{m\pi}{a}\sqrt{1 \pm \frac{k^2 a}{m\pi}}. \qquad (6.628a\text{–}c)$$

The roots (6.628a–c) are two real and distinct symmetric pairs if the condition (6.629a) is met:

$$0 < \frac{k^2 a}{m\pi} < 1: \qquad -P \le \frac{\pi^2 m^2 E h^2}{12\left(1-\sigma^2\right)a^2} \equiv -P_c, \qquad (6.629a, b)$$

implying (6.629b) that: (i) holds for any traction $P > 0$; and (ii) limits a compression $P < 0$ to a critical value P_c. The shape of the directrix of the plate in the case (6.629a, b) of two pairs of distinct symmetric real roots (6.628a–c) of the characteristic polynomial (6.627b) is a linear combination of real exponentials (6.627a) that can be replaced (subsection 1.3.3) by hyperbolic sines and cosines:

$$\Phi_m(y) = C_+ \cosh\left(\vartheta_+ y\right) + C_- \sinh\left(\vartheta_+ y\right) + C^+ \cosh\left(\vartheta_- y\right) + C^- \cosh\left(\vartheta_- y\right), \qquad (6.630)$$

where the constants $\left(C_\pm, C^\pm\right)$ are determined by boundary conditions.

6.8.19 Critical Buckling Stress for a Plate

The boundary conditions (6.624a–c) imply that the function (6.630) must be even (6.631a), and thus the hyperbolic sines in (6.630) are suppressed (6.631b, c), leading (6.625b) to the displacement (6.631d) of the directrix:

$$\Phi_m(y) = \Phi_m(-y): \qquad C_- = 0 = C^-,$$
$$\zeta_{II}(x,y) = \left[C_+ \cosh\left(\vartheta_+ y\right) + C^+ \cosh\left(\vartheta_- y\right)\right]\sin\left(\frac{m\pi x}{a}\right). \qquad (6.631a\text{–}d)$$

Substitution of (6.631d) in the boundary conditions (6.624a–c) leads to:

$$0 = \left(\vartheta_+^2 - \frac{m^2\pi^2\sigma}{a^2}\right)C_+ \cosh\left(\vartheta_+\frac{b}{2}\right) + \left(\vartheta_-^2 - \frac{m^2\pi^2\sigma}{a^2}\right)C^+ \cosh\left(\vartheta_-\frac{b}{2}\right),$$

$$0 = \vartheta_+\left(\vartheta_+^2 - \frac{m^2\pi^2}{a^2}\right)C_+ \sinh\left(\vartheta_+\frac{b}{2}\right) + \vartheta_-\left(\vartheta_-^2 - \frac{m^2\pi^2}{a^2}\right)C^+ \sinh\left(\vartheta_-\frac{b}{2}\right),$$

$$(6.632a, b)$$

that is, equivalent to the matrix system:

$$
\begin{bmatrix}
\left(\mu_+^2-\sigma\right)\cosh\left(\vartheta_+\dfrac{b}{2}\right) & \left(\mu_-^2-\sigma\right)\cosh\left(\vartheta_-\dfrac{b}{2}\right) \\[2ex]
\mu_+\left(\mu_+^2-1\right)\sinh\left(\vartheta_+\dfrac{b}{2}\right) & \mu_-\left(\mu_-^2-1\right)\sinh\left(\vartheta_-\dfrac{b}{2}\right)
\end{bmatrix}
\begin{bmatrix}
C_+ \\[2ex]
C^+
\end{bmatrix}
= 0,
$$

$$(6.633)$$

using the parameters:

$$
\mu_\pm^2 \equiv \left(\frac{\vartheta_\pm a}{m\pi}\right)^2 = 1 \pm \frac{k^2 a}{m\pi} = 1 \pm \sqrt{-\frac{12\left(1-\sigma^2\right)Pa^2}{m^2\pi^2 h^2 E}}.
\qquad (6.634a, b)
$$

A non-trivial solution (6.631d) requires that the integration constants cannot be both zero (6.635a), implying that the determinant of the matrix in (6.633) must be zero (6.635b):

$$
\left(C_+, C^+\right) \neq (0,0): \qquad \mu_-\left(\mu_-^2-1\right)\left(\mu_+^2-\sigma\right)\cosh\left(\vartheta_+\frac{b}{2}\right)\sinh\left(\vartheta_-\frac{b}{2}\right)
$$

$$
= \mu_+\left(\mu_+^2-1\right)\left(\mu_-^2-\sigma\right)\cosh\left(\vartheta_-\frac{b}{2}\right)\sinh\left(\vartheta_+\frac{b}{2}\right).
$$

$$(6.635a, b)$$

Using (6.634b) leads to (6.636a), so that the condition (6.635b) can be rewritten (6.636b):

$$
\mu_+^2-1=1-\mu_-^2: \quad 0=\mu_+\left(\mu_-^2-\sigma\right)\tanh\left(\vartheta_+\frac{b}{2}\right)+\mu_-\left(\mu_+^2-\sigma\right)\tanh\left(\vartheta_-\frac{b}{2}\right).
$$

$$(6.636a, b)$$

Also (6.636a) or (6.634a) imply (6.637a), that confirms that (6.636b) is:

$$
\mu_-^2+\mu_+^2=2: \qquad 0=\mu_+\left(\mu_-^2-\sigma\right)\tanh\left(\frac{m\pi\mu_+ b}{2a}\right)
$$

$$(6.637a, b)$$

$$
+\mu_-\left(2-\mu_-^2-\sigma\right)\tanh\left(\frac{m\pi\mu_- b}{2a}\right)\equiv G(\mu_-),
$$

a function (6.637b) of μ_- only.

From (6.637b) follow the inequalities:

$$G(0) = -\sqrt{2}\,\sigma \tanh\left(\frac{m\pi b}{a\sqrt{2}}\right) \le 0 \le 2\sqrt{\sigma}\,(1-\sigma)\tanh\left(\frac{m\pi b\sqrt{\sigma}}{2a}\right) = G\left(\sqrt{\sigma}\right),$$

$$(6.638)$$

that shows that G has opposite signs at $\mu_- = 0$ and $\mu_- = \sqrt{\sigma}$, so there must be a root in between (6.639a):

$$0 \le \mu_-^2 \le \sigma; \qquad 2 - \sigma \le \mu_+^2 = 1 + \frac{k^2 a}{m\pi} \le 2, \qquad (6.639a, b)$$

the relation (6.637a) then implies (6.639b) that there is another root between $2 - \sigma$ and 2. Substitution of (6.634b) in (6.639a) $\equiv$ (6.640a) leads by (6.627c) to (6.640b):

$$1 - \sigma \le \frac{k^2 a}{m\pi} \le 1: \qquad (1-\sigma)^2 \le -\frac{12\left(1-\sigma^2\right)P a^2}{m^2 \pi^2 h^2\, E} \le 1, \qquad (6.640a, b)$$

showing that the buckling load for a rectangular plate (Figure 6.28b) with sides $x = 0, a\left(y = \pm b/2\right)$ under compression $P < 0$ (free), lies between the bounds:

$$-P_a \equiv \frac{m^2 \pi^2 E h^2}{12\,a^2}\frac{1-\sigma}{1+\sigma} \le -P \le \frac{m^2 \pi^2 E h^2}{12\left(1-\sigma^2\right)a^2} = -P_c\,. \qquad (6.641a, b)$$

The two bounds coincide (6.642c) for a beam (6.642a, b) whose m-th mode has the critical buckling load (6.642d):

$$\sigma = 0,\quad a = L: \qquad -Ph = \frac{\pi^2 E h^3\, m^2}{12\,a^2} = \frac{\pi^2 E I\, m^2}{L^2} = -T_{3,m}\,, \qquad (6.642a\text{–}e)$$

in agreement with (6.642e) $\equiv$ (6.622f) with (6.39d) for the fundamental mode $m = 1$ of a beam pinned at both ends. For a plate the critical buckling load is the lower bound in (6.641a). The upper bound (6.641b) $\equiv$ (6.629b) is a consequence of the assumption (6.629a) of real roots (6.628a–c) of the characteristic polynomial, leading to the buckled shape (6.631d) of the directrix. If the upper bound (6.641b) is exceeded, the shape of the directrix changes (subsection 6.8.20).

6.8.20 Shape of the Directrix of a Buckled Plate

The rectangular plate (Figure 6.29b) with two supported sides under tension and two free sides leads to three cases (Table 6.8) depending on the roots of the characteristic polynomial (6.628a–c) and on the characteristic polynomial (6.627b): (i) in the case I of traction (6.643a) the roots are two distinct complex conjugate pairs and there is no buckling (6.643b) as in the case X of a beam (Table 6.7) supported on continuous springs (subsection 6.3.11); (ii) in the case II of weak compression, (6.629a, b) the roots are two distinct real and symmetric pairs, leading to buckling for compression in the range (6.641a, b) with shape of the directrix specified by (6.631d); and (iii) in the case III of strong compression exceeding (6.643c) the upper bound there is always buckling (6.643d):

$$P > 0: \qquad \zeta_I(x,y) = 0; \qquad -P \ge -P_c; \qquad \zeta_{III}(x,y) \ne 0, \qquad (6.643\text{a–d})$$

as shown next. If the condition (6.629a) is not met (6.644a) the upper bound (6.641b) is exceeded (6.644b) and (6.628c) implies that the characteristic polynomial (6.627b) has (6.644c) one pair of real and symmetric (6.644d) and one pair of imaginary conjugate (6.644e) roots:

$$k^2 a > m\pi: \quad -P \ge -P_c, \quad \vartheta_+^2 > 0 > \vartheta_-^2, \quad \vartheta_{+\pm} = \pm|\vartheta_+|, \quad \vartheta_{-\pm} = \pm i|\vartheta_-|. \quad (6.644\text{a–e})$$

TABLE 6.8

Buckling of a Plate with Mixed Boundary Conditions

Case	I	II	III
Tension	$P > 0$	$-P \le -P_c$	$-P \ge -P_c$
Type	traction	weak compression	strong compression
Squared roots	(6.228a–c) complex	$(\vartheta_\pm)^2 > 0$	$\vartheta_+^2 > 0 > \vartheta_-^2$
		$\vartheta_{\pm\pm} = \pm|\vartheta_\pm|$	$\vartheta_{+\pm} = \pm|\vartheta_+|, \vartheta_{-\pm} = \pm i|\vartheta|$
Condition	$k^4 < 0$	$0 < \dfrac{k^2 a}{m\pi} < 1$	$\dfrac{k^2 a}{m\pi} > 1$
Type	two distinct complex conjugate pairs	two distinct real symmetric pairs	a real symmetric and an imaginary conjugate pair
Buckling load	x	(6.641a, b)	(6.653a, b)
Shape of the directrix	(6.643b)	(6.631d)	(6.646)

$$k^4 \equiv -\frac{12(1-\sigma^2)P}{h^2 E}; \qquad P_c \equiv -\frac{\pi^2 m^2 E h^2}{12(1-\sigma^2)a^2}.$$

Note: In the case (Figure 6.29b) of a rectangular plate clamped on two opposite sides and subject to normal stresses on the two remaining opposite sides, there are three cases of occurrence or non-occurrence of buckling.

The solution of the differential equation (6.626b) is a linear combination of exponentials (6.627a) that may be replaced by circular and hyperbolic cosines and sines:

$$\Phi_m(y) = C_+ \cosh(|\vartheta_+|y) + C_- \sinh(|\vartheta_+|y) + C^+ \cos(|\vartheta_-|y) + C^- \sin(|\vartheta_-|y).$$

(6.645)

The symmetry (6.631a) of the boundary conditions (6.624a–c) again suppresses (6.631b, c) the odd functions in (6.645), leading (6.625b) to the shape of the directrix:

$$\zeta_{III}(x,y) = \left[C_+ \cosh(|\vartheta_+|y) + C^+ \cos(|\vartheta_-|y)\right] \sin\left(\frac{m\pi x}{a}\right),$$

(6.646)

instead of (6.631d).

Substituting (6.646) in the boundary conditions (6.624a–c) yields the homogeneous system of equations:

$$\begin{bmatrix} \left(|\vartheta_+|^2 - \dfrac{m^2\pi^2\sigma}{a^2}\right)\cosh\left(|\vartheta_+|\dfrac{b}{2}\right) & -\left(|\vartheta_-|^2 + \dfrac{m^2\pi^2\sigma}{a^2}\right)\cos\left(|\vartheta_-|\dfrac{b}{2}\right) \\ |\vartheta_+|\left(|\vartheta_+|^2 - \dfrac{m^2\pi^2}{a^2}\right)\sinh\left(|\vartheta_+|\dfrac{b}{2}\right) & |\vartheta_-|\left(|\vartheta_-|^2 + \dfrac{m^2\pi^2}{a^2}\right)\sin\left(|\vartheta_-|\dfrac{b}{2}\right) \end{bmatrix} \begin{bmatrix} C_+ \\ C^+ \end{bmatrix} = 0.$$

(6.647)

A non-trivial solution (6.635a) requires that the determinant of the matrix in (6.647) vanish:

$$0 = (\mu_+^2 - \sigma)|\mu_-|(\mu_+^2 + 1)\cosh\left(|\vartheta_+|\frac{b}{2}\right)\sin\left(|\vartheta_-|\frac{b}{2}\right)$$
$$+ (\mu_-^2 + \sigma)|\mu_+|(\mu_+^2 - 1)\sinh\left(|\vartheta_+|\frac{b}{2}\right)\cos\left(|\vartheta_-|\frac{b}{2}\right);$$

(6.648)

also (6.634a) in the form (6.649a, b) implies (6.649c):

$$\mu_+^2 \equiv \left(\frac{|\vartheta_+|a}{m\pi}\right)^2 = \frac{k^2a}{m\pi} + 1 > 2, \quad \mu_-^2 \equiv \left(\frac{|\vartheta_-|a}{m\pi}\right)^2 = \frac{k^2a}{m\pi} - 1 > 0:$$

(6.649a–c)

$$\mu_+^2 - 1 = \frac{k^2a}{m\pi} = \mu_-^2 + 1 > 1.$$

Substituting (6.649c) simplifies (6.648) to:

$$0 = \left(\mu_+^2 - \sigma\right)|\mu_-|\tan\left(|\vartheta_-|\frac{b}{2}\right) + \left(\mu_-^2 + \sigma\right)|\mu_+|\tanh\left(|\vartheta_+|\frac{b}{2}\right).$$

(6.650)

The second term on the r.h.s. of (6.650) is bounded:

$$0 < \left(\mu_-^2 - \sigma\right)|\mu_+|\tanh\left(|\vartheta_+|\frac{b}{2}\right) \le \left(\mu_-^2 - \sigma\right)|\mu_+|,$$

(6.651a)

whereas the first term varies (Panel 6.1) between $-\infty$ and 0 in the intervals:

$$n = 0,1,....: \qquad \left(n + \frac{1}{2}\right)\pi < |\vartheta_-|\frac{b}{2} < (n+1)\pi;$$

(6.651b, c)

thus there must be a root of (6.650) in each of the intervals (6.651b) and buckling is always possible. The smallest (6.652a) root lies (6.628a) in the range (6.652b):

$$n = 0: \qquad \pi^2 < |\vartheta_-|^2 b^2 = \frac{m^2\pi^2 b^2}{a^2}\left(\frac{k^2 a}{m\pi} - 1\right) < 4\pi^2,$$

(6.652a, b)

that is equivalent (6.649b) to (6.652b) $\equiv$ (6.652c):

$$\frac{m^2\pi^2}{a^2}\left(1 + \frac{a^2}{m^2 b^2}\right)^2 < k^4 = -\frac{12\left(1 - \sigma^2\right)P}{h^2 E} < \left(1 + \frac{4a^2}{m^2 b^2}\right)^2 \frac{m^2\pi^2}{a^2}.$$

(6.652c)

It follows that the lowest critical buckling load lies in the range:

$$-P_b \equiv \frac{h^2 E}{12\left(1 - \sigma^2\right)}\left(\frac{m\pi}{a} + \frac{\pi a}{mb}\right)^2 < -P < \frac{h^2 E}{12\left(1 - \sigma^2\right)}\left(\frac{m\pi}{a} + \frac{4\pi a}{mb}\right)^2 \equiv -P_d.$$

(6.653a, b)

It has been shown that (problem 310) the linear bending of a rectangular plate (Figure 6.29b) under compression at the two supported sides leads (Table 6.8) to three cases: (I) for traction (6.643a) there is (problem 310) no buckling (6.643b); (II/III) for weak (6.629b) [strong (6.444a)] compression [problem 311 (312)] the lowest critical buckling load lies in the range (6.641a, b) [(6.653a, b)] that involves smaller (larger) compressions (6.653c, d):

$$-P_d = -P_c\left(1 + \frac{4a^2}{m^2 b^2}\right) \ge -P_c, \qquad -P_b = -P_a\frac{1 + \sigma}{1 - \sigma}\left(1 + \frac{a^2}{m^2 b^2}\right) \ge -P_a,$$

(6.653c, d)

and the shape of the buckled directrix is specified by (6.631d) [(6.646)] for the m-th mode. The linear bending (section 6.7) with in-plane stresses (section 6.8) is generalized next (section 6.9) to non-linear strong bending that is coupled to in-plane stresses.

6.9 Non-Linear Coupling in a Thick Plate (Foppl 1907, Von Karman 1910)

The linear bending of a plate (section 6.7) causes negligible in-plane stresses, and thus buckling (section 6.8) is due to externally imposed constant stresses as for a membrane (section 6.5). The weak bending (in-plane stresses) in a plate are described [section 6.7 (6.6)] by the transverse displacement (stress function). The non-linear bending corresponds to large slope of the elastica that may be associated with large displacement and non-uniform in-plane stresses, thus also involving strong bending. Thus the non-linear strong bending is described by two variables; namely, the transverse displacement and stress function, that satisfy two differential equations that must be: (i) non-linear due to the large displacements, strains, and stresses; and (ii) coupled because a large bending displacement is associated with non-uniform in-plane stresses and vice-versa. The first non-linear differential equation is the stress balance for the transverse displacement in the weak bending of a plate (section 6.8) that also applies to strong bending (section 6.9) with non-constant in-plane stresses specified by the stress function (subsection 6.9.1). A second coupled equation relating the stress function and transverse displacement is obtained (subsection 6.9.3) from the exact strain tensor. The strain tensor has contributions from (subsection 6.9.2) the transverse displacement and in-plane linear and non-linear stresses. Neglecting the latter, the elastic energy (subsection 6.9.4) has contributions from the transverse and in-plane displacements and their non-linear coupling; equating the variation of the total elastic energy to the work of transverse and in-plane forces leads to the balance equations and boundary conditions (subsection 6.9.5). Simple exact solutions of the non-linear balance equations exist, for example for an elliptic plate (subsection 6.9.6), but the boundary conditions are inaccurate at low-order (subsection 6.9.7). Solutions of the balance equations together with the boundary conditions with high-order accuracy can be obtained using perturbation expansions (subsection 6.9.8); in particular in the axisymmetric case (subsection 6.9.9) the non-linear coupling of bending and stretching (subsection 6.9.10) can be calculated exactly to all orders (subsection 6.9.11). The general method (subsection 6.9.17) is illustrated up to the lowest order of non-linearity (subsection 6.9.12) for a heavy circular plate (subsection 6.9.13) under axial compression (subsection 6.9.14) and clamped at the boundary (subsections 6.9.15–6.9.16).

6.9.1 Transverse Displacement with Non-Uniform In-Plane Stresses

The balance equation (6.530) specifying the transverse displacement for the weak bending of a plate under in-plane stresses also applies to the strong bending of the plate allowing for non-uniform in-plane stresses:

$$f = \nabla^2 \left(D\nabla^2 \zeta \right) - h T_{\alpha\beta} \, \partial_{\alpha\beta} \, \zeta - h \left(\partial_\beta \zeta \right) \left(\partial_\alpha T_{\alpha\beta} \right). \tag{6.654}$$

In the absence of inertia (6.655b) and in-plane (6.655a) volume forces, (6.655c) the momentum equation (6.538) states that the divergence of the stresses is zero (6.655d):

$$\alpha, \beta = 1, 2: \quad f_\alpha = 0 = \frac{\partial}{\partial t} (\rho v_\alpha): \quad \partial_\alpha T_{\alpha\beta} = 0, \left\{ T_{xx}, T_{yy}, T_{xy} \right\} = \left\{ \partial_{yy} \Theta, \partial_{xx} \Theta, -\partial_{xy} \Theta \right\}, \tag{6.655a–e}$$

implying that in (6.654): (i) the last term on the r.h.s. is zero; and (ii) the in-plane stresses (6.655e) derive from a stress function (6.328a–c; 6.329a–d). Assuming a constant bending stiffness for an isotropic plate (6.314d) the **balance equation** (6.654) becomes:

$$\frac{f}{h} = \frac{Eh^2}{12(1-\sigma^2)} \nabla^4 \zeta - \left(\partial_{yy} \Theta \right) \left(\partial_{xx} \zeta \right) - \left(\partial_{xx} \Theta \right) \left(\partial_{yy} \zeta \right) + 2 \left(\partial_{xy} \Theta \right) \left(\partial_{xy} \zeta \right). \tag{6.656}$$

In the balance equation (6.656): (i) the first (bending) term on the r.h.s. is linear for a transverse displacement with small slope (6.410b); and (ii) the second term on the r.h.s. is a non-linear coupling to the in-plane stresses. In order to close the system, a second relation between the transverse displacement and stress function is needed; namely, the **complementary relation** (6.657):

$$E \left[\left(\partial_{xy} \zeta \right)^2 - \left(\partial_{xx} \zeta \right) \left(\partial_{yy} \zeta \right) \right] = \nabla^4 \Theta = \partial_{xyxx} \Theta + \partial_{yyyy} \Theta + 2 \partial_{xxyy} \Theta, \tag{6.657}$$

that will be obtained in the sequel (subsections 6.9.2–6.9.3). Thus the strong non-linear **bending of a plate** *is specified (problem 313) by the biharmonic equation for the transverse displacement (6.656) [stress function (6.657)] with non-linear coupling (Foppl 1907, von Karman 1910) through cross-terms; the coefficients involve the Young modulus E and Poisson ratio σ for an isotropic plate of thickness h, and the transverse force per unit area f appears as a forcing term. If (problem 314) the curvatures are small (6.658a) and the cross product with the stresses also, (6.658b) the transverse displacement (6.658c) [stress function (6.658d)] both satisfy decoupled biharmonic equations:*

$$\left(\partial_{\alpha\beta} \zeta \right)^2 \sim 0 \sim T_{\alpha\beta} \, \partial_{\alpha\beta} \zeta: \qquad \nabla^4 \zeta - f = 0 = \nabla^4 \Theta, \tag{6.658a–d}$$

with forcing by the external transverse force per unit are f (without forcing). The strains and stresses are considered next (subsection 6.9.2) to prove (6.657) including the non-linear terms coupling to (6.656). The extension of (6.656; 6.657) from isotropic to pseudo-isotropic orthotropic elastic plate is considered in the Example E10.15.

6.9.2 Linear and Non-Linear Terms in the Strain Tensor

The total displacement in the strong non-linear bending of a plate consists (6.659b) of a transverse displacement ζ plus an in-plane displacement vector $\vec{u}$:

$$\alpha, \beta = x, y: \qquad \vec{U} - \vec{e}_z\,\zeta(x,y) = \vec{u}(x,y) = \vec{e}_x\,u_x(x,y) + \vec{e}_y\,\vec{u}_y(x,y). \qquad \text{(6.659a, b)}$$

The arc length in the undeflected plane (6.361b) $\equiv$ (6.660a) is increased in a bent plate by the in-plane displacement vector $d\vec{u}$ and transverse displacement (6.659a, b), leading to (6.660b):

$$(ds)^2 = (dx)^2 + (dy)^2, \quad (dL)^2 = (dx + du_x)^2 + (dy + du_y)^2 + (d\zeta)^2. \qquad \text{(6.660a, b)}$$

The difference of square arc lengths (6.660a, b) is a quadratic form (6.661) whose coefficients specify the Cartesian components of the **exact strain tensor**:

$$\frac{(dL)^2 - (ds)^2}{2} = S_{xx}(dx)^2 + S_{yy}(dy)^2 + 2 S_{xy}\,dx\,dy. \qquad \text{(6.661)}$$

From (6.660a, b) follows:

$$\begin{aligned}
(dL)^2 - (ds)^2 &= \left[(1 + \partial_x u_x)dx + (\partial_y u_x)dy\right]^2 - (dx)^2 \\
&+ \left[(\partial_x u_y)dx + (1 + \partial_y u_y)dy\right]^2 - (dx)^2 \\
&+ \left[(\partial_x \zeta)dx + (\partial_x \zeta)dy\right]^2.
\end{aligned} \qquad \text{(6.662)}$$

Thus, equating the coefficients of $(dx)^2$, $(dy)^2$, and $dx\,dy$ in (6.662) and (6.661) leads respectively to (6.663a–c):

$$2 S_{xx} = (\partial_x \zeta)^2 + 2\partial_x u_x + (\partial_x u_x)^2 + (\partial_x u_y)^2, \qquad \text{(6.663a)}$$

$$2 S_{yy} = (\partial_y \zeta)^2 + 2\partial_y u_y + (\partial_y u_x)^2 + (\partial_y u_y)^2, \qquad \text{(6.663b)}$$

$$2 S_{xy} = 2(\partial_x \zeta)(\partial_y \zeta) + (\partial_x u_y + \partial_y u_x) + \left[(\partial_x u_x)(\partial_y u_x) + (\partial_x u_y)(\partial_y u_y)\right]. \qquad \text{(6.663c)}$$

Thus, *the exact non-linear in-plane strains due (6.659a, b) to strong non-linear bending of plate with in-plane stresses are given (problem 315) by (6.663a–c)* ≡ *(6.664a, b):*

$$\alpha,\beta,\gamma = x,y: \quad 2S_{\alpha\beta} = (\partial_\alpha \zeta)(\partial_\beta \zeta) + \partial_\alpha u_\beta + \partial_\beta u_\alpha + (\partial_\alpha u_\gamma)(\partial_\beta u_\gamma), \quad (6.664a, b)$$

where the repeated index in the last term on the r.h.s. of (6.664b) is summed over (6.664a) the two Cartesian coordinates (x,y). The exact non-linear strains (6.663a–c)≡ (6.664a, b) consist of three terms: (i) the product of the gradients of the transverse displacement that is non-linear as for a membrane (6.364a, b); (ii) the symmetrized partial derivatives of the in-plane displacement, that correspond to the strain tensor (6.304c) ≡ (6.555a, b) or symmetric part of the displacement tensor (6.554a); and (iii) the cross-products of the displacement tensor (6.554a) that are non-linear, and are neglected in the sequel (subsection 6.9.3) compared with (ii).

6.9.3 Relation between the Stresses and the In-Plane and Transverse Displacements

The theory of strong non-linear bending of a plate considers in the exact strain tensor (6.663a–c) ≡ (6.664a, b) only the lowest-order terms; that is: (i) the linear in-plane strains (6.665a) omitting the non-linear part (6.665b); and (ii) the gradients of the transverse displacement appear quadratically to lowest order and are retained in (6.665c):

$$\alpha,\beta,\gamma = x,y: \quad (\partial_j u_\alpha)(\partial_j u_\beta) \ll 1: \quad 2S_{\alpha\beta} = (\partial_\alpha \zeta)(\partial_\beta \zeta) + \partial_\alpha u_\beta + \partial_\beta u_\alpha. \quad (6.665a–c)$$

Thus neglecting the non-linear in-plane strains (6.665b) the strain tensor (6.665c) has in-plane components (6.666a–c):

$$\partial_x u_x + \frac{1}{2}(\partial_x \zeta)^2 = S_{xx} = \frac{T_{xx} - \sigma T_{yy}}{E} = \frac{1}{E}(\partial_{yy}\Theta - \sigma\partial_{xx}\Theta), \quad (6.666a)$$

$$\partial_y u_y + \frac{1}{2}(\partial_y \zeta)^2 = S_{yy} = \frac{T_{yy} - \sigma T_{xx}}{E} = \frac{1}{E}(\partial_{xx}\Theta - \sigma\partial_{yy}\Theta), \quad (6.666b)$$

$$\partial_x u_y + \partial_y u_x + (\partial_x \zeta)(\partial_y \zeta) = 2S_{xy} = 2\frac{1+\sigma}{E}T_{xy} = -2\frac{1+\sigma}{E}\partial_{xy}\Theta, \quad (6.666c)$$

where were used in succession: (i) the inverse Hooke law (6.311a, b; 6.306c) with zero out-of-plane normal stresses (6.312e); and (ii) the in-plane components of the stress tensor in terms of the stress function (6.655e). Eliminating the in-plane displacements between (6.666a–c):

$$0 = E\left[\partial_{yy}\left(\partial_x u_x\right) + \partial_{xx}\left(\partial_y u_y\right) - \partial_{xy}\left(\partial_x u_y + \partial_y u_x\right)\right]$$

$$= -\frac{E}{2}\left\{\partial_{yy}\left(\partial_x\zeta\right)^2 + \partial_{xx}\left(\partial_y\zeta\right)^2 - 2\partial_{xy}\left[\left(\partial_x\zeta\right)\left(\partial_y\zeta\right)\right]\right\} \qquad (6.667a)$$

$$+ \partial_{yy}\left(\partial_{yy}\Theta - \sigma\partial_{xx}\Theta\right) + \partial_{xx}\left(\partial_{xx}\Theta - \sigma\partial_{yy}\Theta\right) + 2(1+\sigma)\partial_{xyxy}\Theta,$$

leads to the relation between the transverse displacement and the stress function:

$$E^{-1}\left[\partial_{xxxx}\Theta + \partial_{yyyy}\Theta + 2\partial_{xxyy}\Theta\right] = E^{-1}\nabla^4\Theta$$

$$= \partial_y\left[\left(\partial_x\zeta\right)\left(\partial_{xy}\zeta\right)\right] + \partial_x\left[\left(\partial_y\zeta\right)\left(\partial_{xy}\zeta\right)\right] - \partial_x\left[\left(\partial_{xy}\zeta\right)\left(\partial_y\zeta\right) + \left(\partial_x\zeta\right)\left(\partial_{yy}\zeta\right)\right]$$

$$= \left(\partial_{xy}\zeta\right)^2 - \left(\partial_{xx}\zeta\right)\left(\partial_{yy}\zeta\right),$$

$$(6.667b)$$

proving (6.667b) ≡ (6.657). Thus, *the transverse ζ and in-plane displacement $\left(u_x, u_y\right)$ for the non-linear strong bending of a plate (6.659a, b) specify (problem 316) the strains and stresses by (6.666a–c) to lowest order (6.665a, b) in the exact strains (6.664a, b) ≡ (6.663a–c); the transverse displacement alone specifies the stress function (6.657) in the coupled system (6.656), involving the existence of the elastic* energies of deflection, bending, and in-plane tension (subsection 6.9.4). The balance equations (6.656, 6.657) can be extended (problems 317–320) from isotropic to pseudo-isotropic orthotropic elastic plates (Example 10.16); the boundary conditions (subsection 6.9.5) can be obtained from the principle of virtual work applied to the total elastic energy (subsection 6.9.4).

6.9.4 Elastic Energies of Deflection, Bending, and In-Plane Deformation

The non-linear strong bending of a plate with in-plane stresses involves the total elastic energy per unit area (6.668a) consisting of three terms due to: (i) **bending** (6.668b) ≡ (6.443c) as for an isotropic plate (section 6.7):

$$\bar{E} = \bar{E}_d + \bar{E}_c + \bar{E}_b: \quad 2\bar{E}_d = D\left(\nabla^2\zeta\right)^2 + 2(1-\sigma)\left[\left(\partial_{xy}\zeta\right)^2 - \left(\partial_{xx}\zeta\right)\left(\partial_{yy}\zeta\right)\right], \qquad (6.668a, b)$$

$$2\left(\bar{E}_c + \bar{E}_b\right) = hT_{\alpha\beta}S_{\alpha\beta} = h\left[T_{\alpha\beta}\left(\partial_\alpha\zeta\right)\left(\partial_\beta\zeta\right) + 2T_{\alpha\beta}\,\partial_\alpha u_\beta\right], \qquad (6.668c, d)$$

and (ii–iii) the work of the in-plane elastic stresses (6.589b) on the total strains (6.665a–c) due to the transverse (in-plane) displacement(s) in (6.668c) [(6.668d)] corresponding to **deflection (in-plane deformation)** as for (6.364d) [(6.554b)] a membrane (plate); (iv) in (6.668c, d) the elastic energy per unit volume in square brackets on the r.h.s. must be multiplied by the thickness h of the plate to specify the elastic energy per unit area that appears on the l.h.s. for the elastic membrane (6.364d) [plate (6.554b)]. The principle of virtual work (sections 6.6.2 and 6.7.9) equates the variation of each contribution to the elastic energy to the corresponding form of work: (i–ii) the variation of the elastic energy of bending (6.668b) [deflection (6.668c)] equals the work in a transverse displacement of the contribution (6.528a) [(6.528b)] to the total transverse force per unit area (6.528c, d) that leads to (6.669a, b) for the sum (6.529a) of the corresponding elastic energies:

$$\delta \bar{E}_d + \delta \bar{E}_c = \int_C \left(f_1 + f_2 \right) \delta \zeta \, dA = \int_C f \, \delta \zeta \, dA; \qquad (6.669\text{a, b})$$

(iii) the elastic energy of stretching or in-plane deformation is associated with the work (6.554b) of the in-plane forces in a displacement:

$$\int_C f_\alpha \, \delta u_\alpha \, dA = \delta W_b = \delta \bar{\bar{E}}_b = h \int_C T_{\alpha\beta} \, \delta \left(\partial_\alpha u_\beta \right) dA, \qquad (6.670\text{a–c})$$

multiplied by the thickness h of the plate to convert from unit volume to unit area.

The variation of the elastic energy of in-plane deformation (6.670c) is evaluated by:

$$h^{-1} \delta \bar{\bar{E}}_b = \int_C T_{\alpha\beta} \, \partial_\alpha \left(\delta u_\beta \right) dA = \int_C \left[\partial_\alpha \left(T_{\alpha\beta} \, \delta u_\beta \right) - \delta u_\beta \left(\partial_\alpha T_{\alpha\beta} \right) \right] dA$$
$$= \int_{\partial c} T_{\alpha\beta} \, \delta u_\beta \, n_\alpha \, ds - \int_C \left(\partial_\alpha T_{\alpha\beta} \right) \delta u_\beta \, dA, \qquad (6.671\text{a–d})$$

where: (i) the variation applies only to the displacement tensor, not to the stress tensor (6.671a) due to their linearity (6.563a; 6.589a–e) for an elastic material; (ii) the variation δ commutes with the partial differential ∂ in (6.671b); (iii) an integration by parts (6.450a, b) is performed in (6.671c); and (iv) the divergence theorem (III.9.401a–d) is used in (6.671d) to transform the integral over the surface into one over the boundary. Substituting (6.671d) in (6.670a–c) leads the equality (6.672a):

$$\int_c \left(f_\alpha + h \partial_\beta T_{\alpha\beta} \right) \delta u_\alpha \, dA = h \int_{\partial c} T_{\alpha\beta} n_\alpha \, \delta u_\beta \, ds = 0, \qquad (6.672\text{a, b})$$

between surface and boundary integrals, implying that both must vanish (6.472b). The vanishing of the integrand on the l.h.s. of (6.672a) leads *(problem 321) to the force-stress balance equation (6.538) in the plane (6.673b):*

$$\frac{\partial}{\partial t}\left(\rho\frac{\partial u_\alpha}{\partial t}\right) = 0: \qquad\qquad 0 = h^{-1} f_\alpha + \partial_\beta T_{\alpha\beta}; \qquad\qquad \text{(6.673a, b)}$$

in the absence of inertia force (6.673a) involving the force per unit area f_α converted to unit volume by dividing by the thickness h of the plate.
    The vanishing of the integrand in the r.h.s. of (6.672b) leads to:

$$0 = T_{\alpha\beta}\, n_\alpha\, \delta u_\beta = T_\beta\, \delta u_\beta = \vec{T}\cdot\delta\vec{u}, \qquad\qquad \text{(6.674a–c)}$$

the (problem 322) boundary condition stating that the projection of the in-plane stress vector (6.368a) on the in-plane displacement is zero. This condition (6.674a) can be satisfied similarly to (6.368a–e) by:

$$0 = T_\alpha\,\delta u_\alpha = \vec{T}\cdot\delta\vec{u}\left\{\begin{array}{ll} \vec{T}\perp\delta\vec{u} & \text{orthogonal stress,}\\[4pt] \delta\vec{u}=0 & \text{fixed,}\\[4pt] \vec{T}=0 & \text{free,}\end{array}\right. \qquad \text{(6.675a–d)}$$

corresponding to: (i) orthogonal in-plane displacement and stress vector for the plate (6.675a); or (ii–iii) zero in-plane displacement (6.675b) [stress vector (6.675c)] if the plate is fixed (free) at the boundary. The principle of virtual work applied to the sum of elastic energies of bending, deflection, and in-plane deformation leads to the balance equations and boundary conditions for the strong bending of a thick plate (subsection 6.9.5).

6.9.5 Balance Equations and Boundary Conditions

The total work in the non-linear strong bending of a plate is done by the transverse f (in plane f_α) force(s) on the transverse $\delta\zeta$ (in-plane δu_α) displacements:

$$\delta W = \delta W_d + \delta W_c + \delta W_b = \int_C \left(f\,\delta\zeta + f_\alpha\,\delta u_\alpha \right) dS = \delta\bar{\bar{E}}_d + \delta\bar{\bar{E}}_c + \delta E_b, \qquad \text{(6.676a–c)}$$

and equals the variation of the bending plus deflection (6.668b, c) [in-plane deformation (6.668d)] energies. The variation of the elastic energy is given: (i, ii) for bending (deflection) by (6.453a; 6.454a) [(6.367b)] as for a plate (membrane) in the section 6.6 (6.7) with the transverse force per unit area corresponding to the f_1 (f_2) contribution (6.528a) [(6.528b)] to the total (6.529a) in

(6.669a, b); and (iii) for in-plane deformation by (6.672a). These substitutions in (6.676a–c) lead to (6.677a):

$$\int_C \left\{ f - \nabla^2 \left(D \nabla^2 \zeta \right) + h \partial_\beta \left[T_{\alpha\beta} \left(\partial_\alpha \zeta \right) \right] \right\} \delta\zeta \, dA + \int_C \left(f_\alpha + h \partial_\alpha T_{\alpha\beta} \right) \delta u_\beta \, dA$$

$$= h \int_{\partial C} T_{\alpha\beta} \, \delta u_\beta \, n_\alpha \, ds + h \int_{\partial C} T_{\alpha\beta} \, n_\beta \left(\partial_\alpha \zeta \right) \delta\zeta \, ds + \int_{\partial C} \left[N_n \, \delta\zeta + M_n \, \delta\left(\partial_n \zeta \right) \right] ds = 0,$$

$$\text{(6.677a, b)}$$

using (6.453b) ≡ (6.609a–c) in the third and last term on the r.h.s. of (6.677a). The surface (boundary) integrals on the r.h.s. (l.h.s.) of (6.677a) can be equal only if both vanish (6.677b). Also, both in the r.h.s. and l.h.s. of (6.677a) the variations of the transverse $\delta\zeta$ (in-plane δu_β) displacements are independent, so each must vanish independently. These remarks applied to the r.h.s. (l.h.s.) of (6.677a) lead to the balance equations (boundary conditions) for the strong bending of a thick plate.

From (6.677a, b) follows that *(problem 323) the non-linear strong bending of a plate (section 6.9) involves three terms in the total elastic energy (6.668a) due to bending (6.668b) of a plate (section 6.7) and the work of the in-plane stresses on the transverse (6.668c) [in-plane (6.668d)] displacements [section 6.5 (6.4)] corresponding to deflection (extension, contraction, and/or shear). The variation of the elastic energy of bending and deflection (6.668b, c) [in-plane deformation (6.668d)] is balanced by the work of the transverse f (in-plane f_α) forces per unit area (6.669a, b) [(6.670a–c)] on the transverse $\delta\zeta$ (in-plane δu_α) displacements, leading to the identity (6.677a) where: (i) the surface (boundary) integrals on the l.h.s. (r.h.s) must vanish leading to the balance equations (boundary conditions); and (ii) the transverse $\delta\zeta$ and in-plane δu_α displacements are independent leading to two balance equations (two sets of boundary conditions). The vanishing of the integrand of the: (i) surface integral:*

$$0 = \left[f - \nabla^2 \left(D \nabla^2 \zeta \right) + h T_{\alpha\beta} \, \partial_{\alpha\beta} \zeta \right] \delta\zeta + \left(f_\alpha + h \partial_\alpha T_{\alpha\beta} \right) \left(\partial_\beta \zeta \right) \delta u_\beta, \qquad \text{(6.678)}$$

leads (problem 324) the transverse (6.656) [in-plane (6.673a, b)] balance equation; and (ii) boundary integral:

$$0 = T_{\alpha\beta} \, n_\alpha \, \delta u_\beta + N_n \, \delta\zeta + M_n \, \delta\left(\partial_n \zeta \right) + h T_{\alpha\beta} \, n_\alpha \left(\partial_n \zeta \right) \delta\zeta, \qquad \text{(6.679)}$$

implies that the first (last three) term(s) vanish, leading (problem 325) to:

$$0 = T_{\alpha\beta} \, n_\alpha \, \delta u_\beta = T_\beta \, \delta u_\beta = \vec{T} \cdot \delta\vec{u}, \qquad \text{(6.680a–c)}$$

$$h^{-1} \left[N_n \, \delta\zeta + M_n \, \delta\left(\partial_n \zeta \right) \right] = -T_{\alpha\beta} \, n_\alpha \left(\partial_n \zeta \right) \delta\zeta = -T_\alpha \left(\partial_\alpha \zeta \right) = -\left(\vec{T} \cdot \nabla \zeta \right) \delta\zeta, \qquad \text{(6.681a–c)}$$

the boundary conditions for the in-plane (6.680a–c) [transverse (6.681a–c)] displacements, where was introduced the in-plane stress vector (6.368a).

The first boundary condition (6.680a–c) ≡ (6.674a–c) for the in-plane displacements leads to the same cases (6.675a–d) as for in-plane stresses (subsection 6.9.4). The second set of boundary conditions (6.681a–c) becomes similar to that of weak bending of a plate (6.609a), retaining the normal stress couple (6.609b) and introducing (problem 326) an **augmented normal turning moment:**

$$\bar{N}_n = N_n + hT_{\alpha\beta}\, n_\beta\left(\partial_\alpha\zeta\right) = N_n + hT_\alpha\,\partial_\alpha\zeta = N_n + h\bar{T}.\nabla\zeta, \qquad (6.682a\text{–}c)$$

that adds to the normal component of the turning moment (6.430a, b) the projection of the in-plane stress vector (6.368a) on the gradient of the transverse displacement (6.368b). The second set of boundary conditions (6.681a–c; 6.682a–c) becomes (problem 327) similar (6.683a) to (6.609a):

$$0 = \bar{N}_n\,\delta\zeta + M_n\,\delta\left(\partial_n\zeta\right): \quad \begin{cases} \zeta = 0 = \partial_n\zeta; & clamped, \\ \zeta = 0 = M_n: & pinned\ or\ supported, \\ M_n = 0 = \bar{N}_n: & free, \end{cases} \qquad (6.683a\text{–}g)$$

and includes: (i) the cases of clamped (6.683b, c) ≡ (6.460a, b)/pinned or supported (6.683d, e) ≡ (6.460c, d)/free (6.683f, g) ≡ (6.460e, f) boundaries; (ii) the respective associated boundary conditions (6.472a–d; 6.473a–d; 6.474a–d)/(6.475a–d; 6.476a–d; 6.477a–d)/(6.478a–d; 6.479a–d; 6.480a–d); and (iii) in the last case of free boundary (6.478a–d; 6.479a–d; 6.480a–d) the turning moment must be replaced by the augmented turning moment (6.682a–c). The strong bending is considered next for an elliptic (circular) thick plate [subsections 6.9.6–6.9.7 (6.9.8–6.9.17)] in a low(high)-order approximation.

6.9.6 Bending and Stretching of an Elliptic Plate

It is relatively straightforward to find exact solutions of the non-linear coupled equations (6.656; 6.657) for the strong bending of a plate (subsection 6.9.6), but if the boundary conditions are not met (subsection 6.9.7) the result is strictly not consistent, or at best a low-order approximation. This is illustrated by considering the transverse displacement of a an elliptic plate with half-axis (*a*, *b*) assumed to be specified by (6.684a), ensuring zero displacement at the boundary and implying maximum displacement a the center (6.684 b):

$$\zeta(x,y) = A\left(1 - \frac{x^2}{a^2} - \frac{y^2}{b^2}\right), \qquad A = \zeta(0,0) = \zeta_{max}; \qquad (6.684a, b)$$

from (6.684a, b) follow (6.685a–d):

$$\left\{\partial_x\zeta,\partial_y\zeta\right\}=-2A\left\{\frac{x}{a^2},\frac{y}{b^2}\right\},\quad\left\{\partial_{xx}\zeta,\partial_{yy}\zeta,\partial_{xy}\zeta\right\}=-2A\left\{\frac{1}{a^2},\frac{1}{b^2},0\right\},\quad(6.685\text{a, b})$$

$$\nabla^2\zeta=\partial_{xx}\zeta+\partial_{xx}\zeta=-2A\left(\frac{1}{a^2}+\frac{1}{b^2}\right)=const,\quad\nabla^4\zeta=0.\qquad(6.685\text{c, d})$$

Substitution of (6.685b, d) in (6.656) in the absence of a transverse force (6.686a) leads to (6.686b), implying (6.686c, d):

$$f=0:\quad b^2\,\partial_{yy}\Theta+a^2\,\partial_{xx}\Theta=0,\quad\left\{\partial_{xxxx}\Theta,\partial_{yyyy}\Theta\right\}=-\left\{\frac{b^2}{a^2},\frac{a^2}{b^2}\right\}\partial_{xxyy}\Theta.\quad(6.686\text{a–d})$$

Substituting (6.686c, d) together with (6.685b) in (6.657) yields:

$$\frac{4EA^2}{a^2b^2}=-\nabla^4\Theta=-\partial_{xxxx}\Theta-\partial_{yyyy}\Theta-2\partial_{xxyy}\Theta=\left(\frac{a^2}{b^2}+\frac{b^2}{a^2}-2\right)\partial_{xxyy}\Theta$$

$$\equiv\frac{a^4+b^4-2a^2b^2}{a^2b^2}\partial_{xxyy}\Theta,$$

(6.687a–d)

and (6.687d) ≡ (6.688b) is integrated to specify the stress function (6.688c):

$$a\neq b:\qquad\partial_{xxyy}\Theta=\frac{4EA^2}{\left(a^2-b^2\right)^2}:\qquad\Theta(x,y)=\frac{EA^2x^2y^2}{\left(a^2-b^2\right)^2}.\qquad(6.688\text{a–c})$$

excluding the case (6.688a) of a circular plate; it would be possible to add to (6.688b) a linear function (6.689a) in (x, y), but it would be irrelevant since it would not affect the stresses (6.689b):

$$\Theta(x,y)\to\Theta(x,y)+C_1x+C_2y+C_3:\quad\left\{T_{xx},T_{yy},T_{xy}\right\}=\frac{2EA^2}{\left(a^2-b^2\right)^2}\left\{x^2,y^2,-2xy\right\},$$

(6.689a, b)

that are specified by second-order derivatives (6.655c).

Since the non-zero stresses are (6.689b) in the (x, y) plane, the inverse Hooke law (6.311a–c; 6.306e; 6.313c) specifies the non-zero strains (6.690a–d):

$$\left\{S_{xx},S_{yy},S_{xy},S_{zz}\right\}=\frac{2A^2}{\left(a^2-b^2\right)^2}\left\{x^2-y^2\sigma,y^2-x^2\sigma,-2(1+\sigma)xy,-\sigma\left(x^2+y^2\right)\right\}.$$

(6.690a–d)

The out-of-plane strain (6.690d) ≡ (6.691a) specifies the out-of-plane displacement (6.662b):

$$\partial_z u_z = S_{zz} = -\frac{2A^2\sigma}{\left(a^2 - b^2\right)^2}\left(x^2 + y^2\right); \quad u_z\left(x,y,z\right) = -2A^2\sigma z\frac{x^2 + y^2}{\left(a^2 - b^2\right)^2}. \quad (6.691a, b)$$

The transverse displacement (6.684a) and in-plane strains (6.690a–c) lead (6.666a–c) to (6.692a–c):

$$A^{-2}\partial_x u_x = -2\frac{x^2}{a^4} + A^{-2}S_{xx} = -2\frac{x^2}{a^4} + 2\frac{x^2 - y^2}{\left(a^2 - b^2\right)^2}\sigma, \quad (6.692a)$$

$$A^{-2}\partial_y u_y = -2\frac{y^2}{b^4} + A^{-2}S_{yy} = -2\frac{y^2}{b^4} + 2\frac{y^2 - x^2}{\left(a^2 - b^2\right)^2}\sigma, \quad (6.692b)$$

$$A^{-2}\left(\partial_x u_y + \partial_y u_x\right) = -4\frac{xy}{a^2 b^2} + 2A^{-2}S_{xy} = -4\frac{xy}{a^2 b^2} - 8(1+\sigma)\frac{xy}{\left(a^2 - b^2\right)^2}. \quad (6.692c)$$

The derivatives of the in-plane displacement are specified by (6.692a–c) to within a rotation (6.693a) that substituted in (6.692c) yield (6.693c, d):

$$\partial_x u_y - \partial_y u_x = 2\Omega; \quad B \equiv \frac{1}{a^2 b^2} + \frac{2(1+\sigma)}{\left(a^2 - b^2\right)^2}: \quad \left\{\partial_x u_y, \partial_y u_x\right\} = -2BA^2 xy \pm \Omega, \quad (6.693a–d)$$

involving the constant (6.693b). Thus the four spatial derivatives (6.692a, b; 6.693c, d) of the two components of the in-plane displacement with regard o the in-plane Cartesian coordinates specify the exact differentials:

$$du_x = \left(\partial_x u_x\right)dx + \left(\partial_y u_x\right)dy = 2A^2\left\{\left[\frac{x^2 - y^2}{\left(a^2 - b^2\right)^2}\sigma - \frac{x^2}{a^4}\right]dx - Bxy\,dy\right\} - \Omega dx, \quad (6.694a)$$

$$du_y = \left(\partial_x u_y\right)dx + \left(\partial_y u_y\right)dy = 2A^2\left\{\left[\frac{y^2 - x^2}{\left(a^2 - b^2\right)^2}\sigma - \frac{y^2}{b^4}\right]dy - Bxy\,dx\right\} + \Omega dy. \quad (6.694b)$$

Assuming a uniform rotation (6.695a), the integration of (6.694a, b) specifies the in-plane displacements to within an added constant:

$$\Omega = const: \quad u_x(x,y) = \frac{A^2 x}{3}\left[\frac{2x^2 - 6y^2\sigma}{(a^2 - b^2)} - \frac{2x^2}{a^4} - 3By^2\right] - \Omega x,$$

$$u_y(x,y) = \frac{A^2 y}{3}\left[\frac{2y^2 - 6x^2\sigma}{(a^2 - b^2)} - \frac{2y^2}{b^4} - 3Bx^2\right] - \Omega y.$$

(6.695a–c)

It has been shown that *(problem 328) the non-linear coupled equations for the
strong bending of a isotropic elastic plate (6.656; 6.657) are satisfied for a non-cir-
cular (6.688a) elliptic plate with half-axis (a, b) by: (i) the transverse displacement
(6.684a, b); (ii) the in-plane displacements (6.695b, c) in the case of constant rotation (6.695a); (iii–iv) the stress function (6.688c) and non-zero stresses (6.689b);
and (v) the non-zero total strains (6.690a–d) associated with the transverse and
in-plane displacements.* The boundary conditions and orders of approximation corresponding to these results (subsection 6.9.6) are considered next
(subsection 6.9.7).

6.9.7 Slope, Stress Couples, and Turning Moments

The displacement (6.684a) ≡ (6.696b) vanishes at the boundary (6.696a) of an
elliptic plate with half-axis (a, b):

$$0 = \Phi(x,y) = \frac{x^2}{a^2} + \frac{y^2}{b^2} - 1 = -\frac{\zeta(x,y)}{A}: \quad \{\partial_x\Phi, \partial_y\Phi\} = 2\left\{\frac{x}{a^2}, \frac{y}{b^2}\right\}, \quad (6.696a–c)$$

and the two-dimensional gradient (6.696c) specifies the unit normal:

$$\{n_x, n_y\} = \frac{\nabla\Phi}{|\nabla\Phi|} = C\left\{\frac{x}{a^2}, \frac{y}{b^2}\right\}, \quad C = \left|\frac{x^2}{a^4} + \frac{y^2}{b^4}\right|^{-1/2}. \quad (6.697a–c)$$

The normal derivative of the transverse displacement can be calculated
alternatively by:

$$\partial_n\zeta = \bar{n}.\nabla\zeta = n_x\,\partial_x\zeta + n_y\,\partial_y\zeta = -2AC\left(\frac{x^2}{a^4} + \frac{y^2}{b^4}\right) = -\frac{2A}{C} = -2A\left|\frac{x^2}{a^4} + \frac{y^2}{b^4}\right|^{1/2},$$

(6.698a)

$$\partial_n\zeta = \bar{n}.\nabla\zeta = -A\nabla\Phi.\frac{\nabla\Phi}{|\nabla\Phi|} = -A|\nabla\Phi| = -2A\left|\frac{x^2}{a^4} + \frac{y^2}{b^4}\right|^{1/2}; \quad (6.698b)$$

since (6.698a) ≡ (6.698b) is not zero for (6.696a) the plate is not clamped. Using (6.685b), the stress couples (6.422a–c; 6.423a–c) are given by:

$$\{M_x, M_y, M_z\} = 2AD\left\{\frac{1}{a^2} + \frac{\sigma}{b^2}, \frac{1}{b^2} + \frac{\sigma}{a^2}, 0\right\}, \tag{6.699}$$

leading (6.697a) to the stress couple normal to the boundary:

$$M_n = \bar{M}.\bar{n} = M_x\, n_x + M_y\, n_y = 2ACD\left(\frac{x}{a^4} + \frac{y}{b^4} + \sigma\frac{x+y}{a^2 b^2}\right), \tag{6.700a–c}$$

that is not zero for (6.696a), so the plate is neither supported or pinned nor free.

The constant Laplacian of the transverse displacement (6.685c) implies that the turning moment (6.430a) is zero (6.701a) and thus the augmented turning moment normal to the boundary (6.682c) reduces to the second term (6.701b):

$$\bar{N} = D\nabla\left(\nabla^2\zeta\right) = 0: \qquad h^{-1}\bar{N}_n = \bar{T}.\nabla\zeta = T_x\,\partial_x\zeta + T_y\,\partial_y\zeta, \tag{6.701a, b}$$

and involves the stress vector. From the stresses (6.689b) and outward unit normal (6.697a, b) follow (6.368a) the Cartesian components of the stress vector:

$$T_x = T_{xx}\, n_x + T_{xy}\, n_y = \frac{2EA^2C}{\left(a^2 - b^2\right)^2}\left(\frac{x^3}{a^2} - \frac{2xy^2}{b^2}\right), \tag{6.702a}$$

$$T_y = T_{xy}\, n_x + T_{yy}\, n_y = \frac{2EA^2C}{\left(a^2 - b^2\right)^2}\left(\frac{y^3}{b^2} - \frac{2x^2y}{a^2}\right). \tag{6.702b}$$

The projection of the in-plane stress vector (6.702a, b) on the gradient of the transverse displacement (6.685a) specifies (6.703) the component of the augmented turning moment normal to the boundary:

$$h^{-1}\,\bar{N}_n = -\frac{4EA^3C}{\left(a^2 - b^2\right)^2}\left(\frac{x^4}{a^4} + \frac{y^4}{b^4} - \frac{4x^2y^2}{a^2 b^2}\right) = -\frac{4EA^3C}{\left(a^2 - b^2\right)^2}\left[\left(\frac{x^2}{a^4} - \frac{y^2}{b^2}\right)^2 - \frac{2x^2y^2}{a^2 b^2}\right]$$

$$= -\frac{4EA^3C}{\left(a^2 - b^2\right)^2}\left(\frac{x^2}{a^2} - \frac{y^2}{b^2} - \frac{xy\sqrt{2}}{ab}\right)\left(\frac{x^2}{a^2} - \frac{y^2}{b^2} + \frac{xy\sqrt{2}}{ab}\right), \tag{6.703}$$

that is non-zero but small $O\left(A^3\right)$, thus approximately meeting one (6.683g) of the free boundary conditions.

The assumption of a transverse displacement for a plate (6.684a) ≡ (6.402a) as for a membrane, leads (problem 329) at the elliptic boundary (6.696a) to: (i) exact zero transverse displacement (6.696b); (ii–iii) zero turning moment (6.701a) and small $O(A^3)$ augmented turning moment (6.703); and (iv–v) first order $O(A)$ normal slope (6.698a, b) and stress couple (6.700a–c). Thus, in the general boundary conditions for: (iii) a clamped (6.683b, c) [pinned (6.683d, e)] plate, the first condition is met by zero and the second condition is $O(A)$, showing that it is not met to lowest order; (iii) for a free boundary (6.683f, g) the first condition is $O(A)$ and the second is $O(A^3)$ so again it is not met to lowest order. Of the five distinct boundary conditions in (6.683a–g): (a) only zero displacement (6.683a) ≡ (6.683c) is met exactly (6.696b); (b) the augmented turning moment (6.683g) is not zero (6.703) but is small $O(A^3)$; (c) however the mathematical conditions (a) and (b) are not physically compatible. The displacement (6.684a, b) ≡ (6.403c) applies to a membrane that has no stiffness, and could not be expected to extend to the bending of a stressed plate that has stiffness. This is an example of the risk that an *a priori* choice of transverse displacement (or stress function) that meets the coupled non-linear differential equations (6.656; 6.657) may fail to meet a consistent set (6.683a–g) of boundary conditions; an error in a boundary condition of $O(A)$ indicates that strictly the "solution" is inconsistent, or may "at best" be considered a low-order approximation, an order-of-magnitude estimation, or a dimensional scaling law. To be assured *a priori* to meet both the coupled differential equations (6.656; 6.657) and a consistent set of boundary conditions (6.683a–g) to any order of approximation a perturbation expansion may be used (subsection 6.9.8), for example with radial symmetry (subsection 6.9.9). If the transverse force per unit area and in-plane stresses are polynomials of the radius (subsection 6.9.10), the exact analytical solution can be obtained for all orders (subsection 6.9.11). An example is the non-linear coupling of bending and stretching (subsection 6.9.9) to lowest non-linear order (subsection 6.9.12) of a heavy circular plate under uniform compression (subsection 6.9.13) at its clamped edge (subsection 6.9.14) specifying: (i) the stress function, stresses, strains, and in-plane displacements (subsection 6.9.15); and (ii) the transverse displacement, slope, stress couple, and turning moment (subsection 6.9.16). Thus a comparison is made between an *a priori*, tentative [assured (subsection 6.9.17)] method of considering the strong buckling of a thick plate, with (without) risk of inconsistency in the boundary conditions and low (high) order of approximation, taking as example an elliptic (circular) plate [subsections 6.9.6–6.9.7 (6.9.8–6.9.17)].

6.9.8 Perturbation Expansions for the Transverse Displacement and Stress Function

The **perturbation expansions** for the transverse displacement (6.704a) [stress function (6.704b)]:

$$\{\zeta, \Theta\} = \varepsilon\{\zeta_1, \Theta_1\} + \varepsilon^2\{\zeta_2, \Theta_2\} + \ldots + \varepsilon^n\{\zeta_n, \Theta_n\} + \ldots \qquad \text{(6.704a, b)}$$

assume for small **perturbation parameter** ε either (i) convergence as a series (chapter I.21) or (ii) a reasonably accurate approximation by truncation to some order $n \geq 2$. Substitution of the perturbation expansions (6.704a, b) in the coupled equations (6.656; 6.657) for the strong bending of a plate leads at: (i) order one (6.705a) to decoupled stress function (6.705b) $\equiv$ (6.658d) [transverse displacement (6.705c) $\equiv$ (6.658c)] satisfying unforced (forced) biharmonic equations:

$$f \sim O(\varepsilon): \qquad\qquad \nabla^4 \Theta_1 = 0, \qquad \nabla^4 \zeta_1 = f, \qquad\qquad (6.705a\text{–}c)$$

where the forcing in (6.705c) is due to the transverse force per unit area that is assumed to be of the lowest order (6.705a); (ii) two (6.706a) starts the non-linear coupling with biharmonic operators (6.706b, c) forced by order one terms:

$$O(\varepsilon^2): \qquad\qquad \frac{1}{E}\nabla^4 \Theta_2 = \left(\partial_{xy}\zeta_1\right)^2 - \left(\partial_{xx}\zeta_1\right)\left(\partial_{yy}\zeta_1\right), \qquad\qquad (6.706a, b)$$

$$\frac{D}{h}\nabla^4 \zeta_2 = \left(\partial_{yy}\Theta_1\right)\left(\partial_{xx}\zeta_1\right) + \left(\partial_{xx}\Theta_1\right)\left(\partial_{yy}\zeta_1\right) - 2\left(\partial_{xy}\Theta_1\right)\left(\partial_{xy}\zeta_1\right); \qquad (6.706c)$$

(iii) order n to (6.707a) biharmonic equations (6.707b, c) forced by all lower orders up to $n-1$:

$$O(\varepsilon^n): \qquad \frac{1}{E}\nabla^4 \Theta_n = \sum_{m=1}^{n}\left[\left(\partial_{xy}\zeta_m\right)\left(\partial_{xy}\zeta_{n-m}\right) - \left(\partial_{xx}\zeta_m\right)\left(\partial_{yy}\zeta_{n-m}\right)\right], \qquad (6.707a, b)$$

$$\frac{D}{h}\nabla^4 \zeta_n = \sum_{m=1}^{n}\left[\left(\partial_{yy}\Theta_m\right)\left(\partial_{xx}\zeta_{n-m}\right) + \left(\partial_{xx}\Theta_m\right)\left(\partial_{yy}\zeta_{n-m}\right) - 2\left(\partial_{xy}\Theta_m\right)\left(\partial_{xy}\zeta_{n-m}\right)\right].$$

$$(6.707c)$$

Thus, *(problem 330) the perturbation expansions (6.704a, b) substituted in a system of non-linear coupled differential equations (6.656; 6.657) lead to a sequence of linear differential equations that are: (i) decoupled (6.705b, c) at the lowest order (6.705a); (ii) become coupled (6.706b, c) first at second order (6.706a); and (iii) at order n are coupled (6.707a–c) by all lower orders as in a* **generalized Markov chain***;* that is, a sequence of problems in which each iteration depends only on all the preceding and not on the following. The perturbation expansions (subsection 6.9.8) are applied next (subsection 6.9.9) to the strong bending of a circular plate with axial symmetry.

6.9.9 Non-Linear Coupling of Bending and Stretching with Axial Symmetry

The relation between the Laplacian in the plane in Cartesian coordinates (I.11.28a) ≡ (6.708a) and in polar coordinates (I.11.28b) with radial symmetry:

$$\partial_{xx} + \partial_{yy} \equiv \nabla^2 = r^{-1} \partial_r (r \partial_r) = \partial_{rr} + r^{-1} \partial_r:$$

$$\{\partial_x, \partial_y\} \leftrightarrow \{d_r, 0\}, \quad \{\partial_{xx}, \partial_{yy}, \partial_{xy}\} = \{d_{rr}, r^{-1} dr, 0\}, \qquad \text{(6.708a–c)}$$

suggests the transformation from Cartesian coordinate in the plane to axisymmetric polar coordinates for the first (6.708b) [second (6.708c)] order derivatives; the second-order derivatives (6.708c) agree with (6.486a, c) and also with (6.470e, f) with (x, y) interchanged because y rather than x was placed in the radial direction. Substituting (6.708a–c) in the non-linear bending equations (6.657) [(6.656)] leads to (6.709) [(6.710)]:

$$\frac{1}{E} \nabla^4 \Theta = -\zeta'' \frac{\zeta'}{r} = -\frac{\left(\zeta'^2\right)'}{2r}, \qquad \text{(6.709)}$$

$$D \nabla^4 \zeta - f = \frac{h}{r} \left(\Theta' \zeta'' + \Theta'' \zeta' \right) = \frac{h}{r} \left(\Theta' \zeta' \right)'. \qquad \text{(6.710)}$$

In the case of axial symmetry: (i) the stress function specifies (6.334b–d) the stresses (6.711a–c):

$$\{T_{rr}, T_{\phi\phi}, T_{r\phi}\} = \left\{ \frac{\Theta'}{r}, \Theta'', 0 \right\}; \qquad \text{(6.711a–c)}$$

(ii–iii) the inverse Hooke law (6.311a, b; 6.306c; 6.313c) specifies the strains (6.713a–c):

$$E \{S_{rr}, S_{\phi\phi}, S_{r\phi}, S_{zz}\} = \left\{ T_{rr} - \sigma T_{\phi\phi}, T_{\phi\phi} - \sigma T_{rr}, (1+\sigma) T_{r\phi}, -\frac{\sigma}{1-\sigma} \left(S_{rr} + S_{\phi\phi} \right) \right\}, \qquad \text{(6.712a–d)}$$

$$= \left\{ \frac{\Theta'}{r} - \sigma \Theta'', \Theta'' - \frac{\sigma}{r} \Theta', 0, -\frac{\sigma}{1-\sigma} \left(\Theta'' + \frac{\Theta'}{r} \right) \right\} \qquad \text{(6.713a–d)}$$

$$\{S_{rr}, S_{\phi\phi}, S_{r\phi}, S_{zz}\} = \left\{ u' + \frac{\zeta'^2}{2}, \frac{u}{r}, 0, -\frac{\sigma}{1-\sigma} \left(u' + \frac{u}{r} + \frac{\zeta'^2}{2} \right) \right\}, \qquad \text{(6.714a–d)}$$

(iv) the strains are given by (6.665a–c) ≡ (6.666a–c) and (6.313c) using also (6.354a–c) with radial symmetry (6.708a) leading to (6.714a–d); (v) the radial component of the stress couple (6.471d) ≡ (6.715a) is unaffected by in-plane stresses:

$$M_r = -D\left(\zeta'' + \frac{\sigma}{r}\zeta'\right); \quad \bar{N}_r = D\left(\nabla^2\zeta\right)' + hT_{rr}\zeta' = D\left[\frac{(\zeta'r)'}{r}\right]' + \frac{h}{r}\Theta'\zeta', \quad (6.715a\text{--}c)$$

(vi) the radial component of the augmented turning moment (6.682c) ≡ (6.715b) consists of two terms (6.715c); namely, (vi-1) due to bending in the turning moment (6.465a); (vi-2) augmented by the in-plane stresses (6.682a–c). Thus *(problem 331) the axial symmetry; that is, the dependence only on the distance from the axis, leads to: (i–ii) the stresses (6.711a–c) and strains (6.712a–c) ≡ (6.713a–c) ≡ (6.714a–d); and (iii–iv) the radial stress couple (6.715a) [augmented turning moment (6.715b, c)]. All four (i–iv) depend on the stress function and transverse displacement that satisfy the system (6.709; 6.710) of coupled non-linear differential equations that specify the strong bending of a thick isotropic plate.* The solution for a clamped (subsection 6.9.12) heavy circular plate under axial compression (subsection 6.9.11) is obtained as an example of the use of perturbation expansion (subsection 6.9.8) with radial symmetry (subsection 6.9.10).

6.9.10 Strong Bending of a Circular Plate by Transverse Loads

Consider (Figure 6.30a) a circular plate under strong bending (6.657; 6.656) by a transverse force per unit area (6.716a) with radial symmetry (6.708a–c) leading to (6.709; 6.710) ≡ (6.716b, c):

$$f(r) = \frac{dF}{ds}: \quad \nabla^4\Theta = -\frac{E}{2r}\left(\zeta'^2\right)', \quad f = D\nabla^4\zeta - \frac{h}{r}\left(\Theta'\zeta'\right)'. \quad (6.716a\text{--}c)$$

The perturbation expansion (6.704a, b) substituted in the coupled nonlinear strong bending equations (6.716b, c) lead to the generalized Markov chain of differential equations that: (i–ii) are decoupled (6.717b, c) [first coupled (6.718b, c)] at order one (6.716a) [two (6.718a)]:

$$O(\varepsilon): \quad \nabla^4\Theta_1 = 0, \quad \nabla^4\zeta_1 = f; \quad (6.717a\text{--}c)$$

$$O(\varepsilon): \quad \nabla^4\Theta_2 = -\frac{E}{2r}\left(\zeta_1'^2\right)', \quad \nabla^4\zeta_2 = \frac{h}{Dr}\left(\Theta_1'\zeta_1'\right)'; \quad (6.718a\text{--}c)$$

$$O(\varepsilon^n): \quad \nabla^4\Theta_n = -\frac{E}{2r}\sum_{m=1}^{n}\left(\zeta_m'\zeta_{n-m}'\right)', \quad \nabla^4\zeta_n = \frac{h}{Dr}\sum_{m=1}^{n}\left(\Theta_m'\zeta_{n-m}'\right)', \quad (6.719a\text{--}c)$$

(iii) the order *n* coupled (6.719a) all lower orders (6.719b, c). Thus, *(problem 332) the non-linear strong bending of a circular plate with axial symmetry (6.708a–c) is*

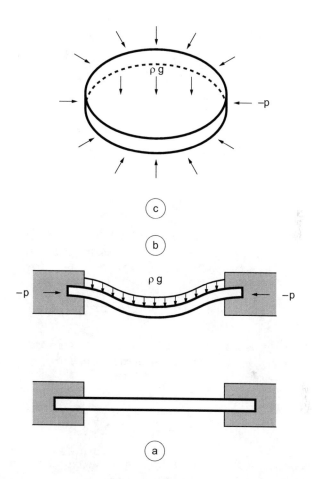

FIGURE 6.30
The non-linear (strong) bending with large slope (deflection) is associated with in-plane stresses, for example for a flat circular plate (Figure 6.24b) that is (a) clamped on the boundary and subject to (b) its own weight and (c) axial compression.

specified (6.716a–c) by the perturbation expansions (6.704a, b), whose terms are the solutions of the generalized Markov chain of differential equations decoupled at order one (6.717a–c), first coupled at order two (6.718a–c), and increasingly coupled at higher orders (6.719a–c). This system is readily solved in the case of forcing by powers, polynomial, or series of the radius (subsection 6.9.11).

6.9.11 Radially Symmetric Biharmonic Equation Forced by a Power

In the case of a radially symmetric biharmonic equation (6.501c) ≡ (6.720b) forced by a power (6.720a):

$$C r^k = \nabla^4 \zeta = \zeta'''' + 2 r^{-1} \zeta''' - r^{-2} \zeta'' + r^{-3} \zeta',$$

(6.720a, b)

a particular integral may be sought in the form (6.721a) leading to (6.721b):

$$\zeta = J r^{k+4}: \qquad C r^k = \nabla^4 \left(J r^{k+4} \right) = J r^k P_4(k), \qquad (6.721a\text{–}c)$$

involving the quartic polynomial:

$$
\begin{aligned}
P_4(k) &= (k+4)(k+3)(k+2)(k+1) \\
&\quad + 2(k+4)(k+3)(k+2) - (k+4)(k+3) + k + 4 \\
&= (k+4)(k+2)\left[(k+3)(k+1) + 2(k+3) - 1 \right] \qquad (6.722a\text{–}d) \\
&= (k+4)(k+2)\left[(k+3)^2 - 1 \right] = (k+4)^2 (k+2)^2 ,
\end{aligned}
$$

that is similar to (6.506a–d) setting $n = k + 4$. Thus, *(problem 333) a radially symmetric biharmonic equation forced by a power (6.720a, b) $\equiv$ (6.723a) has the particular integral (6.721a–c; 6.722d) $\equiv$ (6.723b):*

$$\nabla^4 \zeta = C r^k: \qquad \zeta(r) = \frac{C r^{k+4}}{(k+4)^2 (k+2)^2}. \qquad (6.723a, b)$$

This result can be used to obtain (problem 334) by superposition the particular integral (6.724b) of a radially symmetric biharmonic equation forced by a polynomial (6.724a):

$$\nabla^4 \tilde{\zeta} = \sum_{k=0}^{K} C_k r^k: \qquad \tilde{\zeta}(r) = \sum_{k=0}^{K} \frac{C_k r^{k+4}}{(k+4)^2 (k+2)^2}, \qquad (6.724a, b)$$

and is applied next (subsection 6.9.12) to a heavy circular plate under axial compression.

6.9.12 Heavy Circular Plate under Axial Compression

At order one (6.717a–c) there is decoupling of: (i) the transverse deflection (6.512a) $\equiv$ (6.725d) of a circular plate of radius a under its own weight (6.725a) that is the solution of (6.501b) $\equiv$ (6.725b) with coefficient (6.413d) $\equiv$ (6.725c):

$$f = \rho g, \quad D \nabla^4 \zeta_1 = \rho g, \quad H \equiv \frac{\rho g}{64 D} = \frac{3 \rho g \left(1 - \sigma^2 \right)}{16 E h^3}: \quad \zeta_1(r) = H \left(r^2 - a^2 \right)^2 ;$$

$$(6.725a\text{–}d)$$

$$T_{rr} = -p, \qquad \nabla^4 \Theta_1 = 0: \qquad \Theta_1 = -\frac{1}{2} p r^2, \qquad (6.726a\text{–}c)$$

(ii) a uniform axial compression (6.726a) with pressure p, for which the biharmonic equation for the stress function (6.717b) $\equiv$ (6.726b) has solution

(6.358d) ≡ (6.726c). With the substitutions (6.725d; 6.726c) the perturbation equations (6.718a–c; 6.719a–c) are biharmonic with forcing (6.724a) by polynomials, so the particular integral (6.724b) can be applied to all orders. For the purpose of illustrating the method it is sufficient to consider the second order; that is, the lowest for which non-linear coupling of bending and in-plane deformation occurs (subsection 6.9.13).

6.9.13 Non-Linear Coupling of Bending and Compression

The first order stress function (6.725c) [transverse displacement (6.726d)] has first order radial derivative (6.727a) [(6.727b)]:

$$\Theta_1'(r) = -pr, \qquad \zeta_1'(r) = 4Hr(r^2 - a^2), \qquad \text{(6.727a, b)}$$

that appear in the second-order forced biharmonic equation (6.718b) ≡ (6.728a) [(6.718c) ≡ (6.728b)]:

$$\nabla^4 \Theta_2 = -\frac{8EH^2}{r}\left[r^2\left(r^2 - a^2\right)^2\right]' = -16EH^2\left(3r^4 - 4a^2r^2 + a^4\right), \qquad \text{(6.728a)}$$

$$\nabla^4 \zeta_2 = -\frac{4pHh}{Dr}\left[r^2\left(r^2 - a^2\right)\right]' = -\frac{8pHh}{D}\left(2r^2 - a^2\right). \qquad \text{(6.728b)}$$

The biharmonic equation (6.728b) [(6.728a)] is forced by a polynomial (6.724a) and its particular integral (6.724b) specifies the second-order stress function (6.729a) [transverse displacement (6.729b)]:

$$
\begin{aligned}
\Theta_2(r) &= -16EH^2\left(\frac{3r^8}{8^2 6^2} - \frac{4a^2 r^6}{6^2 4^2} + \frac{a^4 r^4}{4^2 2^2}\right) \\
&= -\frac{16EH^2 r^4}{8^2 6^2}\left(3r^4 - 4.2^2 a^2 r^2 + 6^2 a^4\right) \qquad \text{(6.729a)} \\
&= -\frac{EH^2 r^4}{144}\left(3r^4 - 16a^2 r^2 + 36a^4\right),
\end{aligned}
$$

$$
\begin{aligned}
\zeta_2(r) &= -\frac{8pHh}{D}\left(\frac{2r^6}{6^2 4^2} - \frac{a^2 r^4}{4^2 2^2}\right) \\
&= -\frac{8pHhr^4}{6^2 4^2 D}\left(2r^2 - 3^2 a^2\right) \qquad \text{(6.729b)} \\
&= -\frac{pHhr^4}{72D}\left(2r^2 - 9a^2\right).
\end{aligned}
$$

The total stress function (6.730a) [transverse displacement (6.730b)] for (problem 335) the non-linear strong bending of a heavy (Figure 6.30c) circular plate (Figure 6.30a) under compression (Figure 6.30b) is given by the sum of: (i) the general integral of the unforced biharmonic equation (6.503b) corresponding to (6.503e) that coincides with the last four terms on the r.h.s. of (6.502e) with arbitrary constants $B_{1-4}(C_{1-4})$:

$$\Theta(r) = B_4\, r^2 \log r + B_3\, r^2 + B_2 \log r + B_1 - \frac{1}{2}p r^2 - \frac{EH^2 r^4}{144}\left(3r^4 - 16a^2\, r^2 + 36a^4\right),$$
$$(6.730a)$$

$$\zeta(r) = C_4\, r^2 \log r + C_3\, r^2 + C_2 \log r + C_1 + H\left(r^2 - a^2\right)^2 - \frac{pHhr^4}{72D}\left(2r^2 - 9a^2\right),$$
$$(6.730b)$$

(ii–iii) the lowest decoupled (6.726c) [(6.725d)] and next coupled (6.729a) [(6.729b)] order that introduces coupling to the lowest order 2 in the particular integral; and (iii) the complete integral is the sum of (i) and (ii). The two sets of four arbitrary constants of integration $B_{1-4}(C_{1-4})$ are determined from boundary conditions, for example for a clamped plate under axial compression at the boundary (subsection 6.9.14).

6.9.14 Transverse Displacement and Stress Function with Clamping

The stress function (6.730a) leads (6.711b) to the tangential stress (6.731):

$$T_{\phi\phi}(r) = B_4\left(2\log r + 3\right) + 2B_3 - \frac{B_2}{r^2} - p - \frac{EH^2 r^2}{6}\left(7r^4 - 20a^2 r^2 + 18a^4\right).$$
$$(6.731)$$

A finite stress at the center (6.732a) implies (6.732b, c), leading (6.730a) to the stress function (6.732d):

$$T_{\phi\phi}(0) < \infty: \quad B_4 = 0 = B_2: \quad \Theta(r) = B_3\, r^2 - \frac{1}{2}p r^2 - \frac{EH^2 r^4}{144}\left(3r^4 - 16a^2\, r^2 + 36a^4\right),$$
$$(6.732a–d)$$

where the constant (6.733a) can be omitted because it does not affect the stress (6.711a–c), either tangential (6.731) or radial (6.733b):

$$B_1 = 0: \qquad T_{rr}(r) = 2B_3 - p - \frac{EH^2 r^2}{6}\left(r^4 - 4a^2\, r^2 + 6a^4\right). \qquad (6.733a, b)$$

The boundary condition specifying the compression (6.734a):

$-p = T_{rr}(a)$:

$$B_3 = \frac{EH^2a^6}{4}, \Theta(r) = -\frac{1}{2}pr^2 - \frac{EH^2r^2}{144}\left(3r^6 - 16a^2r^4 + 36a^4r^2 - 36a^6\right),$$

(6.734a–c)

determines the remaining constant of integration (6.734b) that, substituted in (6.732d), determines the stress function (6.734c).

In the transverse displacement (6.730b), two constants are zero (6.508b) ≡ (6.735a) [(6.508d) ≡ (6.735b)] because the transverse displacement must be finite (6.508a) [there is no concentrated force (6.508c)] at the center:

$$C_2 = 0 = C_4: \quad \zeta(r) = C_3 r^2 + C_1 + H\left(r^2 - a^2\right)^2 - \frac{pHhr^4}{72D}\left(2r^2 - 9a^2\right), \quad (6.735\text{a–c})$$

leading to (6.735c). The slope (6.736a) [displacement (6.736c)] vanish on the boundary:

$$0 = \zeta'(a) = 2C_3 a + \frac{pHha^5}{6D}: \qquad\qquad C_3 = -\frac{pHha^4}{6D}, \qquad (6.736\text{a, b})$$

$$0 = \zeta(a) = C_1 + C_3 a^2 + \frac{7pHha^6}{72D}: \qquad C_1 = -\frac{19pHha^6}{72D}, \qquad (6.736\text{c, d})$$

determining the two remaining constants of integration (6.736b) [(6.736d)].

Substituting (6.736b, d) in (6.735c) specifies the transverse displacement (6.737):

$$\zeta(r) = H\left(r^2 - a^2\right)^2 - \frac{pHh}{72D}\left(2r^6 - 9a^2 r^4 + 12a^4 r^2 + 19a^6\right). \qquad (6.737)$$

A clamped heavy (Figure 6.30b) circular plate (Figure 6.30a) under axial compression at the boundary (Figure 6.30c) has (problem 336) stress function (6.734c) [transverse displacement (6.737)] to the second or lowest non-linear approximation of transverse bending and in-plane deformation leading to the stresses, strains, and in-plane displacements (slope, stress couple, and augmented turning moment) that are obtained next [subsection 6.9.15 (6.9.16)].

6.9.15 Stresses, Strains, and Radial Displacement

The stress function (6.734c) specifies (6.711a–c) the non-zero stresses, namely radial (6.733b; 6.734b) ≡ (6.738a) [tangential (6.731; 6.732b, c; 6.733a) ≡ (6.738b)]:

$$T_{rr}(r) = -p - \frac{EH^2}{6}\left(r^6 - 4a^2 r^4 + 6a^4 r^2 - 3a^6\right), \tag{6.738a}$$

$$T_{\phi\phi}(r) = -p - \frac{EH^2}{6}\left(7r^6 - 20a^2 r^4 + 18a^4 r^2 - 3a^6\right). \tag{6.738b}$$

The radial (6.738a) [tangential (6.738b)] stresses: (i) differ at the boundary where it equals (6.739a) [is less than (6.739b)] the compression:

$$T_{rr}(a) = -p > -p - \frac{EH^2 a^6}{3} = T_{\phi\phi}(a); \tag{6.739a, b}$$

$$T_{rr}(0) = -p + \frac{EH^2 a^6}{2} = T_{\phi\phi}(0) > -p, \tag{6.739c, d}$$

(ii) coincide (6.739c) [≡(6.739d)] and are higher than the compression at the center. The non-zero stresses (6.738a, b) specify (6.712a–d) the non-zero strains; for example, (6.714b) the tangential strain (6.740b) specifies (6.714b; 6.738a, b) the radial displacement (6.740a):

$$\frac{u_r(r)}{r} = S_{\phi\phi}(r)$$

$$= -\frac{1-\sigma}{E}p - \frac{H^2}{6}\left[(7-\sigma)r^6 - 4(5-\sigma)a^2r^4 + 6(3-\sigma)a^4 r^2 - 3(1-\sigma)a^6\right], \tag{6.740a–c}$$

where on the r.h.s. of (6.740a): (i) the first term is the linear approximation (6.359b); and (ii) the second term is the lowest order non-linear correction. The tangential strain (6.740b) [radial displacement (6.740a)]: (i) is non-zero (zero) at the center (6.741a) [(6.741b)]:

$$S_{\phi\phi}(0) = (1-\sigma)\left(-\frac{p}{E} + \frac{H^2 a^6}{2}\right), \qquad u_r(0) = 0; \tag{6.741a, b}$$

$$S_{\phi\phi}(a) = \frac{u_r(a)}{a} = -\frac{1-\sigma}{E}p + \frac{H^2 a^6}{3}, \tag{6.741c, d}$$

and (ii) at the boundary both are non-zero (6.741c) [(6.741d)] with the non-linear effect increasing the strain and displacement in all non-zero cases.

The remaining non-zero strains are radial (6.712a) ≡ (6.742a) [out of the plane (6.712d) ≡ (6.742c)] that specifies the normal displacement (6.742b)]:

$$S_{rr}(r) = -\frac{1-\sigma}{E}p - \frac{H^2}{6}\left[(1-7\sigma)r^6 - 4(1-5\sigma)a^2r^4 + 6(1-3\sigma)a^4r^2 - 3(1-\sigma)a^6\right],$$

(6.742a)

$$\frac{u_z(r)}{z} = S_{zz}(r) = \frac{2\sigma}{E}p - \frac{H^2\sigma}{3}\left(4r^6 - 12a^2r^4 + 12a^4r^2 - 3a^6\right), \qquad (6.742b, c)$$

where on the r.h.s. of (6.742a) [(6.742c)] the: (i) first term is the linear approximation (6.359a) [(6.357d)]; and (ii) second term is the lowest order non-linear correction. The radial strain (6.742a) equals the tangential strain (6.741a) ≡ (6.743b) at the center and is distinct (6.671d) at the boundary (6.743c, d):

$$S_{rr}(0) = (1-\sigma)\left(-\frac{p}{E} + \frac{H^2a^6}{2}\right) \equiv S_{\phi\phi}(0) > S_{rr}(a) = -\frac{1-\sigma}{E}p + \frac{H^2a^6\sigma}{3} \neq S_{\phi\phi}(a);$$

(6.743a–d)

the transverse displacement is specified on axis (6.743e) by the out-of-plane strain (6.742b) that is larger at the center (6.743f) than on the boundary (6.743g):

$$\frac{u_z(0)}{z} = S_{zz}(0) = \frac{2\sigma}{E}p + H^2\sigma a^6 > \frac{2\sigma}{E}p - \frac{H^2\sigma a^6}{3} \equiv S_{zz}(a). \qquad (6.743e–g)$$

The area (6.744a) [volume (6.744b)] change:

$$D_2(r) = S_{rr}(r) + S_{\phi\phi}(r) = -\frac{\sigma}{1-\sigma}S_{zz}(r), \qquad (6.744a)$$

$$D_3(r) = D_2(r) + S_{zz}(r) = \frac{1-2\sigma}{1-\sigma}S_{zz}(r), \qquad (6.744b)$$

follow from (6.740c; 6.742a, c). The boundary conditions are checked next (subsection 6.7.16).

6.9.16 Slope, Stress Couple, and Augmented Turning Moment

From transverse displacement (6.737) follows the slope (6.745a) that vanishes both at the boundary (6.736a) ≡ (6.745b) and center (6.745c):

$$\zeta'(r) = 4Hr(r^2 - a^2) - \frac{pHhr}{6D}(r^4 - 3a^2r^2 + 2a^4): \qquad \zeta'(a) = 0 = \zeta'(0).$$

(6.745a–c)

The radial (6.486a) [tangential (6.486c)] curvature is given by (6.746a) [(6.746b)]:

$$k_r(r) = \zeta''(r) = 4H(3r^2 - a^2) - \frac{pHh}{6D}(5r^4 - 9a^2 r^2 + 2a^4), \quad (6.746a)$$

$$k_\phi(r) = \frac{\zeta'(r)}{r} = 4H(r^2 - a^2) - \frac{pHh}{6D}(r^4 - 3a^2 r^2 + 2a^4), \quad (6.746b)$$

does not (does) vanish on the boundary (6.747b) [(6.747a)]:

$$k_\phi(a) = 0 \neq k_r(a) = Ha^2\left(8 + \frac{pa^2 h}{3D}\right); \quad (6.747a, b)$$

$$k_\phi(0) = -Ha^2\left(\frac{pha^2}{3D} + 4\right) = k_r(0), \quad (6.747c, d)$$

and coincide (6.747d) [$\equiv$ (6.747c)] at the center.

The radial stress couple (6.715a) is given (6.746a, b) by (6.748a, b):

$$M_r(r) = -D\left[k_r(r) + \sigma k_\phi(r)\right] = -4HD\left[(3+\sigma)r^2 - (1+\sigma)a^2\right]$$
$$+ \frac{pHh}{6}\left[(5+\sigma)r^4 - 3(3+\sigma)a^2 r^2 + 2(1+\sigma)a^4\right], \quad (6.748a, b)$$

is: (i) non-zero at the center (6.749a):

$$M_r(0) = -(1+\sigma)a^2 H\left(4D + \frac{pha^2}{3}\right); \qquad M_r(a) = -H^2 a\left(\frac{pha^2}{3} + 8D\right), \quad (6.749a, b)$$

(ii) on the boundary is non-zero (6.749b) because the plate is clamped; and (iii) has a lowest-order non-linear correction in both cases (6.749a, b).

The Laplacian of the transverse displacement (6.750a) is the sum of the radial (6.746a) and tangential (6.746b) curvatures (6.750b) and is given by (6.750c):

$$\nabla^2\zeta = \zeta'' + \frac{\zeta'}{r} = k_r(r) + k_\phi(r) = 8H(2r^2 - a^2) - \frac{pHh}{3D}(3r^4 - 6a^2 r^2 + 2a^4); \quad (6.750a-c)$$

$$N_r(r) = (D\nabla^2\zeta)' = D\left(\zeta''' + \frac{\zeta''}{r} - \frac{\zeta'}{r^2}\right) = 32HDr - 4pHhr(r^2 - a^2), \quad (6.751a-c)$$

the turning moment (6.465a) is specified by the radial derivative of the bending stiffness multiplied by the Laplacian (6.751a), and in the case of constant
bending stiffness, (6.751b) is specified by (6.751c). The augmented turning
moment (6.715c) adds to the turning moment (6.751c) a term (6.752a) involving
the derivatives (6.745a) [(6.738a) multiplied by r in (6.711a)] of the transverse
displacement (6.737) [stress function (6.734c)] leading to (6.752a, b):

$$\bar{N}_r(r) - N_r(r) = \frac{h}{r}\Theta'\zeta' = hT_{rr}\zeta',\qquad (6.752a, b)$$

where may be substituted (6.745a) and (6.738a). At the center the turning
moment (6.751c) vanishes (6.753a) and also (6.745c) the augmented turning
moment (6.753b):

$$N_r(0) = 0 = \bar{N}_r(0); \qquad \bar{N}_r(a) = N_r(a) = 32\,H\,D\,a,\qquad (6.753a-d)$$

on the boundary (6.745b) the turning moment and augmented turning
moment (6.752b) coincide (6.753c) and (6.751c) so do not vanish (6.753d)
because the plate is clamped. The bending of a thick heavy clamped circular plate to the lowest order of non-linearity (subsections 6.9.9–6.9.16) is an
example of the method of perturbation expansions (subsection 6.9.8) that in
the axisymmetric case with transverse force and in-plane stress polynomial
functions applies exactly to all orders of non-linearity (subsection 6.9.17).

6.9.17 Method for Axisymmetric Strong Bending

It has been shown that *the strong bending (6.656; 6.657) with radius symmetry (6.708a–c) of (Figure 6.30a) a heavy plate (6.725a) under uniform axial compression (6.739a) at (Figure 6.30b) its circular clamped (6.736a, c) boundary with
radius a is specified to second order; that is, the lowest order of non-linearity, by
the stress function (6.734c) and transverse displacement (6.737) that lead (problem
337) in the interior of the plate (respectively at the center and boundary) to the:
(i) stresses (6.738a, b) [(6.739a–d)]; (ii) strains (6.740a–c; 6.742a, c) [(6.741a, c, d;
6.743a, b, c, d, f, g)]; (iii) in-plane (6.740a) [(6.741b, d)] and out-of-plane (6.742b)
[(6.743e)] displacements; (iv) area (6.744a) and volume (6.744b) change; (v) radial
stress couple (6.748a, b) [(6.749a, b)]; and (vi) unaugmented (augmented) radial
turning moment (6.751a–c) [(6.752a, b; 6.738a; 6.745a)] do not coincide in general,
except at the center where they vanish (6.753a, b) and at the boundary (6.753c, d)
where they are non-zero.*

*This case is an example of (problem 338) the general method of solution of the
non-linear equations (6.656; 6.657) for the strong bending of plates via perturbation expansions (6.704a, b): (i) leading to the generalized Markov chain of linear
differential equations (6.705a–c; 6.706a–c; 6.707a–c) in which each depends on all
the preceding; (ii) in the case of radial symmetry (6.708a–c) the equations for non-
linear bending (6.716a–c) lead to the perturbation sequence (6.717a–c; 6.718a–c;*

6.719a–c); (iii) if the transverse force per unit area and in-plane stresses at the lowest linear order (6.717a–c) are polynomials of the radius, the solutions (6.724a, b) apply to all higher orders (6.718a–c; 6.719a–c) specifying the stress function (6.704b) and transverse displacement (6.704a) to any order of accuracy; (iv) from (iii) can be calculated the stresses (6.711a–c), strains (6.712a, d; 6.713a–d), and in-plane (6.714b) and out-of-plane (6.714a) displacements, and the radial stress couple (6.715a) and augmented turning moment (6.715b, c); and (v) from (vi) can be applied any boundary conditions, such as (6.683a–g) [(6.675a–d)] for the transverse (in-plane) displacement (s).

NOTE 6.1: One/Two/Three-Dimensional Elasticity

The classification of a number of problems in elasticity is made in Lists 6.1–6.3 (pp. 344–347), Tables 6.9–6.11, and Diagrams 6.1–6.3. The main subjects addressed in this and preceding volumes of the series (List 6.1 and Table 6.9) include: (i) plane elasticity (chapter II.4) as a particular case of general three dimensional elasticity: (ii) linear and non-linear deflection of a string (chapter III.2); (iii) deflection of membranes under isotropic (sections II.6.1–II.6.2) and anisotropic (section 6.6) stresses; (iv–vi) torsion of rods (sections II.6.5–II.6.8), bending of bars (section III.4) and buckling of beams (sections 6.1–6.3); and (vii–x) in-plane deformation (section 6.6) and transverse bending (section 6.7) and their combination for linear (non-linear) cases [section 6.8 (6.9)]. Other problems concern curved rods, shells, and three-dimensional bodies and non-elastic constitutive relations in rheology.

The cases of one- and two-dimensional elastic bodies are reconsidered (List 6.2, Table 6.9, and Diagram 6.1) by type of deformation: (i) torsion for straight rods (sections II.6.5–II.6.8); (ii) compression/traction for (ii-1) straight rods (section 6.4; notes III.2.5–III.2.6 and III.4.4–III.4.7) and (ii-2) flat plates (section 6.5); (iii) transverse deflection without bending stiffness

TABLE 6.9

One- and Two-Dimensional Elastic Bodies without Curvature

Dimension	One	Two
Body	string, bar, beam	membrane, plate, stressed plate
Plane elasticity	–	II.4
Longitudinal tension	bar: 6.4	plane: 6.5
Transverse deformation without stiffness: deflection of	string: III.2	membrane II.6.1–II.6.2; 6.6
With stiffness: bending of	bar: III.4	plate: 6.7
With stiffness and longitudinal tension	beam 6.1–6.3	coupled bending: 6.8–6.9
Torsion	bar: II.6.5–II.6.8	–

Note: Classification of one(two)-dimensional elastic bodies without curvature in the undeformed state including strings (membranes), bars and rods (plates), and beams (stressed plates).

Elastic deflection and bending

	One - dimensional	Two - dimensional
without bending stiffeness	**strings** III.2	**membrane** III.6.1 – III.6.2; 6.6
combined: elastic stability	**beams** 6.1 – 6.3	**stressed plates** 6.8 – 6.9
with bending stiffeness	**bars** III.4	**plates** 6.7

DIAGRAM 6.2
Elastic deflection and bending (Table 6.10) on one- and two-dimensional elastic bodies with and without stiffness.

for (iii-1) strings (chapter III.2) and (iii-2) membranes (sections II.6.1–II.6.3 and 6.5); (iv) bending with stiffness of (iv-1) straight bars (chapter III.4) and (iv-2) flat plates (section 6.6); (v) the combination of (iii) and (iv) in the buckling of (v-1) straight beams (sections 6.1–6.3) and (v-2) flat plates (sections 6.8–6.9).

The transverse deflection bending or buckling are more detailed (List 6.3 and Diagram 6.2) including linear (non-linear) cases for: (i) the deflection of elastic strings [sections III.2.1–III.2.5 (III.2.6–III.2.9)]; (ii) the deflection of an elastic membranes [sections II.6.1 and 6.6 (sections II.6.1–II.6.2); (iii) the bending of a straight bar [sections III.4.1–III.4.5 (III.4.7–III.4.9)]; (iv) the straight beam under axial tension, including buckling under compression [sections III.4.6 and 6.1–6.3 (6.1)]; and (v) the flat plate with in-plane stresses including buckling [sections 6.7–6.8 (6.9)]. This variety of problems, including (a) linear (non-linear) cases of small (large) displacements, slopes, strains, and stresses and (b) homogeneous (inhomogeneous) media with properties not depending (depending) on position have common methods of solution (note 6.2).

NOTE 6.2: Spatial, Temporal, and Wave Problems

The methods presented in this and preceding volumes of the series to solve problems of elasticity (chapters II.4, III.2, III.4 and IV.6) in one (two) dimensions [strings, bars, beams, and rods (membranes, plates, and plane elasticity)] lead to: (i) ordinary (partial) differential equation if there is one (more than one) independent variable (position and/or time); (ii) the steady problems, that is (A) independent of time, use only spatial variables, and the unicity of solution requires boundary conditions. The vibration problems lead to linear (non-linear) ordinary differential equations with unicity of solution requiring initial conditions. The inclusion in the elastic force-stress balance (A) of the inertia force (B) leads to wave problems specified by partial differential equations in space-time (notes 6.3–6.23) for which the unicity of solution requires both initial and boundary conditions.

The wave equations, starting with the simplest, apply to: (i) linear and non-linear transverse vibrations of an elastic string (membrane) allowing for non-uniform density and tangential (in-plane anisotropic) stresses [notes 6.3 (6.4)]; (ii) a straight elastic rod may also have decoupled torsional (longitudinal) vibrations [notes 6.5 (6.6)]; and (iii) tangential tension (in-plane anisotropic stresses) affect the transversal vibrations of beams (stressed plates) combining [note 6.7 (6.8)] the phenomena associated with string and bars (membranes and plates). There are analogies (note 6.9) among the six types (i–ii) of vibrations and waves, and the applied external forces can include (note 6.10) damping, translational, and rotational springs, as well as others such as gravity.

An example combining several of the preceding phenomena is the vibrations of a beam; that is, a bar with bending stiffness subject to tangential tension, in the presence of damping and supported on translational springs; this leads to a linear wave equation with stiffness combining a beam in space with a damped harmonic oscillator in time; they are coupled by the mode frequency in the separation (note 6.11) of space and time variables. Concerning the spatial part, the boundary conditions specify the wavelengths of modes (note 6.12), and the spatial differential equation leads to the dispersion relation (note 6.13), specifying the modal frequencies. The propagating waves may be non-dispersive (dispersive) with a permanent (changing) waveform [note 6.14 (6.16)], and the superposition of waves with the same amplitude propagating in opposite directions leads to standing modes (note 6.15). The temporal part specifies the damping and effective frequencies of the modes (note 6.17), whose amplitudes are determined by the initial conditions for the displacement and velocity (note 6.18). The waves may be generated either by initial conditions out-of-equilibrium (note 6.18) or by external applied forces (note 6.19). In the case of forcing (note 6.19), the amplitude and phase of the responses (note 6.20) depends on the presence (absence) of damping [note 6.21 (6.22)] and is distinct in non-resonant and resonant cases (note 6.23).

NOTE 6.3: Transverse Waves along an Elastic String

The exact non-linear balance equation for the non-linear deflection of an elastic string under non-uniform tension subject to a shear stress or transverse force per unit length (6.752b) omits in (6.8) the bending stiffness $EI = 0$, and thus corresponds (6.752c) to the second term on the r.h.s. of (6.8):

$$\zeta' \equiv \partial_x \zeta \equiv \frac{\partial \zeta}{\partial x}: \qquad \frac{dF}{dx} = f = -\left\{T\zeta'\left|1+\zeta'^2\right|^{-1/2}\right\}', \qquad (6.752a\text{–}c)$$

where prime denotes derivative with regard to position (6.752a) that is the only variable in the steady case. In the unsteady case, when the transverse displacement depends also on time (6.753a): (i) the time derivative specifies the velocity (6.753b); (ii) the product by the mass density per unit length (6.753c) specifies the linear momentum (6.753d):

$$z = \zeta(x,t): \qquad v = \dot{\zeta} \equiv \partial_t \zeta \equiv \frac{\partial \zeta}{\partial t}, \qquad \rho_1 = \frac{dm}{dx}, \qquad p = \rho_1 v = \rho_1 \dot{\zeta}; \qquad (6.753a\text{–}d)$$

and (iii) the time derivative of the linear momentum (6.753d) specifies the inertia force (6.538) ≡ (6.754a, b):

$$f_i = \dot{p} = \left(\rho_1 \dot{\zeta}\right)^{\cdot}: \qquad f(x,t) = f_a(x,t) - f_i, \qquad (6.754a\text{–}c)$$

that is subtracted from the forcing term in (6.752c) to separate the external applied forces (6.754c) that may depend on position and time. Substituting (6.754b, c) in (6.752c) leads to:

$$\left(\rho_1 \dot{\zeta}\right)^{\cdot} - \left\{T\zeta'\left|1+\zeta'^2\right|^{-1/2}\right\}' = f_a(x,t); \qquad (6.755)$$

that is, the exact, non-linear **wave equation** for (Figure 6.31) the transverse displacement of vibrations along an elastic string, with mass density per unit length ρ_1, tangential tension T, and external applied force per unit length f_a generally functions of position and time.

The mass density may be a function of: (i) position for a non-uniform string of variable thickness (Examples E.III.10.2–E.III.10.3); or (ii) time for a collapsible tube; say, containing a liquid. The tangential stress may be a function of: (i) position in an external forced field, for example a heavy string hanging in the gravity field (Example E.III.10.7); or (ii) time if the string is subject to an unsteady pull from one (two) end(s). In addition to the dependence of the (a) mass density and/or (b) tangential tension on position and/or time, the (c) problem is linear (non-linear) for small (large) slope [sections III.2.1–III.2.5 (III.2.6–III.2.9)]. These three criteria (a, b, c) allow several simplifications of the general wave equation (6.755), of which four are mentioned: (i) if the

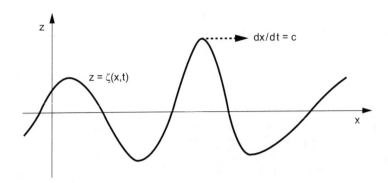

FIGURE 6.31
The unsteady generalization of the deflection of an string (Figures III.2.1–III.2.22) or bending of a bar (Figures III.4.1–III.4.15) or beam (Figures 6.1–6.7) leads to transversal elastic waves with propagation speed c.

mass density (6.753c) is constant (6.756a) the **transversal elastic wave speed** (6.756b) appears in the wave equation (6.756c):

$$\rho_1 = const; \quad c_e(x,t) = \sqrt{\frac{T(x,t)}{\rho_1}}: \quad \ddot{\zeta} - \left\{ c_e^2\, \zeta'\left|1 + \zeta'^2\right|^{-1/2} \right\}' = \frac{f_a(x,t)}{\rho_1}; \quad (6.756a\text{–}c)$$

(ii) in the linear case of small slope (6.757a) the wave equation (6.755) simplifies to (6.757b):

$$\zeta'^2 \ll 1: \qquad\qquad \left(\rho_1 \dot{\zeta}\right)^{\!\cdot} - \left(c_e^2\, \zeta'\right)' = f_a(x,t); \qquad\qquad (6.757a, b)$$

and (iii) combining (i) and (ii) in the linear case (6.758a) with constant mass density (6.758b) simplifies the wave equation (6.755) to (6.758c):

$$\zeta'^2 \ll 1, \qquad \rho_1 = const: \qquad \ddot{\zeta} - \left(c_e^2\, \zeta'\right)' = \rho_1^{-1} f_a(x,t). \qquad (6.758a\text{–}c)$$

All the preceding wave equations (6.755; 6.756c; 6.757b; 6.758d) are more general than the classical wave equation.

The **classical one-dimensional wave equation** (6.759e) applies in the linear case (6.759a), with (6.759b) [(6.759c)] the mass density (tangential tension) a function of position (time), in which case the elastic wave speed can depend on position and time (6.759d):

$$\zeta'^2 \ll 1, \quad \rho_1 = \rho_1(x), \quad T = T(t): \quad c_e(x,t) = \sqrt{\frac{T(t)}{\rho_1(x)}}, \quad \ddot{\zeta} - c_e^2\, \zeta'' = \frac{f_a(x,t)}{\rho_1}.$$

$$(6.759a\text{–}e)$$

Thus the classical wave equation (6.759e) applies to the linear vibrations (6.759a) of an elastic string of variable thickness (6.759b) subject to an unsteady tangential tension (6.759c); the classical wave equation (6.759e) applies in particular to a uniform string under constant tension when the elastic wave speed (6.759d) is constant. Thus *(6.755) is (problem 339) the general wave equation specifying (Figure 6.31) the transverse displacement of an elastic string with tangential tension T and mass density ρ_1 (external applied transverse force f_a) per unit length, all functions of position and time. The particular cases include: (i) for constant mass density (6.756a) the wave operator (6.756c) has only one coefficient, namely the elastic wave speed (6.756b) involving also the tangential tension; (ii) the linear case (6.757b) of small slope (6.757a); (iii) the combination (i–ii) of (6.758c) linearity (6.758a) and constant mass density (6.758b); and (iv) the classical wave equation (6.759e) in the linear case (6.759a) with mass density (tangential tension) a function of position (6.759b) [time (6.759c)] allowing for an elastic wave speed (6.759d) depending on both.* The equation of transversal waves can be extended from one (to two) dimension(s) for [note 6.3 (6.4)] an elastic string (membrane).

NOTE 6.4: **Waves in a Membrane under Isotropic Tension**

The equation for the transverse waves along an elastic membrane under isotropic tension can be obtained by two equivalent and alternative methods: (a) start with the steady deflection of an elastic membrane under tension (section 6.5) and include the inertia force as for an elastic string (note 6.3); (b) generalize the wave equation (6.755) of an elastic string from one to two dimensions to apply to an elastic membrane. Since method (a) has already been illustrated (note 6.3), method (b) is used next in the "transformation" from [Figure 6.31 (6.32)] an elastic string (to a membrane): (i) the transverse displacement (6.760a) is a function of time and one (two) spatial coordinates; and (ii) time derivatives are unchanged and first(second)-order spatial derivatives are replaced by the gradient (6.760b) [Laplace (6.760c)] operator:

$$z = \zeta(x,t) \leftrightarrow z = \zeta(x,y,t), \quad \partial_x \leftrightarrow \nabla = \vec{e}_x \partial_x + \vec{e}_y \partial_y, \partial_{xx} \leftrightarrow \nabla^2 = \partial_{xx} + \partial_{yy}.$$

$$(6.760a\text{--}c)$$

Applying the transformations (6.760a–c) to (6.755) leads to:

$$\left(\rho_2 \dot{\zeta} \right)^{\cdot} - \nabla \cdot \left\{ T \left| 1 + (\nabla \zeta . \nabla \zeta) \right|^{-1/2} \nabla \zeta \right\} = f_a(x,y,t); \qquad (6.761a)$$

that is, the exact, non-linear general wave equation for the transverse displacement of vibrations along an elastic membrane with mass density

(6.761b) [applied external transverse force (6.761c)] per unit area and isotropic tangential tension (6.761d):

$$\rho_2(x,y,t)=\frac{dm}{dA}, \qquad f_a(x,y,t)=\frac{dF}{dA}, \qquad T_{\alpha\beta}=T(x,y,t)\delta_{\alpha\beta}, \qquad (6.761b\text{–}d)$$

that may all depend on position and time.

The particular cases include: (i) constant mass density (6.762a) leading to the wave equation (6.762c) with the same transverse elastic wave speed (6.756b) ≡ (6.762b):

$$\rho_2 = const:\ c_e(x,y,t)=\sqrt{\frac{T(x,y,t)}{\rho_2}}:\ \ddot{\zeta}-\nabla\cdot\left\{c_e^2\left|1+(\nabla\zeta.\nabla\zeta)\right|^{-1/2}\nabla\zeta\right\}=\rho_2^{-1}f_a(x,y,t);$$

$$(6.762a\text{–}c)$$

(ii) linear wave equation (6.763b) for small slope (6.763a):

$$|\nabla\zeta|^2 \ll 1: \qquad\qquad \left(\rho_2\dot{\zeta}\right)^{\bullet}-\nabla.\left(T\nabla\zeta\right)=f_a(x,y,t); \qquad (6.763a, b)$$

(iii) combining (i–ii) linear (6.764a) wave equation (6.764c) with constant mass density (6.764b):

$$(\nabla\zeta.\nabla\zeta)\ll 1, \qquad \rho_2=const: \qquad \ddot{\zeta}-\nabla.\left(c_e^2\nabla\zeta\right)=\rho^{-1}f_a(x,y,t); \qquad (6.764a\text{–}c)$$

and (iv) the **two-dimensional classical wave equation** (6.765e) in the linear case (6.765a) with mass density (6.765b) [isotropic tangential tension (6.765c)] a function of position (time) only, so that the elastic wave speed (6.765d) may depend on position and time:

$$|\nabla\zeta|^2 \ll 1, \qquad \rho_2=\rho_2(x,y), \quad T_{\alpha\beta}=\delta_{\alpha\beta}T(t):$$

$$(6.765a\text{–}e)$$

$$c_e(x,y,t)=\sqrt{\frac{T(t)}{\rho_2(x,y)}}, \qquad \ddot{\zeta}-c_e^2\nabla^2\zeta=\rho_2^{-1}f_a(x,y,t).$$

Thus *(6.761a) is (problem 340) the general wave equation specifying (Figure 6.32) the transverse displacement of an elastic membrane (6.760a) with isotropic tangential tension (6.761d) and mass density (6.761a) [transverse external applied force (6.761b)] per unit area that may all depend on position and time. The particular*

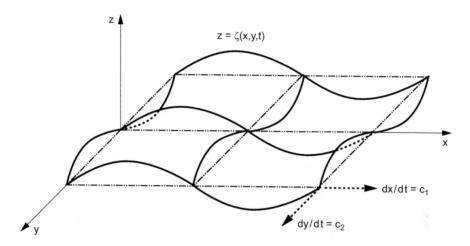

FIGURE 6.32
The unsteady generalization of the deflection of membranes (Figures II.6.1–III.6.4 and 6.14–6.18) and bending of plates (Figures 6.19–6.29) leads to transversal elastic waves in two dimensions that may have different propagating speeds in orthogonal principal directions.

cases include: (i) the wave equation (6.762c) for constant mass density (6.762a) with the transverse elastic wave speed (6.762b) as the sole parameter involving the isotropic tangential tension; (ii) the linear case (6.763b) of small slope (6.763a); (iii) the combination (6.764c) of (ii) linearity (6.764a) and (i) constant mass density (6.764b); and (vi) the two-dimensional classical wave equation (6.765e) in the linear case (6.765a) with mass density per unit area (6.765b) [isotropic tangential tension (6.765c)] that depends only on position (time), leading to a transverse elastic wave speed (6.765d) that may depend on both. The one-dimensional elastic body without (with stiffness) is the string (rod), that may have transversal vibrations [Note 6.3 (6.7)]; a rod may also have longitudinal (torsional) vibrations [Note 6.6 (6.5)].

NOTE 6.5: Torsional Vibrations of a Straight Rod

The steady torsion of a straight rod (sections II.6.5–II.6.8) is specified (Figure 6.33) by the angle ϕ of rotation along the longitudinal x-axis, whose spatial derivative is the **torsion** (III.6.129a) $\equiv$ (6.766a, b) that is related to the **axial torque** by (II.6.149a) $\equiv$ (II.6.171b) $\equiv$ (6.766c) where the **torsional stiffness** C may be non-uniform:

$$\tau = \phi' \equiv \partial_x \phi: \qquad \left(C\phi'\right)' = M_x = M_a + M_i. \qquad \text{(6.766a–d)}$$

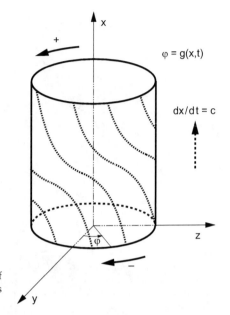

FIGURE 6.33
The unsteady generalization of the torsion of
rods (Figures II.6.10–II.6.14) is torsional waves
propagating along the axis.

In the unsteady case, axial torque is separated from the external applied
axial torque (6.766d) and the **inertia torque**: (i) inertia torque is (6.767a) the
time derivative of the **angular momentum**; (ii) the angular momentum is the
product (6.767b) of the **moment of inertia** I of the cross-section by the angular velocity Ω_x of rotation around the x-axis; and (iii) the angular velocity is
(6.767c) the time derivative of the angle of rotation:

$$M_i = \dot{L}_x, \qquad L_x = I\Omega_x, \qquad \Omega_x = \dot{\phi}; \qquad M_i = (I\Omega)^{\bullet} = \left(I\dot{\phi}\right)^{\bullet} ; \qquad \text{(6.767a–e)}$$

from (6.767a–c) follows the inertia torque (6.767d) ≡ (6.767e) that substituted
in (6.766d) leads to:

$$\phi = g(x,t): \qquad \left(I\dot{\phi}\right)^{\bullet} - \left(C\phi'\right)' = M_a(x,t), \qquad \text{(6.768a, b)}$$

as the **torsional wave equation** (6.768b) for the angle of rotation around the
axis (6.768a). Thus *(6.768b) is (problem 341) the torsional wave equation specifying the angle of rotation around the axis (6.768a) for a straight elastic rod with
applied axial torque M_a, that may depend on position and time, as well as the
moment of inertia I and torsional stiffness C of the cross-section. The particular*

cases include: (i) the simplification (6.769c) involving the **torsional wave speed** (6.769b) in the case of constant moment of inertia of the cross-section (6.769a):

$$I = const: \qquad c_t = \sqrt{\frac{C(x,t)}{I}}: \qquad \ddot{\phi} - \left(c_t^2 \phi' \right)' = I^{-1} M_a(x,t); \qquad \text{(6.769a–c)}$$

and (ii) the one-dimensional classical wave equation (6.770d) for moment of inertia (6.770a) [torsional stiffness (6.770b)] of the cross-section depending only on position (time), so that the torsional wave speed (6.770c) may depend on both:

$$I = I(x), \quad C = C(t): \qquad c_t(x,t) = \sqrt{\frac{C(t)}{I(x)}}: \qquad \ddot{\phi} - c_t^2 \, \phi'' = I^{-1} M_a(x,t).$$

$$\text{(6.770a–d)}$$

The torsional (longitudinal) vibrations of an elastic rod satisfy a second-order wave equation in space and time [note 6.5 (6.6)].

NOTE 6.6: Longitudinal Compressive/Tractive Vibrations of a Rod

The steady longitudinal deformation, either an extension or a compression (Figure 6.34) of an elastic rod (section 6.4) specifies the longitudinal displacement (6.290d) ≡ (6.771a):

$$\left(E u' \right)' = -F = -\left(F_a - F_i \right); \qquad F_i = \dot{p} = \left(\rho_1 \dot{u} \right)^{\bullet}, \qquad \text{(6.771a–e)}$$

In the unsteady case, the external applied force (6.771b) is separated from the inertia force that is the time derivative of the linear momentum (6.754a) ≡ (6.771d). The linear momentum is the product (6.771e) of the mass density per unit length (6.753c) by the velocity; that is, the

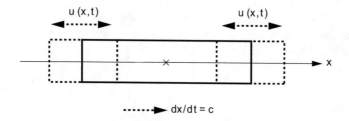

FIGURE 6.34
The unsteady generalization of the compression and extension of rods (Figures 6.8–6.10) is longitudinal waves propagating along the rod.

time derivative of the longitudinal displacement. Substituting (6.771e) in (6.771a) leads to:

$$u = u(x,t): \qquad \left(\rho \dot{u}\right)^{\cdot} - \left(E u'\right)' = F_a(x,t), \qquad (6.772a, b)$$

which is a linear wave equation because a linear relation between stresses and strains (6.290a) was assumed for an elastic material with Young modulus E.

Thus (6.672b) is the **wave equation** *specifying (problem 342) the longitudinal displacement (6.772a) of a straight elastic rod (Figure 6.34) under an axial external applied force F_a that may depend on position and time, as well as the Young modulus E of the material and the mass density per unit length (6.753c). The particular cases include: (i) constant mass density (6.773a) leading to the wave equation (6.773c) whose sole coefficient is the* **longitudinal wave speed** *(6.773b):*

$$\rho_1 = const: \qquad c_\ell(x,t) = \sqrt{\frac{E(x,t)}{\rho_1}}, \qquad \ddot{u} - \left(c_\ell^2 u'\right)' = \rho_1^{-1} F_a(x,t); \qquad (6.773a\text{--}c)$$

and (ii) the one-dimensional classical wave equation (6.774d) in the case of mass density per unit length (6.774a) [Young modulus (6.774b)] depending only on position (time), implying that the torsional wave speed may depend on both (6.774c):

$$\rho_1 = \rho_1(x), \quad E = E(t): \quad c_\ell(x,t) = \sqrt{\frac{E(t)}{\rho(x)}}, \quad \ddot{u} - \left(c_\ell^2 u'\right)' = \rho^{-1} F_a(x,t). \qquad (6.774a\text{--}d)$$

The torsional (note 6.5) and longitudinal (note 6.6) [transversal or bending vibrations] of a straight elastic rod (bar without or beam with axial tension) lead to a wave equation that is: (i) of the second-order in time; (ii) of the second(fourth)-order in space.

NOTE 6.7: **Non-Linear Bending Vibrations of a Beam**

In the steady case the non-linear transverse deflection (bending) of an elastic string (bar) is given by the first (second) term on the r.h.s. of (6.8), that is (6.752c) ≡ (6.775a) [(6.775b)]:

$$-f_1 = \left\{ T \zeta' \left|1 + \zeta'^2\right|^{-1/2} \right\}', \qquad f_2 = \left\{ EI \zeta'' \left|1 + \zeta'^2\right|^{-3/2} \right\}'', \qquad (6.775a, b)$$

that: (i) replace the tangential tension (6.776a) by the bending stiffness (6.776b) ≡ (6.9a) that is the product of the Young modulus of the material by the moment of inertia of the cross-section; (ii–iii) replace first- by second-order derivatives (6.776c) leading to opposite signs for the shear stress or trans-verse force per unit length (6.776d); and (iv) change the exponent of the arc length per unit distance along the x-axis (6.776e) from the slope (6.2a, b) [cur-vature (6.3a–c)]:

$$T \quad \leftrightarrow \quad B = EI, \quad \partial_x \quad \leftrightarrow \quad \partial_{xx}, -f_1 \quad \leftrightarrow \quad f_2, \quad \left|1 + \zeta'^2\right|^{-\nu/2}: \quad \nu = 1 \quad \leftrightarrow \quad \nu = 3$$

$$(6.776a\text{–}f)$$

The transverse force per unit length adds (6.777b) in the steady case (6.8) $\equiv$ (6.775a, b) $\equiv$ (6.777a):

$$\left\{B\zeta''\left|1+\zeta'^2\right|^{-3/2}\right\}'' - \left\{T\zeta'\left|1+\zeta'^2\right|^{-1/2}\right\}' = f_1 + f_2 = f = f_a - f_i = f_a - \left(\rho\dot{\zeta}\right)^{\!\cdot},$$

$$(6.777a\text{–}e)$$

and in the unsteady case the inertia force (6.754b) $\equiv$ (6.777e) is subtracted from the external transversal applied force (6.754c) $\equiv$ (6.777d).

Thus *(problem 343) the exact, non-linear general one-dimensional bending wave equation (6.777e)* $\equiv$ *(6.778)*:

$$\left(\rho\dot{\zeta}\right)^{\!\cdot} - \left\{T\zeta'\left|1+\zeta'^2\right|^{-1/2}\right\}' + \left\{B\zeta''\left|1+\zeta'^2\right|^{-3/2}\right\}'' = f_a(x,t), \qquad (6.778)$$

specifies the transverse displacement of an elastic bar with bending stiffness (6.9a) under tangential tension T, with mass density ρ_1 per unit length (6.753c) subject to a shear stress, that is transverse external applied force per unit length f_a all generally functions of position and time. The particular cases include: (i) for constant mass density (6.779a) the simplified wave equation (6.779c) involving only two param-eters, namely the transversal elastic wave speed (6.756b) and the **stiffness disper-sion parameter** *(6.779b)*:

$$\rho_1 = const: \quad b(x,t) = \sqrt{\frac{B(x,t)}{\rho_1}}:$$

$$(6.779a\text{–}c)$$

$$\ddot{\xi} - \left\{c_e^2\,\zeta'\left|1+\zeta'^2\right|^{-1/2}\right\}' + \left\{b^2\,\zeta''\left|1+\zeta'^2\right|^{-3/2}\right\}'' = \frac{f_a(x,t)}{\rho_1};$$

(ii) in the linear case (6.780a) of small slope (6.780b):

$$\zeta'^2 \ll 1: \qquad \left(\rho\dot{\zeta}\right)^{\!\cdot} - \left(T\zeta'\right)' + \left(B\zeta''\right)'' = f_a(x,t); \qquad (6.780a, b)$$

(iii) combining (i–ii) for (6.781c) the linear case (6.781a) with constant mass density (6.781b):

$$\zeta'^2 \ll 1; \quad \rho_1 = const: \qquad \ddot{\zeta} - \left(c_e^2\,\zeta'\right)' + \left(b^2\,\zeta''\right)'' = \rho^{-1} f_a(x,t); \qquad (6.781a\text{--}c)$$

and (iv) the **classical wave equation with stiffness** *(6.782f) in the linear case (6.782a) with mass density (6.782b) [tangential tension (6.782c) and bending stiffness (6.782d)] function(s) only of position (time) implying a transverse elastic wave speed (6.759d) [stiffness dispersion parameter (6.782e) that generally depend on position and time:*

$$\zeta'^2 \ll 1, \quad \rho_1 = \rho_1(x), \quad T = T(t), \quad B = B(t):$$

$$b(x,t) = \sqrt{\frac{B(t)}{\rho_1(x)}}, \quad \ddot{\zeta} - c_e^2\,\zeta'' + b^2\,\zeta'''' = \rho_1^{-1} f_a(x,t). \qquad (6.782a\text{--}f)$$

The method of extension from transverse waves [note 6.3 (6.4)] from an elastic string (to an elastic membrane) also applies [note 6.7 (6.8)] to the extension from a beam (to a stressed plate).

NOTE 6.8: Bending Vibrations of a Stressed Plate

The method (6.760a–c) of extension of the transverse waves from the elastic string (to the elastic membrane) also applies [notes 6.3 (6.4)] to the passage [note 6.7 (6.8)] from a beam (to a plate) under axial tension (in-plane stresses) with two additions: (i) replacing the bending stiffness (6.783a) of a bar (6.9a) ≡ (6.776b) ≡ (6.783b) [plate (6.413d) ≡ (6.783d) implying (6.783e):

$$EI = B \quad \leftrightarrow \quad D = \frac{E h^3}{12\left(1-\sigma^2\right)} = \frac{E I}{1-\sigma^2}, \qquad \left(B\zeta''\right)'' \quad \leftrightarrow \quad \nabla^2\left(D\nabla^2\zeta\right);$$

$$(6.783a\text{--}e)$$

$$\left(T\zeta'\right)' \quad \leftrightarrow \quad \nabla.\left(T\nabla\zeta\right) \quad \leftrightarrow \quad \partial_\alpha\left(T_{\alpha\beta}\,\partial_\beta\zeta\right), \qquad (6.784a\text{--}c)$$

and (ii) replacing the tangential tension along a string (6.784a) by the isotropic tension in a membrane (6.784b) or more generally (6.673b) by the anisotropic in-plane stresses in a plate (6.784c). Substitution of the transformations (6.760a–c; 6.783a–e; 6.784a, c) leads from the linear (6.780a) [(6.785a)] equation of bending waves in a beam (6.780b) [to a stressed plate (6.785b)]:

$$(\partial_\alpha \zeta)(\partial_\beta \zeta) \ll 1: \qquad \left(\rho_2 \dot{\zeta} \right)^{\!\bullet} - \partial_\alpha \left(T_{\alpha\beta} \, \partial_\beta \zeta \right) + \nabla^2 \left(D \nabla^2 \zeta \right) = f_a \left(x_1, x_2, t \right),$$

$$(6.785a, b)$$

that is considered next in the general and particular cases.

Thus *(6.785b) is (problem 344) the linear (6.785a) bending wave equation speci-fying the transverse displacement (6.760a) of an elastic plate with bending stiffness (6.314d) ≡ (6.783b) subject to in-plane stress $T_{\alpha\beta}$ with mass density per unit area (6.761b) subject to an external transverse applied force per unit area (6.761c) that may all depend on position and time. The particular cases include: (i) isotropic stresses (6.786a) leading to (6.786b):*

$$T_{\alpha\beta} = \delta_{\alpha\beta} \, T(x,y,t): \qquad \left(\rho_2 \dot{\zeta} \right)^{\!\bullet} - \nabla . (T \nabla \zeta) + \nabla^2 \left(D \nabla^2 \zeta \right) = f_a \left(x,y,t \right);$$

$$(6.786a, b)$$

(ii) constant mass density (6.787a) leading from (6.785b) to (6.787c) involving the stiffness dispersion parameter (6.787b):

$$\rho_2 = const: \qquad \bar{b} = \sqrt{\frac{D(x,y,t)}{\rho_2}}: \qquad \ddot{\zeta} - \partial_\alpha \left(\rho_2^{-1} T_{\alpha\beta} \, \partial_\beta \zeta \right) + \nabla^2 \left(\bar{b}^2 \, \nabla^2 \zeta \right)$$

$$= \rho_2^{-1} f_a (x,y,t);$$

$$(6.787a-c)$$

(iii) in the reference frame of principal stresses may be introduced two transverse elastic wave speeds (6.788b, c) in orthogonal directions appearing in the wave equation (6.788d):

$$\rho_2 = const: \qquad c_{1,2}(x,y,t) = \sqrt{\frac{T_{11,22}(x,y,t)}{\rho_2}}:$$

$$(6.788a-d)$$

$$\ddot{\zeta} - \partial_1 \left(c_1^2 \, \partial_1 \zeta \right) - \partial_2 \left(c_1^2 \, \partial_2 \zeta \right) + \nabla^2 \left(\bar{b}^2 \, \nabla^2 \zeta \right) = \rho^{-1} f_a (x_1, x_2, t);$$

(iv) in the reference frame of principal stresses depending only on time (6.789b, c) with mass density depending only on position (6.789a) leading to the wave equation (6.789d):

$$\rho_2 = \rho_2(x,y), \quad T_{11,22} = T_{11,22}(t):$$

(6.789a–d)

$$\ddot{\zeta} - c_1^2 \, \partial_{11} \zeta - c_2^2 \, \partial_{22} \zeta + \bar{b}^2 \left(\partial_{11} + \partial_{22} \right)^2 \zeta = \rho^{-1} f_a(x_1, x_2, t);$$

and (v) in the case of mass density (6.790a) [isotropic in-plane stress (6.790b)] depending only on position (time) is obtained the **classical two-dimensional wave equation with stiffness** *(6.790e):*

$$\rho_2 = \rho_2(x,y), \quad T_{\alpha\beta} = \delta_{\alpha\beta} \, T(t): \quad c_e(x,y,t) = \sqrt{\frac{T(t)}{\rho_2(x,y)}}, \quad \bar{b}(x,y,t) = \sqrt{\frac{T(t)}{\rho_2(x,y)}},$$

(6.790a–d)

$$\ddot{\zeta} - c_e^2 \nabla^2 \zeta - \bar{b}^2 \nabla^4 \zeta = \rho^{-1} f_a(x_1, x_2, t),$$

(6.790e)

involving the transverse elastic wave speed (6.790c) and dispersive stiffness parameter (6.790d). The six sets of wave equations (notes 6.3–6.8) are compared (Table 6.11) next (note 6.9).

NOTE 6.9: Comparison of Wave Variables, Speeds, and Equations

The six sets of waves are compared in Table 6.10 in three pairs of vertical columns: (i–ii) the transversal waves in elastic strings (membranes) that have no stiffness [note 6.3 (6.4)]; (iii–iv) the torsional (longitudinal) vibrations of rods [note 6.5 (6.6)]; (v–vi) the bending vibrations of beams (stressed plates) that [note 6.7 (6.8)] include tangential tension (i) [in-plane stresses (ii)]. For each of the six waves (i–vi) there are four sets of information in lines: (a) type of wave; (b) wave variables; (c) wave speeds; and (d) wave equations. Concerning *(problem 345)* the *wave variables* they are: (a-1, 2) one(two)-dimensional transverse displacements (6.791a) [(6.791b)] for strings, membranes, beams, and plates; (a-3, 4) longitudinal displacement (6.791c) [angle of rotation around the axis (6.791d)] for longitudinal (torsional) oscillations of rods:

$$z = \zeta(z,t) \quad \leftrightarrow \quad z = \zeta(x,y,t) \quad \leftrightarrow \quad u = u(x,t) \quad \leftrightarrow \quad \phi = \phi(x,t); \quad (6.791a\text{–}d)$$

$$v = \dot{\zeta} \quad \leftrightarrow \quad v = \dot{u} \quad \leftrightarrow \quad \Omega = \dot{\phi}, \quad (6.792a\text{–}c)$$

$$\zeta', \; \nabla \zeta \quad \leftrightarrow \quad s = u' \quad \leftrightarrow \quad \tau = \phi', \quad (6.793a\text{–}c)$$

TABLE 6.10

Comparison of Wave Variables, Speeds, and Equations

Case	I	II	III	IV	V	VI
Medium	elastic string	elastic membrane	elastic rod	elastic rod	bar/beam	stressed plate
Note	6.3	6.4	6.5	6.6	6.7	6.8
Figure	3.1	6.32	6.33	6.34	–	–
Oscillation	transversal	transversal	torsional	longitudinal	transversal	transversal
Variable	displacement ζ	displacement ζ	angle ϕ	longitudinal displacement u	displacement ζ	displacement ζ
Time derivative	velocity: $\dot{\zeta}$	velocity: $\dot{\zeta}$	angular velocity: $\dot{\phi}$	velocity: $\dot{u}$	velocity: $\dot{\zeta}$	velocity: $\dot{\zeta}$
Spatial derivative	slope: ζ'	slope: $\nabla\zeta$	torsion: ϕ'	strain: u'	slope: ζ'	slope: $\nabla\zeta$
Inertia	mass density per unit length: ρ_1	mass density per unit area: ρ_2	moment of inertia of the cross-section: I	mass density per unit length: ρ_1	mass density per unit area: ρ_2	mass density per unit area: ρ_2
Restoring effect	tangential tension: T	tangential tension: T	torsional stiffness: C	Young modulus: E	tangential tension: T	bending stiffness: D and in-plane stresses $T_{\alpha\beta}$
Wave speed	$c_e = \sqrt{T/\rho_1}$	$c_e = \sqrt{T/\rho_2}$	$c_t = \sqrt{C/I}$	$c_\ell = \sqrt{E/\rho_1}$	$c_e = \sqrt{T/\rho_1}$	$c_e = \sqrt{T/\rho_2}$
Dispersion parameter	–	–	–	–	$b = \sqrt{B/\rho_1}$	$\bar{b} = \sqrt{D/\rho_2}$
General wave equation	(6.755)	(6.761a–d)	–	–	(6.778)	–
Linear wave equation	(6.757a, b)	(6.763a–c)	(6.768a, b)	(6.772a, b)	(6.780a, b)	(6.785a, b)
Constant mass density	(6.756a–c)	(6.762a–c)	(6.769a–c)	(6.773a–c)	(6.779a–c)	(6.787a–c)
Classical wave	(6.759a–e)	(6.765a–e)	(6.770a–d)	(6.774a–d)	(6.782a–f)	(6.790a–e)

Note: Comparison of the transverse waves in elastic (i) strings and (ii) membranes, the (iii) torsional and (iv) longitudinal vibrations of straight rods, and the transverse vibrations of (i) beams and (vi) stressed plates.

TABLE 6.11

Non-Dispersive versus Dispersive Waves

	Non-Dispersive	Dispersive
Dispersion relation	linear	non-linear
Phase speed and group velocity	$u \equiv \dfrac{\omega}{k} = \dfrac{\partial \omega}{\partial k} \equiv w$	$u \equiv \dfrac{\omega}{k} \neq \dfrac{\partial \omega}{\partial k} \equiv w$
Waveform	maintained	dispersed
Figure	6.38b	6.38a, c

Note: Comparison of dispersive and non-dispersive waves in terms of (i) dispersion relation, (ii) phase speed, (iii) group velocity, and (iv) evolution of the waveform.

*the **temporal (spatial) derivatives** are: (b-1) the velocity (6.792a) [slope (6.793a)] for transverse displacements; (b-2) the velocity (6.792b) [strain (6.793b)] for longitudinal displacements; and (b-3) the angular velocity (6.792c) [torsion (6.793c)] for rotation around an axis.*

*The **inertia effect** is represented by: (c-1) the mass density per unit length (6.794a) for strings, beams, and longitudinal vibrations of rods; (c-2) the mass density per unit area (6.794b) for membranes and plates; and (c-3) the moment of inertia of the cross-section (6.794c) for the torsion of rods:*

$$\rho_1 = \frac{dm}{ds} \quad \leftrightarrow \quad \rho_2 = \frac{dm}{dA} \quad \leftrightarrow \quad I = \int r^2 \, dm; \qquad (6.794a{-}c)$$

$$T \quad \leftrightarrow \quad T_{\alpha\beta} \quad \leftrightarrow \quad C \quad \leftrightarrow \quad E, \qquad (6.795a{-}d)$$

*the **restoring effect** is: (d-1) the tangential tension (6.795a) for elastic strings and beams and isotropic membranes and plates; (d-2) the in-plane stresses (6.795b) for anisotropic membranes and stressed plates; and (d-3, 4) the torsional stiffness of the cross-section (6.795c) [Young modulus of the elastic material (6.795d)] for the longitudinal (torsional) vibrations of rods. The square root of restoring effect divided by inertia effect specifies the **wave speeds**: (e-1) the transverse elastic wave speed (6.796a) for strings, membranes, beams, and plates; (e-2, 3) the longitudinal (6.796b) [torsional (6.796c)] wave speed for the longitudinal (torsional) vibrations of rods:*

$$c_e = \sqrt{\frac{T}{\rho_{1,2}}} \quad \leftrightarrow \quad c_\ell = \sqrt{\frac{T}{\rho_1}} \quad \leftrightarrow \quad c_t = \sqrt{\frac{C}{I}}; \quad b = \sqrt{\frac{B}{\rho_1}} \quad \leftrightarrow \quad \bar{b} = \sqrt{\frac{D}{\rho_2}}, \qquad (6.796a{-}e)$$

*the two cases of dispersive waves, namely transverse vibrations of bars (plates) involve the **dispersion stiffness** parameter (6.796d) [(6.796e)] that is the square root of the bending stiffness divided by the mass density. For each of the six types of waves (i–vi) are (notes 6.3–6.8; Table 6.11) indicated three to five (three or four) wave* equations from: (α) the most general non-linear with parameters depending on position and time for inhomogeneous unsteady media; (β) the classical that are linear and in some cases allow limited dependence of the parameters on position or time or both. The wave equations are put next (note 6.10) in two general forms for more detailed subsequent analysis (notes 6.11–6.23).

NOTE 6.10: Damping and Translational and Rotary Springs

In the linear (6.780a) [(6.785a)] general one(two)-dimensional bending wave equation for a beam (6.780b) [stressed plate (6.785b)], in the external transverse applied force per unit length (6.797a) [(6.798a)] may be separated: (i) force of resistance f_1 depending on the velocity causing dissipation; (ii–iii) restoring forces $f_2(f_3)$ depending on the displacement (slope) due to a translational (rotary) spring; and (iv) the remaining external applied forces f_e:

$$f_a(x,t) - f_e(x,t) = f_1(\dot{\zeta}) + f_2(\zeta) + f_3(\zeta') = -\mu\dot{\zeta} - \nu\zeta - \vartheta\zeta', \tag{6.797a, b}$$

$$f_a(x,y,t) - f_i(x,y,t) = f_1(\dot{\zeta}) + f_2(\zeta) + f_3(\nabla\zeta) = -\mu\dot{\zeta} - \nu\zeta - \vec{\vartheta}.\nabla\zeta. \tag{6.798a, b}$$

Assuming that the three forces $f_{1,2,3}$ are (6.797b) [(6.798b)] linear: (i) the force of resistance is proportional and opposite to the velocity through the **friction coefficient** μ; (ii) the restoring force due to a linear translational spring is proportional to the displacement through the **resilience** ν; and (iii) the restoring force due to the rotary spring is proportional to the slope $\zeta'(\nabla\zeta)$ through the **rotary resilience scalar** ϑ (**vector** $\vec{\vartheta}$).
Substituting (6.797b) [(6.798b)] in (6.780b) [(6.785b)] leads to the **linear general bending wave equation** *in one (6.799) [two (6.800)] dimensions*:

$$\left(\rho_1\dot{\zeta}\right)^{\cdot} - \left(T\zeta'\right)' + \left(B\zeta''\right)'' + \mu\dot{\zeta} + \nu\zeta + \vartheta\zeta' = f_e(x,t), \tag{6.799}$$

$$\left(\rho_2\dot{\zeta}\right)^{\cdot} - \partial_\alpha\left(T_{\alpha\beta}\,\partial_\beta\,\zeta\right) + \nabla^2\left(D\nabla^2\zeta\right) + \mu\dot{\zeta} + \nu\zeta + \vec{\vartheta}.\nabla\zeta = f_e(x,y,t), \tag{6.800}$$

consisting [problem 346 (347)] of the following seven terms from left to right: (i) the inertia force (6.754a) involving the velocity (6.753b) and the mass density per unit length (6.753c) [area (6.761b)]; (ii) the tangential stress (in-plane stresses) leading to the classical one-dimensional (two-dimensional anisotropic) wave equation; (iii) the bending stiffness for a beam B (plate D); (iv) the linear resistance with friction coefficient μ; (v) the linear restoring force due to a translational spring with resilience ν; (vi) the linear restoring force due to a rotational *spring with scalar ϑ (vector $\vec{\vartheta}$) resilience; and (vii) the remaining transverse applied force f_e per unit length (area).*

The **classical bending wave equation** in one (6.801d) [two (6.802d)] dimensions with [problem 348 (349)] all coefficients in (6.799) [(6.800)] out of the derivatives:

$$\dot{\rho}=0=T'=B': \qquad \ddot{\zeta}+2\chi\dot{\zeta}+\omega_t^2\,\zeta+\omega_r^2\,\zeta'-c_e^2\,\zeta''+b^2\,\zeta''''=\rho_1^{-1}f_e\left(x,t\right),$$

$$(6.801a\text{–}d)$$

$$\dot{\rho}=0=\partial_\gamma\,T_{\alpha\beta}=\partial_\gamma\,D: \qquad \ddot{\zeta}+2\chi\dot{\zeta}+\omega_t^2\,\zeta+\omega_{r1}^2\,\partial_1\zeta+\omega_{r2}^2\,\partial_2\zeta-c_1^2\,\partial_{11}\zeta$$

$$-c_2^2\,\partial_{22}\zeta+\overline{b}^2\left(\partial_{11}+\partial_{22}\right)^2\zeta=\rho_2^{-1}\,f_e\left(x,y,t\right),$$

$$(6.802a\text{–}d)$$

holds for: (i) mass density independent of time (6.801a) [(6.802a)]; (ii) damping coefficient (6.803a) $\equiv$ (2.23b) as for a linear oscillator:

$$\chi\equiv\frac{\mu}{2\rho_{1,2}};\qquad \omega_t=\sqrt{\frac{\nu}{\rho_1}},\qquad \omega_r=\sqrt{\frac{\vartheta}{\rho_2}},\qquad \omega_{r1,2}=\sqrt{\frac{\vartheta_{1,2}}{\rho_2}},\qquad (6.803a\text{–}e)$$

(iii) natural frequency (6.803b) $\equiv$ (2.23a) for a translational spring as for an harmonic oscillator; (iv) natural frequency (6.803c) [frequencies (6.803d, e)] for a one (two)-dimensional translational (rotary) spring; (v) transverse elastic wave speed (6.804a) $\equiv$ (6.759d) [speeds (6.804b, c) $\equiv$ (6.788b, c)] for the tangential tension (in-plane stresses in the principal reference frame):

$$c_e=\sqrt{\frac{T}{\rho_1}},\qquad c_{1,2}=\sqrt{\frac{T_{11,22}}{\rho_2}},\qquad b=\sqrt{\frac{B}{\rho_1}},\qquad \overline{b}=\sqrt{\frac{D}{\rho_1}},\qquad (6.804a\text{–}e)$$

(vi) dispersive stiffness parameter (6.804c) $\equiv$ (6.782e) [(6.804d) $\equiv$ (6.790d)] for a beam (plate); and (vii) other transversal external applied forces per unit mass. The simpler one-dimensional case (6.801a–d) with constant coefficients is chosen for analysis of **free (forced) waves** [notes 6.11–6.17 (6.18–6.23)] that is in the absence $f_e=0$ (presence $f_e\neq 0$) of external forces.

NOTE 6.11: **Separation of Variables in a Partial Differential Equation**

Consider (Figure 6.35) the one-dimensional (6.799) unforced (6.805a) linear (6.805b) bending wave equation (6.805i) with constant coefficients, namely the mass density (6.805c), friction coefficient (6.805d), resilience for the

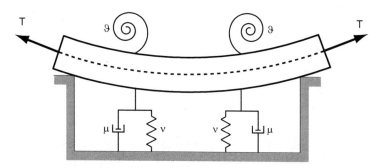

FIGURE 6.35
A combination of the preceding cases is the transverse waves in a beam, that is an elastic bar
under tangential tension like an elastic string (Figure 6.32) adding: (i) dissipation by damping
proportional to the velocity; and (ii–iii) restoring forces due to translational (rotational) springs
proportional to the displacement (slope).

translational (6.805e) and rotational (6.805f) spring, tangential stress (6.805g),
and bending stiffness (6.805h):

$$f_e = 0, \quad \zeta'^2 \ll 1, \quad const = \rho_1, \mu, \nu, \vartheta, T, B: \quad \rho_1 \ddot{\zeta} + \mu \dot{\zeta} + \nu \zeta + \vartheta \zeta' - T \zeta'' + B \zeta'''' = 0.$$

$$(6.805a\text{–}i)$$

The wave equation (6.805i) for free modes (6.805a) is a linear partial differential equation in space-time with constant coefficients (6.805b–h) that can
be solved by **separation of variables**; that is, a solution exists as the product
of two functions (6.806a) one depending only on position and the other only
on time:

$$\zeta(x,t) = X(x)Y(t): \quad \frac{\rho_1 \ddot{Y} + \mu \dot{Y}}{Y} = -\nu + \frac{T X'' - B X'''' - \vartheta X'}{X} = -\rho_1 \omega^2;$$

$$(6.806a\text{–}c)$$

substitution of (6.806a) in (6.805i) and division by (6.806a) leads to (6.806b)
where the r.h.s (l.h.s.) depends only on time (position) so both must be constant (6.806c). The constant in (6.806c) is chosen so that ω has the dimensions
of inverse of time, corresponding to an **natural frequency** in the linear ordinary differential equation with constant coefficients specifying the temporal
(6.807a) [spatial (6.807b)] dependence:

$$\rho_1 \ddot{Y} + \mu \dot{Y} + \rho_1 \omega^2 Y = 0 = B X'''' - T X'' + \vartheta X' + \left(\nu - \rho_1 \omega^2 \right) X. \quad (6.807a, b)$$

Thus, *the solution of the linear (6.805b) unforced (6.805a) bending wave equation (6.805i) with constant coefficients (6.805c–h) can be obtained (problem 350) by*

separation of variables as the product (6.806a) of a function of position (by a func-
tion of time), satisfying a linear ordinary differential equation with constant coeffi-
cients (6.807b) [(6.807a)] with the oscillation frequency ω as the separation constant.
The solution of the spatial (6.807b) [temporal (6.807a)] factor in the space-
time transverse displacement is considered next [notes 6.12–6.16 (6.17–6.18)],
involving boundary (initial) conditions.

NOTE 6.12: Boundary Conditions, Fundamental Mode, and Harmonics

Considering a beam of length L supported (Figure 6.23b) [or pinned
(Figure 6.23c)] at both ends [Figure 6.35 (6.36)], the boundary conditions
are zero displacement (6.808a, b) and curvature (6.808c, d):

$$\zeta(0,t)=0=\zeta(L,t), \quad \partial_{xx}\zeta(0,t)=0=\partial_{xx}\zeta(L,t): \quad X_n(x)=\sin\left(\frac{n\pi x}{L}\right),$$

$$(6.808\text{a–e})$$

that are satisfied by the spatial dependence (6.808e) in the transverse displacement (6.806a). The solution (6.808e) = (6.809c) is periodic (6.809d) with
wavelength (6.809a) that specifies the **wavenumber** (6.809b) in (6.809e):

$$\lambda_n=\frac{2L}{n}=\frac{2\pi}{k_n}: \quad X_n(x)=\sin\left(\frac{n\pi x}{L}\right)=\sin\left(\frac{2\pi x}{\lambda_n}\right)=\sin(k_n x). \quad (6.809\text{a–e})$$

The **fundamental mode** corresponds (Figure 6.37a) to the longest wavelength (6.810a) that has **nodes** or zeros at the boundary points $x=0,L$, and
corresponds (6.810b) to the smallest wavenumber:

$$\lambda_1=2L, \quad k_1=\frac{2\pi}{\lambda_1}=\frac{\pi}{L}; \quad \lambda_n=\frac{2L}{n}=\frac{\lambda_1}{n}, \quad k_n=\frac{2\pi}{\lambda_n}=\frac{n\pi}{L}=k_1 n,$$

$$(6.810\text{a–d})$$

the successive **harmonics** $n=2,3,4$ in the (6.810a–d) have (Figure 6.37b, c, d):
(i) shorter wavelength (6.810c) ≡ (6.809a) with $(n-1)$ nodes inside the $0<x<L$,
for a total of $(n+1)$, including the boundaries $x=0,L$; and (ii) the wavenumber of the n-th harmonic is a multiple of the fundamental wavenumber given
by (6.809b) ≡ (6.810d). It has been shown that for *(problem 351) a beam of length L*
supported (Figure 6.23b) or pinned (Figure 6.23c) at both ends [Figure 6.34 (6.35)]
the boundary conditions (6.808a–d) are satisfied by a sinusoidal dependence on
position (6.808e) corresponding to the wavelength (6.810a) [(6.810b)] and wave-
number (6.810c) [(6.810d)] for the fundamental mode (Figure 6.37a) [harmonics

(Figures 6.37b, c, d) of orders n = 2,3,4,...]. The spatial dependence (6.808e) must satisfy not only the boundary conditions (6.808a–d) but also the differential equation (6.807b), leading to the dispersion relation (note 6.13).

NOTE 6.13: Dispersion Relation and Oscillation Frequencies

Omitting (Figure 6.36) the rotary spring (6.811a) the spatial dependence (6.808e) satisfies the differential equation (6.807b) if (6.811b) holds:

$$\vartheta = 0: \qquad 0 = \left[B\left(\frac{n\pi}{L}\right)^4 + T\left(\frac{n\pi}{L}\right)^2 + v - \rho_1\,\omega_n^2 \right]\sin\left(\frac{n\pi x}{L}\right). \qquad (6.811a, b)$$

The vanishing of (6.811b) at all positions leads to the **dispersion relation** (6.812a):

$$\omega_n = \pm\left|\frac{B}{\rho_1}\frac{n^4\pi^4}{L^4} + \frac{T}{\rho_1}\frac{n^2\pi^2}{L^2} + \frac{v}{\rho_1}\right|^{1/2} = \pm\left|b^2\,k_n^4 + c_e^2\,k_n^2 + \omega_0^2\right|^{1/2} = \frac{2\pi}{\tau_n}, \qquad (6.812a\text{–}c)$$

specifying (problem 352) the frequency (6.812a, b) [period (6.812b, c)] of the mode(s) in three cases: (I) for (6.813a, b) a translational spring there is only one natural frequency of the harmonic oscillator (6.813c) ≡ (2.23a):

$$T = 0 = B: \qquad\qquad \omega_n = \sqrt{\frac{v}{\rho_1}} \equiv \omega_0; \qquad (6.813a\text{–}c)$$

$$v = 0 = B: \qquad\qquad \omega_n = \pm c_e\,\frac{n\pi}{L} = \pm c_e\,k_n, \qquad (6.814a\text{–}d)$$

$$v = 0 = T: \qquad\qquad \omega_n = \pm b\,\frac{n^2\,\pi^2}{L^2} = \pm b\,k_n^2, \qquad (6.815a\text{–}d)$$

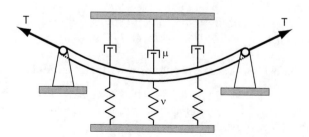

FIGURE 6.36
Omitting in Figure 6.35 the rotational spring, the boundary conditions of support or pinned at both ends $x = 0, L$ of the vibrating bar leads to the modes indicated in Figure 6.37.

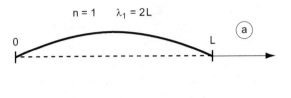

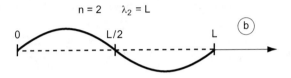

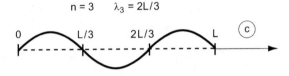

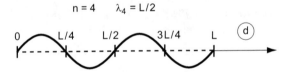

FIGURE 6.37
The standing modes of a transversal elastic wave in a beam pinned at both ends consist of:
(i) a fundamental mode with wavelength equal to twice the length of the beam, so that the
nodes or points of zero displacement are the supports (a); (ii) the harmonics of first (b), second
(c), third (d), and higher *n* order divide the fundamental wavelength by *n* and have $n - 1$ $(n + 1)$
nodes excluding (including) the two supports.

*(II–III) for an elastic string (6.814a, b) [bar (6.815a, b)] the natural frequencies of
the fundamental mode and harmonics (6.814c) [(6.815c)]: (a) involve as coefficient
the transversal elastic wave speed (6.804a) [stiffness dispersion parameter (6.804c)];
(b) are linear (6.814d) [non-linear (6.815d)] functions of the wavenumber, leading to
non-dispersive (dispersive) waves [notes 6.14–6.15 (6.16)].*

NOTE 6.14: **Non-Dispersive Propagation with Permanent Waveform**

*In the case II of an elastic string (6.814a, b) ≡ (6.816a, b) the dispersion relation
(6.814c, d) leads (problem 353) to the frequency (6.816c, d) and **period** (6.816e–g)
of oscillation of the n-th mode:*

$$v = 0 = B: \qquad \omega_n = \pm c_e \frac{n\pi}{L} = \pm c_e\, k_n, \qquad \tau_n \equiv \frac{2\pi}{\omega_n} = \pm \frac{2\pi}{c_e\, k_n} = \pm \frac{2L}{c_e\, n}. \qquad \text{(6.816a–g)}$$

The **fundamental frequency** (6.817a) is given (6.816: 6.804a) by (6.817b–f):

$$n = 1: \qquad \pm\omega_1 = c_e \frac{\pi}{L} = \frac{\pi}{L}\sqrt{\frac{T}{\rho_1}} = c_e\,k_1 = \frac{2\pi}{\tau_1} = \frac{2\pi c_e}{\lambda_1}, \qquad (6.817\text{a–f})$$

implying that, for example in a piano: (i) the bass (treble) notes, that is with low (high) frequency correspond to long (short) strings with thick (thin) cross-section for larger (smaller) mass density per unit length; (ii) each string of the piano is tuned for higher (lower) pitch, that is increasing (decreasing) the frequency, by tightening (loosening) a screw holding the string for a larger (smaller) tangential tension. The **harmonic frequencies** (6.818a) are multiplies of the fundamental frequency (6.817a–d) [corresponding to submultiples (6.818b) of the fundamental period (6.817e, f)]:

$$\pm\omega_n = c_e\,k_n = n\omega_1 = \frac{n\pi}{L}c_e = \frac{n\pi}{L}\sqrt{\frac{T}{\rho_1}}, \qquad (6.818\text{a})$$

$$\tau_n = \frac{2\pi}{\omega_n} = \frac{\tau_1}{n} = \pm\frac{2L}{c_e\,n} = \pm\frac{2L}{n}\sqrt{\frac{\rho_1}{T}} = \frac{\lambda_n}{c_e}, \qquad (6.818\text{b})$$

and the waveperiod is the time-taken to travel at the wavespeed a distance equal to the wavelength.

The transverse vibrations of an elastic string (6.819a) with constant elastic wave speed (6.819b) satisfy the classical wave equation (6.819c) ≡ (6.819d):

$$B = 0, \qquad c = \sqrt{\frac{T}{\rho}} = const: \qquad 0 = \ddot{\zeta} - c^2\zeta'' = \partial_{tt}\zeta - c^2\,\partial_{xx}\zeta; \qquad (6.819\text{a–d})$$

a sinusoidal solution (6.820a) in position (time) with wavenumber k (frequency ω) substituted in (6.819d) leads to:

$$\zeta(x,t) = A\exp\left[i(kx - \omega t)\right]: \qquad 0 = c^2 k^2 - \omega^2 \rightarrow \omega = \pm kc, \qquad (6.820\text{a–d})$$

the linear (6.820d) ≡ (6.814d) dispersion relation (6.820c). Since wave equation (6.819d) is linear, the principle of superposition holds for the transverse displacement (6.820a) of non-dispersive waves (6.820d) leading to (6.821a):

$$\zeta_\pm(x,t) = \int_{-\infty}^{+\infty} A(k)\exp\left[ik(x \mp ct)\right]dk = \zeta_\pm(x \mp ct); \qquad (6.821\text{a, b})$$

from (6.821a) ≡ (6.821b) it follows that *(problem 354) the general transverse displacement* (6.822c) *of waves in an elastic string that satisfy the mechanical wave* *equation (6.819a–d) is the sum of two arbitrary twice differentiable functions (6.822a) of the **phases** (6.822b):*

$$\zeta_{\mp} \in \mathcal{D}^2(|R): \qquad \varphi_{\pm}(x,t) = x \mp ct, \qquad \zeta(x,t) = \zeta_{+}(\varphi_{+}) + \zeta_{-}(\varphi_{-}).$$

$$(6.822a-c)$$

*The phases $\varphi_{+}(\varphi_{-})$ are constant (6.823a) for an observer (6.823b) travelling in the positive (negative) x-direction (Figure 6.31) at the **phase speed** (6.823c) equal to the elastic wave speed:*

$$const = \varphi_{\pm}(x,t) = x \mp ct \quad \Rightarrow \quad dx = \pm c\,dt \quad \Rightarrow \quad \frac{dx}{dt} = \pm c. \qquad (6.823a-c)$$

*Thus a linear relation between the frequency and wavenumber (6.820d) corresponds to non-dispersive waves that propagate at the same phase speed (6.823c) for all wavelengths and thus have a **permanent waveform** that does not change during propagation (Figure 6.38b).* It remains to explain (note 6.15) how waves travelling in opposite directions (note 6.14) can form standing modes (note 6.15).

NOTE 6.15: Unidirectional Propagating Waves and Bidirectional Standing Modes

In the case of a constant wave speed (6.824a), the classical wave operator (6.819d) ≡ (6.824b) can be split into two factors (6.824c):

$$c = const: \qquad 0 = \left(\partial_{tt} - c^2\,\partial_{xx}\right)\zeta = \left(\partial_t - c\,\partial_x\right)\left(\partial_t + c\,\partial_x\right)\zeta. \qquad (6.824a-c)$$

Each factor in (6.824c) is a linear first-order partial differential equation with constant coefficients (6.825a):

$$0 = \partial_t \zeta_{\pm} \pm c\,\partial_x \zeta_{\pm}; \qquad \zeta_{\pm}(x,t) = const \quad \Rightarrow \quad (\partial_t \zeta_{\pm})dt + (\partial_x \zeta_{\pm})dx = 0, \qquad (6.825a-c)$$

specifying a **unidirectional propagating** wave since: (i) the wave field is constant (6.825b) for (6.825c); (ii) the **implicit differentiation theorem** (6.825c) ≡ (6.826a):

$$\left(\frac{dx}{dt}\right)_{\zeta_{\pm}} = -\frac{\partial_t \zeta_{\pm}}{\partial_x \zeta_{\pm}} = \pm c, \qquad \varphi_{\pm} = x \mp ct, \qquad \zeta_{\pm}(x,t) = f(\varphi_{\pm}), \qquad (6.826a-c)$$

shows by (6.825a) that the wave travels at the wave speed c in the positive or negative x direction (6.826b); (iii) the wave field thus can depend (6.826d) only on the phases (6.826c) ≡ (6.822b); and (iv) the two unidirectional waves

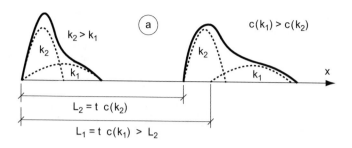

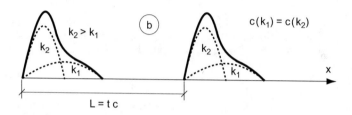

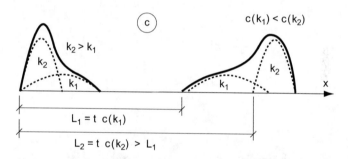

FIGURE 6.38
The propagating waves are non-dispersive if the frequency is proportional to the wavenumber, so that the propagating speed is independent of the wavenumber, and a "wave packet" consisting of different wavenumber remains together while propagating and the total waveform does not change (b). If the ratio of frequency to wavenumber is not constant, and increases (a) [decreases (c)] with the wavenumber, shorter waves propagate faster (more slowly) and the wave packet spreads out during propagation, so that the total wave form of dispersive waves changes during propagation until all components with different wavelengths separate.

propagating at the same speed in opposite directions (6.826c, d) ≡ (6.821b) add (Figure 6.39) in the general solution (6.827c) ≡ (6.822a–c):

$$c = const: \qquad \partial_{tt}\zeta = c^2 \partial_{xx}\zeta \quad \Rightarrow \quad \zeta(x,t) = \zeta_+(x-ct) + \zeta_-(x+ct), \qquad \text{(6.827a–c)}$$

of the classical wave equation (6.827b) ≡ (6.824b, c) with constant wave speed (6.827a) ≡ (6.824a).

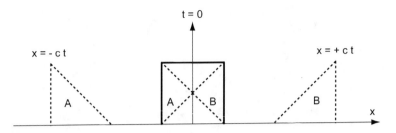

FIGURE 6.39
The classical wave equation that is of the second-order can be decomposed in two first-order wave equations representing waves propagating in opposite directions, for example $B(A)$ in the positive (negative) x-direction. The superposition $A + B$ of the undirectional waves propagating in opposite directions is: (a) still a propagating wave if the amplitudes are unequal; (b) a standing mode, with fixed nodes, if the amplitudes are equal, for example due to reflections at fixed boundaries (Figure 6.40).

Consider two sinusoidal waves with amplitudes A (B) propagating in opposite positive (negative) x-directions:

$$\zeta(x,t) = A\sin(kx - \omega t) + B\sin(kx + \omega t);$$ (6.828)

using the identities (II.5.47b) ≡ (6.829):

$$\sin(kx \mp \omega t) = \sin(kx)\cos(\omega t) \mp \cos(kx)\sin(\omega t),$$ (6.829)

leads to:

$$\zeta(x,t) = (A + B)\sin(kx)\cos(\omega t) + (B - A)\cos(kx)\sin(\omega t).$$ (6.830)

If the amplitudes are different, $A \neq B$, the transverse displacement (6.830) does not vanish at fixed points; that is, it has no nodes and the wave is propagating. If the amplitudes are the same (6.831a) for two sinusoidal waves propagating in opposite directions (6.828), their superposition is a **standing mode** (6.831b) with fixed **nodes** (6.831d) at the positions (6.831c):

$$A = B: \quad \zeta(x,t) = 2A\sin(kx)\cos(\omega t): \quad kx = n\pi \to \zeta\left(\frac{n\pi}{k}, t\right) = 0,$$
$$\text{(6.831a–d)}$$

in agreement with $k_n L = n\pi$ in (6.810d) ≡ (6.831d). Thus *(problem 355) the solution of the classical wave equation (6.827b) ≡ (6.824b) ≡ (6.819c, d) with constant* *wave speed (6.824a) ≡ (6.827a) consists of the superposition (6.827c) ≡ (6.822b, c) of two **unidirectional waves propagating** (6.825a–c) at the same wave speed in opposite directions (6.826a–c). The sinusoidal (6.828) ≡ (6.830) case with the same amplitude (6.831a) propagating in opposite directions leads (6.831b) to **standing modes** (6.831c, d).* The free propagation without forcing can be considered for dispersive (non-dispersive) waves [note(s) 6.16 (6.14–6.15)].

NOTE 6.16: Phase Speed and Group Velocity

The phase of a wave propagating (problem 356) in the positive x-direction is given by (6.832b) taking into account the dispersion relation (6.832a) relating frequency and wavenumber:

$$\omega = \omega(k): \qquad\qquad \varphi(x,t) = k\,x - \omega(k)t = const\,; \qquad\qquad (6.832\text{a–c})$$

*if the phase is taken as constant (6.832c) for constant wavenumber (6.833a) [position (6.834a)] it leads (6.833b) [(6.834b)] to the **phase speed** (6.834c) [**group velocity** (6.834c)] that is the velocity of wave crests (wave particles):*

$$k = const: \qquad k\,dx - \omega(k)dt = 0: \qquad \frac{dx}{dt} = \frac{\omega(k)}{k} = u(k), \qquad (6.833\text{a–c})$$

$$x = const: \qquad\qquad x - \frac{\partial\omega}{\partial k}t = 0, \qquad \frac{x}{t} = \frac{\partial\omega}{\partial k} = w(k). \qquad (6.834\text{a–c})$$

   In the case of non-dispersive waves (6.835a), the phase speed (6.835b) and group velocity (6.835d) coincide with the wave speed (6.835b):

$$\omega = ck: \qquad\qquad u \equiv \frac{\omega}{k} = c = \frac{\partial\omega}{\partial k} = w. \qquad\qquad (6.835\text{a–d})$$

   In the case of dispersive waves [for example bending waves (6.815d) ≡ (6.836a) in an elastic bar] the phase speed (6.836b) and group velocity (6.836a) are different:

$$\omega = bk^2: \qquad\qquad u = \frac{\omega}{k} = bk \neq 2bk = \frac{\partial\omega}{\partial k} = w = 2u, \qquad (6.836\text{a–d})$$

[in this case the former is one-half of the latter (6.836d)].
   The combination of (i) non-dispersive [(ii) dispersive] waves in an elastic string (6.814a–d) [bar (6.815a–d)] is (problem 357) dispersive for a beam, and including also (iii) the natural frequency of a translational spring (6.813a–c), leads to an

oscillation frequency (6.812b) ≡ (6.837a) implying the distinct phase speed (6.837b)
and group velocity (6.837c):

$$\omega(k) = \pm \left| \omega_0^2 + c_e^2 k^2 + b^2 k^4 \right|^{1/2} ; \tag{6.837a}$$

$$u \equiv \frac{\omega}{k} = \pm \left| \frac{\omega_0^2}{k^2} + c_e^2 + b^2 k^2 \right|^{1/2} , \tag{6.837b}$$

$$w \equiv \frac{\partial \omega}{\partial k} = \pm \frac{\left| 2 c_e^2 k + 4 b^2 k^3 \right|^{1/2}}{2\omega}. \tag{6.837c}$$

Considering (Table 6.11) a **wave packet** consisting (problem 358) of non-dispersive (dispersive) waves with different wave numbers, the phase speed of wave crests and group velocity of wave particles are: (i) equal (distinct); (ii) do not (do) depend on the wavelength; thus (iii) the wave packet stays together, preserving (disperses changing) the waveform [Figure 6.38b; 6.38a, c]. The consideration of the boundary (initial) conditions [notes 6.11–6.16 (6.17–6.18)] specifies the dispersion relation (the amplitudes) of the free wave modes.

NOTE 6.17: **Eigenvalues for the Wavenumber and Frequency and Eigenfunctions**

For each **eigenvalue**; that is, wavenumber (6.810d) [wavelength (6.810c)] and corresponding mode frequency (6.812a, b) [period (6.812b, c)], there is an **eigenfunction** or wave mode (6.806a) that is the product of: (i) a spatial part (6.808e) obtained before (notes 6.12–6.17); and (ii) a temporal part that is the solution of (6.806b) ≡ (6.838b):

$$\chi \equiv \frac{\mu}{2\rho_1} : \qquad\qquad \ddot{Y}_n + 2\chi \dot{Y}_n + \omega_n^2 Y_n = 0, \tag{6.838a, b}$$

that is similar to the damped harmonic oscillator (6.838b) ≡ (2.22) with a similar decay (6.838a) ≡ (2.23b) for each natural frequency (6.812b). Since (6.838b) is a linear second-order differential equation with constant coefficients, its solutions are exponential (6.839a) where α is a root of the characteristic polynomial (6.839b) of the second degree:

$$Y_n(t) = e^{\alpha t} : \qquad\qquad 0 = \alpha^2 + 2\chi\alpha + \omega_n^2. \tag{6.839a, b}$$

The cases of supercritical and critical damping have been considered (section 2.3), together with subcritical damping (section 2.4), that is taken in the sequel (6.840a) leading to the roots (6.840b) of the characteristic polynomial (6.839b):

$$\omega_n^2 > \chi^2: \qquad \alpha_\pm = -\chi \pm i\bar{\omega}_n, \qquad \bar{\omega}_n \equiv \left|\omega_n^2 - \chi^2\right|^{1/2}, \qquad (6.840a\text{–}c)$$

where $(6.840c) \equiv (2.105d)$ is the **modal frequency** of the n-th mode.

The general integral of (6.838b) is $(6.841a) \equiv (6.841b)$:

$$Y_n(t) = e^{-\chi t}\left(C_n^+ e^{i\bar{\omega}_n t} + C_n^+ e^{-i\bar{\omega}_n t}\right) = e^{-\chi t} A_n \cos(\bar{\omega}_n t) + B_n \sin(\bar{\omega}_n t), \qquad (6.841a, b)$$

that is substituted in (6.806a) to specify the **eigenfunctions:**

$$\zeta(x,t) = e^{-\chi t} \sum_{n=1}^{\infty} \sin(k_n x)\left[A_n \cos(\bar{\omega}_n t) + B_n \sin(\bar{\omega}_n t)\right], \qquad (6.842)$$

whose superposition is (problem 359) the general standing wave field involving: (i) the wavenumbers (6.810d) and corresponding natural (6.812b) and oscillation (6.840c) frequencies that coincide (6.843b) for weak damping (6.843a):

$$\chi^2 \ll \omega_n^2 \quad \Rightarrow \quad \bar{\omega}_n = \omega_n; \qquad \{A_n, B_n\} \neq \{0,0\}, \qquad (6.843a\text{–}c)$$

*(ii) the **wave modes** that have at least one non-zero **amplitude**, determined [note(s) 6.18 (6.19–6.21)] by initial conditions (or forcing by an external force).*

NOTE 6.18: **Amplitudes and Initial Displacement and Velocity**

The wave equation with stiffness (6.805i) is of the fourth (second) order in position (time) and thus a unique solution requires (section 9.1) four boundary (two initial) conditions; for example, (6.808a–d) for supported (Figure 6.35) or pinned (Figure 6.36) ends [the displacement (6.842) and velocity (6.844) at an initial time $t = 0$]:

$$v(x,t) \equiv \partial_t\left[\zeta(x,t)\right]$$

$$= e^{-\chi t} \sum_{n=1}^{\infty} \sin(k_n x)\left[(B_n\bar{\omega}_n - A_n\chi)\cos(\bar{\omega}_n t) - (A_n\bar{\omega}_n + B_n\chi)\sin(\bar{\omega}_n t)\right]. \qquad (6.844)$$

The two **initial conditions** specify (problem 360) the initial **displacement** (6.842) [**velocity** (6.844)] at (6.845a) [(6.845b)] time $t = 0$:

$$\{\zeta(x,0), v(x,0)\} = \sum_{n=1}^{\infty} \sin\left(\frac{n\pi x}{L}\right)\{A_n, B_n\bar{\omega}_n - A_n\chi\}, \qquad (6.845a, b)$$

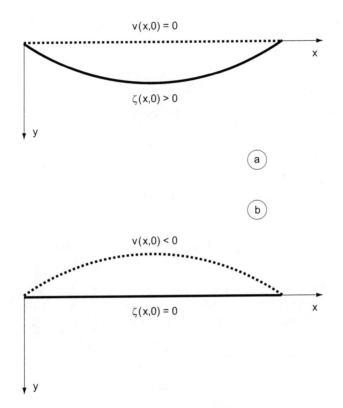

FIGURE 6.40
The wave equation for the transverse vibrations of a beam under axial tension supported on springs and in the presence of linear damping (Figure 6.36) is of the fourth (second) order in space (time), and thus unicity of solution requires four (two) boundary (initial) conditions; for example, supported or pinned [specifying the initial (a) displacement and (b) velocity].

*showing that: (i) the **wave generation** can be due to an initial displacement from [or an initial velocity imparted from] the equilibrium position [Figure 6.40a(b)] or both; (ii) the **mode amplitudes** are specified by:*

$$\left\{A_n, B_n\bar{\omega}_n - A_n\chi\right\} = \frac{1}{L}\int_0^L \left\{\zeta(x,0), v(x,0)\right\}\sin\left(\frac{n\pi x}{L}\right)dx, \quad (6.846a, b)$$

that are the coefficients (II.5.170a, b;II.5.171b) of the Fourier (subsection II.5.7.6) sine series (6.845a, b). Using the identities (II.5.88c) ≡ (6.847a) [(II.5.88b) ≡ (6.847b)]:

$$2\sin\left(k_n x\right)\cos\left(\bar{\omega}_n t\right) = \sin\left(k_n x + \bar{\omega}_n t\right) + \sin\left(k_n x - \bar{\omega}_n t\right), \qquad (6.847a)$$

$$2\sin\left(k_n x\right)\sin\left(\bar{\omega}_n t\right) = \cos\left(k_n x - \bar{\omega}_n t\right) - \cos\left(k_n x + \bar{\omega}_n t\right), \qquad (6.847b)$$

in (6.842) leads to:

$$\zeta(x,t) = \frac{e^{-\chi t}}{2} \sum_{n=1}^{\infty} \left\{ \begin{array}{l} A_n \left[\sin(k_n x - \bar{\omega}_n t) + \sin(k_n x - \bar{\omega}_n t) \right] \\ + B_n \left[\cos(k_n x - \bar{\omega}_n t) - \cos(k_n x + \bar{\omega}_n t) \right] \end{array} \right\}, \qquad (6.848)$$

confirming (note 6.15) that the standing modes (6.831b–d) are the superposition (6.848) of waves with the same amplitude (6.831a) propagating in opposite directions. The wave modes can be generated either (i) by initial condition for free waves (notes 6.11–6.18) or (ii) by external forcing (notes 6.19–6.22).

NOTE 6.19: Wave Generation by Forcing in Space-Time

The wave equation (6.805i) is reconsidered in homogeneous and steady media (6.805b–h) in the presence (6.849), instead of absence (6.805a), of forcing that may be a function of position and time:

$$\rho_1 \ddot{\zeta} + \mu \dot{\zeta} + \nu \zeta - T \zeta'' + B \zeta'''' = \rho_1 f_e(x,t). \qquad (6.849)$$

In the r.h.s. of (6.849), the external force per unit mass is assumed to be: (i) a function of position of bounded oscillation (subsection I.27.9.5 and note 1.9) over the length L of the beam (6.850a), that vanishes at the two ends (6.850c, d) and has (subsection II.5.7.8) a Fourier sine series (II.5.188b) $\equiv$ (6.850b) with coefficients (II.5.190b) $\equiv$ (6.850e):

$$f_a(x,t) \in \mathcal{F}(0,L): \qquad f_a(x,t) = \cos(\omega_a t) \sum_{n=1}^{\infty} f_n \sin\left(\frac{n\pi x}{L}\right) \qquad (6.850a, b)$$

$$f_a(0,t) = 0 = f_a(L,t): \qquad f_n = \frac{1}{L} \int_0^L \frac{f_a(x,t)}{\cos(\omega_a t)} \sin\left(\frac{n\pi x}{L}\right) dx; \qquad (6.850c\text{–}e)$$

and (ii) a sinusoidal function of time with **applied frequency** ω_a. *The forcing* (6.850b) $\equiv$ (6.851a) *is (problem 361) the real part of the **complex representation*** (6.851a):

$$\{f_a(x,t), \zeta_*(x,t)\} = \mathrm{Re}\left[\exp(i\omega_a t)\right] \sum_{n=1}^{\infty} \{f_n, g_n\} \sin\left(\frac{n\pi x}{L}\right), \qquad (6.851a, b)$$

*and the **response** (6.851b) or particular integral of the forced wave equation (6.849) is sought as a similar superstition (6.851b) of **normal modes** with amplitudes g_n to be determined (note 6.21). The free wave solution (6.842) due to initial conditions (6.846a, b) can be added in the complete integral to the forced solution obtained next (notes 6.20–6.22).*

NOTE 6.20: **Amplitude and Phase of the Forced Response**

Substituting the forcing (6.851a) and the response (6.851b) in the forced wave equation (6.849) leads to the algebraic relation (6.852a) between the known (unknown) forcing (6.850e) [response (6.851b)] coefficients:

$$
f_n = g_n \left(\frac{v}{\rho_1} + 2 i \omega_a \chi - \omega_n^2 + \frac{T}{\rho_1} \frac{n^2 \pi^2}{L^2} + \frac{B}{\rho_1} \frac{n^2 \pi^2}{L^2} \right)
$$

$$
= g_n \left(\omega_0^2 + c_e^2 k_n^2 + b^2 k_n^4 - \omega_a^2 + 2 i \omega_a \chi \right) \tag{6.852a–c}
$$

$$
= g_n \left(\omega_n^2 - \omega_a^2 + 2 i \omega_a \chi \right),
$$

where: (i) were introduced (6.852b) the natural frequency of the translational spring (6.803b), the decay (6.803a), the transverse elastic wave speed (6.804a), and the dispersive stiffness parameter (6.804c) in addition to the wavenumber (6.810d) of the n-th mode; and (ii) using (6.812a, b) mode frequency simplifies (6.852b) to (6.852c). Provided that the factor in brackets on the r.h.s. of (6.852c) does not vanish (6.853a), the amplitudes g_n can be obtained by division (6.853b):

$$
\omega_n - \omega_a \neq 0 \neq \chi : \qquad g_n = \frac{f_n}{\omega_n^2 - \omega_a^2 + 2 i \omega_a \chi} = f_n E_n e^{i\phi_n} ; \tag{6.853a–c}
$$

the result (6.853b) ≡ (2.193) is analogous to the response of a damped harmonic oscillator to sinusoidal forcing at the applied frequency ω_a replacing the single natural frequency ω_0 by the mode frequencies ω_n with amplitudes (6.854a) and phases (6.854b, c):

$$
\frac{1}{E_n} = \left| (\omega_n - \omega_a)^2 + 2 i \omega_a \chi \right| = \left| (\omega_n^2 - \omega_a^2)^2 + 4 \omega_a^2 \chi^2 \right|^{1/2}, \tag{6.854a}
$$

$$
\phi_n = - arc \tan \left(\frac{2 \omega_a \chi}{\omega_n^2 - \omega_a^2} \right) = arc \cot \left(\frac{\omega_n^2 - \omega_a^2}{2 \omega_a \chi} \right). \tag{6.854b, c}
$$

Substitution of (6.853a–c; 6.854a–c) in (6.851b) specifies the responses with (without) damping [note 6.21 (6.22)].

NOTE 6.21: **Non-Resonant and Resonant Forcing with Damping**

The particular integral of the wave equation (6.849) with forcing sinusoidal in time (6.850b) and of bounded fluctuation is space (6.850a, e) is the forcing specified equivalently: (i) by substituting (6.853b) in (6.851a, b) leading to (6.855a):

$$\zeta_*(x,t) = \sum_{n=1}^{\infty} f_n \sin\left(\frac{n\pi x}{L}\right) \ \mathrm{Re}\left\{\frac{e^{i\omega_a t}}{\omega_n^2 - \omega_a^2 + 2i\omega_a t}\right\}$$

$$= \sum_{n=1}^{\infty} f_n \sin(k_n x) \ \mathrm{Re}\left\{\frac{\left(\omega_n^2 - \omega_a^2 - 2i\omega_a \chi\right)e^{i\omega_a t}}{\left(\omega_n^2 - \omega_a^2\right)^2 + 4\omega_a^2 \chi^2}\right\},$$

$$(6.855a\text{--}c)$$

where multiplication by the complex conjugate of the denominator gives $(6.855b) \equiv (6.856)$:

$$\zeta_*(x,t) = \sum_{n=1}^{\infty} f_n \sin(k_n x)\frac{\left(\omega_n^2 - \omega_a^2\right)\cos(\omega_n x) + 2\omega_a \chi \sin(k_n x)}{\left(\omega_n^2 - \omega_a^2\right)^2 + 4\omega_a^2 \chi^2}; \qquad (6.856)$$

(ii) by substituting (6.853c) in (6.851b) leading to (6.857a, b):

$$\zeta_*(x,t) = \sum_{n=1}^{\infty} f_n \sin\left(\frac{n\pi x}{L}\right)\mathrm{Re}\left\{E_n e^{i\omega_a t + i\phi_n}\right\}$$

$$(6.857a, b)$$

$$= \sum_{n=1}^{\infty} f_n \sin(k_n x) E_n \cos(\omega_a t + \phi),$$

that is equivalent to (6.858):

$$\zeta_*(x,t) = \sum_{n=1}^{\infty} f_n E_n \sin(k_n x)\left[\cos\phi_n \cos(\omega_n t) - \sin\phi_n \sin(\omega_n t)\right]; \qquad (6.858)$$

(iii) from (6.853b, c) or (6.854a–c) follow:

$$E_n\{\cos\phi_n, \sin\phi_n\} = \frac{\{\omega_n^2 - \omega_n^2, 2\omega_a \chi\}}{E_n^2} = \frac{\{\omega_n^2 - \omega_n^2, 2\omega_a \chi\}}{\left(\omega_n^2 - \omega_0^2\right) + 4\omega_a^2 \chi^2}, \qquad (6.859a, b)$$

that prove the coincidence of $(6.856) \equiv (6.858)$.

Thus *the wave equation with stiffness (6.849) with an external applied force per unit mass (6.850b) that is sinusoidal in time with applied frequency ω_a and a function of bounded fluctuation (6.850a) along the length L of the beam, has particular integral or response to forcing given in the general case I (problem 362) without resonance and with damping: (i) explicitly by (6.856); (ii) alternatively by (6.858) with the amplitudes (6.854a) and phases (6.854b, c). In the case II (problem 363) of damping (6.860a) with **resonance** (6.860b) that is the applied frequency equal to the* *m-th modal frequency: (i) the response simplifies for the m-th mode and is unchanged for the remaining modes (6.860c):*

$$\chi \neq 0, \quad \omega_a = \omega_m: \quad \zeta_*(x,t) = \frac{f_m}{2\omega_a \chi} \sin(k_m x)\sin(\omega_a t)$$

$$+ \sum_{\substack{n=1 \\ n \neq m}}^{\infty} f_n \sin(k_n x) \frac{\left(\omega_n^2 - \omega_a^2\right)\cos(\omega_n x) + 2\omega_n \chi \sin(k_n x)}{\left(\omega_n^2 - \omega_a^2\right)^2 + 4\omega_n^2 \chi^2},$$

$$\text{(6.860a–c)}$$

corresponding to the amplitudes (6.854a) [(6.861c)] and phases (6.854b, c) [(6.861d)] for the n ≠ m non-resonant (n = m resonant) mode:

$$\chi \neq 0, \quad \omega_a = \omega_m: \qquad\qquad 2E_m \omega_a \chi = 1, \qquad \phi_m = \frac{\pi}{2}, \qquad \text{(6.861a–d)}$$

implying that the resonant mode is in out-of-phase (6.861d) with the forcing. The remaining resonant (non-resonant) cases III (VI) without damping are considered next (Note 6.22).

NOTE 6.22: Undamped Non-Resonant and Resonant Response

In the case III (problem 364) of absence of damping (6.862a) and no resonance (6.862b); that is, applied frequency distinct from all mode frequencies, the response (6.856) is given by (6.862c):

$$\chi = 0, \qquad \omega_a \neq \omega_n: \qquad \zeta_*(x,t) = \sum_{n=1}^{\infty} \frac{f_n}{\omega_n^2 - \omega_a^2} \sin(k_n x)\cos(\omega_n t), \qquad \text{(6.862a–d)}$$

corresponding to amplitudes (6.863c) with zero phase (6.863d):

$$\chi = 0, \qquad \omega_a \neq \omega_n: \qquad \left(\omega_n^2 - \omega_a^2\right)E_n = 1, \qquad \phi_n = 0. \qquad \text{(6.863a–d)}$$

In the case IV (problem 365) of resonance at the m-th mode (6.864b) without damping (6.864a) the response (6.864c):

$$\chi = 0, \omega_a = \omega_m:$$

$$\zeta_*(x,t) = \frac{f_m t}{2\omega_a} \sin(k_n x)\sin(\omega_a t) + \sum_{\substack{n=1 \\ n \neq m}}^{\infty} \frac{f_n}{\omega_n^2 - \omega_a^2} \sin(k_n x)\cos(\omega_n t),$$

$$\text{(6.864a–c)}$$

consists of: (i) the same sum as (6.862c) for non-resonant modes n ≠ m; and (ii) the undamped resonant mode has amplitude increasing linearly with time (6.865c) and is out of phase (6.865d) relative to the forcing:

$$\chi = 0, \qquad \omega_a = \omega_m: \qquad\qquad 2\omega_a E_m = t, \qquad \phi_m = \frac{\pi}{2}. \qquad\qquad \text{(6.865a–d)}$$

The results (6.864a–c; 6.865a–d) concerning the undamped resonant mode are proved next.

The condition (6.853a) that allows division in (6.852c) to obtain (6.853b) is valid in cases I, II, and III, but not in case IV of undamped resonance (6.864a, b), so (6.855c) fails only in this case. The undamped resonant mode is:

$$\zeta_{*m}(x,t) = \lim_{\omega_m \to \omega_a} f_m \sin(k_m x) \operatorname{Re}\left\{ \frac{e^{i\omega_a t} - e^{i\omega_m t}}{\omega_m^2 - \omega_a^2} \right\}, \qquad\qquad \text{(6.866)}$$

where: (i) in the absence of damping (6.864a) the m-th term in (6.855c) reduces to (6.866); and (ii) a free wave with the same amplitude and frequency ω_m was subtracted, since this remains a solution of the forced differential equation. Both the numerator and denominator in curly brackets in (6.866) have simple zeros for $\omega_a = \omega_m$, and this 0:0 indetermination is resolved by the L'Hospital rule (I.19.35) differentiating separately the numerator and denominator with regard to ω_m before taking the limit:

$$\lim_{\omega_m \to \omega_a} \operatorname{Re}\left\{ \frac{e^{i\omega_a t} - e^{i\omega_m t}}{\omega_m^2 - \omega_a^2} \right\} = \lim_{\omega_m \to \omega_a} \operatorname{Re}\left\{ \frac{\dfrac{\partial}{\partial \omega_m}\left(e^{i\omega_a t} - e^{i\omega_m t} \right)}{\dfrac{\partial}{\partial \omega_m}\left(\omega_m^2 - \omega_a^2 \right)} \right\}$$

$$= \lim_{\omega_m \to \omega_a} \operatorname{Re}\left\{ \frac{-it\, e^{i\omega_m t}}{2\omega_m} \right\} \qquad\qquad \text{(6.867)}$$

$$= \frac{t}{2\omega_a} \operatorname{Re}\left(-i e^{i\omega_a t} \right)$$

$$= \frac{t}{2\omega_a} \sin\left(\omega_a t \right).$$

Substituting (6.867) in (6.866) proves the first term on the r.h.s. of (6.864a). The physical interpretation of cases I to IV of forcing is made together with the case of free waves in a summary review of the solution of the wave equation (note 6.23).

NOTE 6.23: **Wave Equation with Boundary and Initial Conditions**

Diagram 6.3 illustrates the method of solution of a wave equation with boundary and initial conditions in the case (6.849) of (Figure 6.36) the linear (6.805b) transverse vibrations of a beam with bending stiffness B, under tangential tension T, with mass density ρ_1 per unit length, supported on translational springs with resilience v, and with dissipation by damping μ. The vibrations can be: (i) free modes due to initial conditions out of equilibrium; (ii) forced modes due to a transverse external applied force. The unforced wave equation (6.805i) can be solved by separation of variables (6.806a) as the product of functions of position (time) that satisfy separate differential equations with a common separation constant, in this case the frequency. Since the wave equation is a linear partial differential equation with constant coefficients of order 4 (2) on position (time), the spatial (temporal) part satisfies a linear ordinary differential equation with constant coefficients of order 4 (2), so that unicity of solution (section 9.1) requires 4 (2) independent and compatible boundary (initial) conditions.

Starting with the spatial part A of free waves I there are four steps: (I.A.1) determine the four boundary conditions, in this case for a beam supported or pinned at both ends (6.808a–d), which specify the spatial eigenvalues, that is, the wavenumbers (6.810d) or wavelengths (6.810c); (I.A.2) match each spatial eigenvalue to a spatial eigenfunction (6.808e), in this case the fundamental mode (Figure 6.37a) and harmonics (Figure 6.37b, c, d) of all orders; (I.A.3) substitute the spatial eigenfunctions (6.808e) in the spatial differential

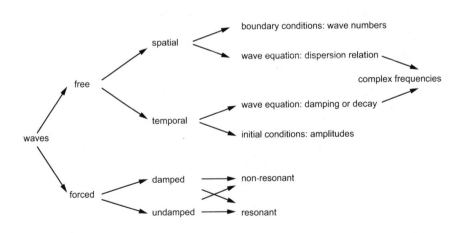

Free modes and forced waves

DIAGRAM 6.3
The solution of a wave equation by separation of variables involves a sequence of steps for the spatial and temporal part of the free wave modes that are also used in the construction of forced solutions.

equation (6.806c), which leads to the dispersion relation (6.812a, b); and (I.A.4) use the dispersion relation to specify the temporal eigenvalues, that is, the frequencies or periods of the wave modes. This completes the spatial part A for free waves (I), and allows the determination of the temporal part B: (I.B.1) the mode frequencies appear in the temporal differential equation (6.806b) that is thus completely specified; (I.B.2) the solution of the temporal differential equation (6.838a, b) specifies the temporal eigenfunctions (6.841a, b); (I.B.3) the general free wave solution (6.842) is a superposition of products of spatial and temporal eigenfunctions for each mode with two sets of arbitrary amplitudes; and (I.B.4) the two sets of amplitudes are determined (6.846a, b) by two initial conditions specifying the shape of the beam (Figure 6.40a) and its transverse velocity (Figure 6.40b) at a fixed time.

The free wave modes (I) are used to obtain the forced modes (II) in four steps (II.A) as follows: (II.A.1) the forcing function is expanded (6.851a) in a series of normal modes, with known (6.850e) coefficients (forcing harmonics); (III.A.2) the response is represented by (6.851b) a similar modal decomposition with unknown coefficients (response harmonics); (II.A.3) substitution of the forcing and response in the wave equation (6.849) relates (6.852a–c) the response harmonics to the forcing harmonics; (I.A.4) this relation is used to determine the response harmonics that specify the general response (6.855a–c). These are (II.B) as for the damped harmonic oscillator with sinusoidal forcing (section 2.7–2.8) four cases: (II.B.1) in the non-resonant case with damping (6.856) ≡ (6.858), the phase (6.859b, c) is such that the work of the external applied force is balanced by dissipation and the amplitude is constant (6.859a); (II.B.2) in the case of resonance with damping (6.860a–c; 6.861a–d), the phase difference between the forcing and the response is maximum at $\pi/2$, so that dissipation is most effective at limiting the constant amplitude; (II.B.3) in the absence of damping outside resonance (6.862a–c; 6.863a–d) the forcing is in-phase with the displacement, and thus out-of-phase with the velocity, so no work is done on average over a period and the amplitude is constant as in the two preceding cases; (II.B.4) in the case of resonance without damping (6.864a–c; 6.865a–d), the forcing is out-of-phase with the displacement, hence in-phase with the velocity, and since the work of the external force cannot be dissipated in the absence of damping, the amplitude increases linearly with time.

Conclusion 6

The bending of an elastic beam (Figure 6.1) is due to a bending moment M (Figure 6.1c) associated with tranverse force F (Figure 6.1d) and tangential tension (Figure 6.1e) that may be [Figure 6.1a(b)] a traction (compression). The bending moment is proportional to the local curvature of the elastica or neutral fiber of the beam (Figure 6.2b) corresponding to the tangent circle whose radius (Figure 6.2a) best approximates the elastica. The case of a compression can lead to buckling if it exceeds a critical value that depends on the way the beam is supported: the critical buckling load is largest (smallest) for a beam [Figure 6.3a(d)] with clamped ends (cantilever with one clamped and one free end), and takes intermediate larger (smaller) values for a beam [Figure 6.3c (b)] with one clamped and one pinned end (two pinned ends). The buckling may be opposed in the four cases of cantilever (clamped and/or pinned) beams [Figure 6.3d (a, b, c)] by a translational spring [Figure 6.4d (a, b, c)]; for example, at the free end (mid position); reversing the position of the spring decreases (Figure 6.5a–d) instead of increases (Figure 6.4a–d) the critical buckling load. The critical buckling load is the same (Table 6.1) for weak (strong) bending, but the shape of the buckled elastica is different (Panel 6.2). The buckling can be opposed or facilitated by translational (rotary) springs (Table 6.3 (6.4)]. The resilience of the spring can be chosen (Panel 6.1) to cause buckling without an axial load (Table 6.2). The critical buckling load corresponds to the first of an infinite discrete sequence of buckling modes (Panels 6.3–6.7). The beam; that is, a bar with bending stiffness under axial traction or compression, can also be continuously supported on springs; for example, translational springs (Table 6.5), in the absence (presence) of transverse loads [Figure 6.6 (6.7)].

The axial traction (compression) of a straight rod [Figure 6.8a(b)] causes an extension (compression) associated with a longitudinal force (Figure 6.9). The resistance to stretching (compression) depends on the Young modulus of the material, that may be non-uniform (Figure 6.10), affecting the longitudinal displacement. The two-dimensional analog of longitudinal deformation of a rod is in-plane stresses in a plate, such as: (i) a torque applied to drill a hole (Figure 6.11); or (ii/iii) stress concentration near a hole ion an infinite plate due to stresses at infinity (Figure 6.12) [compression at the hole (Figure 6.13)]. The case of transverse loads with large in-plane tension leads to the deflection (Figure 6.14b) of a plane membrane (Figure 6.14a) that may be subject to anisotropic stresses consisting of compressions/tractions and shears (Figure 6.16). The shears are eliminated by a rotation (Figure 6.15a, b) to principal stress axis (Figure 6.17). The shape of the membrane under transverse loads implies a constant displacement along two characteristic lines (Figure 6.17); the unequal principal stresses leads to the equilibrium of an elliptical membrane under its own weight (Figure 6.18).

A two-dimensional elastic body that is flat (Figure 6.19a) in the undeformed state and has bending stiffness, when under load (Figure 6.19b) has a neutral surface or directrix (Figure 6.20) that is neither stretched nor shortened: the surfaces on the inner (outer) side are shortened (stretched) due to bending by transverse forces associated with turning moments (Figure 6.21b) and stress couples (Figure 6.21a). The shape of the directrix is determined by the balance of the work of the transverse forces against the elastic energy of the plate (Figure 6.22) that also specifies the boundary conditions (Table 6.6) including clamped (Figure 6.23a), supported (Figure 6.23b), pinned (Figure 6.23c), and free boundary (Figure 6.23d). These boundary conditions (Table 6.7) apply in general to a plate whose boundary is an arbitrary closed regular curve (Figure 6.24a) and in particular to circular (Figure 6.24b) and rectangular (Figure 6.24c) plates. The bending of a circular plate under its own weight is considered with [Figure 6.25a(b)] with the edge clamped (supported or pinned) and also suspended from the center with free edge (Figure 6.25c). As for the axial tension in a beam, the in-plane stresses in a plate do not (do) cause buckling in the case of tractions (compressions beyond a critical load overcoming tractions). For example, a rectangular plate supported on all sides (Figure 6.29a) buckles under compression or if the compressions overcome the tractions; in the case of a rectangular plate clamped on two sides and supported on the other (Figure 6.29b) there is (Table 6.8) no buckling (two cases of buckling) under traction (compression). The strong non-linear bending of a plate with large slope couples non-linearly the transverse displacement and in-plane stresses, for example for a clamped circular plate (Figure 6.30a) subject to its own weight (Figure 6.30b) and axial compression (Figure 6.30c).

The cases of one(two)-dimensional elastic bodies (Tables 6.9–6.10, Lists 6.1–6.3 and Diagrams 6.1–6.2) include; (i) strings (membranes) without bending stiffness; (ii) bars (plates) with bending stiffness; and (iii) the combination of (i) and (ii) in beams (stressed plates) under tangential tension (in-plane stresses). The rods and plates may have deformation in bending, torsion and extension and contraction. The deformations of elastic bodies, result from the balance of forces and stresses and depend on material properties that may be isotropic (anisotropic); that is, independent (dependent) direction, for example, for a plate without (with) reinforcements [Figure 6.26a (b, c)]. In the anisotropic case there may be symmetries; for example, with regard to one plane (three orthogonal planes) in the case of a homoclinic (orthotropic) material [Figure 6.28b(c)]. Including the inertia force in the force stress balance (Figure 6.27) leads to waves, such as: (i) the transverse vibrations of [Figure 6.31 (6.32)] elastic strings and beams (membranes and plates); and (ii) the torsional (longitudinal) oscillations of rods [Figure 6.33 (6.34)]. Considering the transverse vibrations of beams under tangential tension, for example, additional effects include damping and support on translational (and rotational) springs [Figure 6.36 (6.35)]. In the case of an infinite plate, there are free waves propagating in opposite directions (Figure 6.39); if the wave speed does not (does) depend on the wavelength the different wavelengths propagate together (disperse) leading [Figure 6.38b(a, c)] to a permanent (changing) waveform. The superposition of waves propagating in opposite directions with the same amplitude; for example, due to reflexion at fixed ends, leads to standing modes, consisting of a fundamental (Figure 6.37a) and harmonics (Figures 6.37b, c, d). The generation of wave modes; that is, the amplitude of each mode, is determined by: (i) the initial shape (Figure 6.40a) and velocity (Figure 6.40b) out-of-equilibrium; and (ii) the external forcing (Diagram 6.3) by a transverse force per unit length.

List 6.1 Elasticity

a. *Three-dimensional*: II.4.3–II.4.4.

b. *Plane*: II.4.

c. *Without bending stiffness*:

  C.a One-dimensional: elastic string: see list III.2.

  C.b Two-dimensional: elastic membrane:

    C.b.α Linear isotropic: section II.6.1;

    C.b.β Non-linear isotropic: section II.6.2;

    C.b.γ Linear anisotropic: section 6.6.

d. *With bending stiffness, one-dimensional, straight rod:*

  D.a Torsion of rod: sections II.6.4–II.6.8;

  D.b Traction/compression of rod:

    D.b.α Linear and homogeneous: notes III.2.5 and III.4.4;

    D.b.β Non-linear and homogeneous: notes III.2.6 and III.4.5–III.4.7;

    D.b.γ Linear and inhomogeneous: section 6.4.

  D.c Bending of bars and buckling of beams: see list 6.3.

e. *With bending stiffness, two-dimensional flat plate;*

  E.a In-plane stresses: section 6.5;

  E.b Weak bending: section 6.7;

  E.c Elastic stability: section 6.8;

  E.d Strong bending: section 6.9.

List 6.2 Twenty-One Instances of One- and Two-Dimensional Elasticity

a. *Transverse deflection of elastic string:* sections III.2.1–III.2.2:

  1 – Linear: sections III.2.3–III.2.5, examples III.10.3–III.10.7;

  2 – Non-linear: sections III.2.6–III.2.9, examples III.10.5–III.10.7.

b. *Transverse deflection of a membrane:* sections II.6.1–II.6.2; 6.6:

  3 – Linear isotropic: section II.6.1;

  4 – Non-linear isotropic: sections II.6.2–II.6.3;

  5 – Linear anitropic: section 6.6.

c. *In-plane deformations:*

6 – Plane elasticity: chapter II.4;

7 – In-plane stresses in a plate: section 6.5.

d. *Straight elastic bar (without axial tension):*

8 – Torsion: sections II.6.4–II.6.8;

9 – Extension/contraction: notes III.2.5–III.2.6, III.4.4–III.4.7, section 6.4;

10 – Bending: sections III.4.1–III.4.2;

11 – Linear bending: sections III.4.3–III.4.5, examples III.10.10–III.10.11;

12 – Non-linear bending: sections III.4.7–III.4.9.

e. *Straight beam (with axial tension):*

13 – Linear and non-linear buckling under compression: section 6.1;

14 – Linear buckling with discrete support by translational or rotary springs: section 6.2;

15 – Bending/buckling with continuous support by translational springs: section 6.3;

16 – Tangential stresses due to bending by transverse loads: section III.4.6;

17 – Bending by transverse loads in the presence of translational springs: subsection 6.3.14;

18 – Linear bending by transverse loads: example 10.10.

f. *Bending of flat plate:*

19 – Linear without in-plane stresses: section 6.7;

20 – Linear with in-plane stresses: section 6.8;

21 – Non-linear: section 6.9.

List 6.3 Thirty-One Cases of Deflection of a Beam

a. Linear buckling of uniform *beam* without transverse loads, under axial compression and without springs: subsections 6.1.1–6.1.4:

1 – Clamped beam: subsection 6.1.5;

2 – Clamped-pinned beam: subsection 6.1.7;

3 – Pinned beam: subsection 6.1.6;

4 – Cantilever beam: subsections 6.1.7–6.1.12.

b. Linear buckling of a uniform beam without transverse loads, under axial compression and with a *point translational spring*: subsections 6.2.1–6.2.5, 6.2.11–6.2.13, 6.2.15–6.2.17:

    5 – At the middle of a clamped beam: subsection 6.2.3;

    6 – At the middle of a clamped-pinned beam: subsection 6.2.5;

    7 – At the middle of a pinned beam: subsection 6.2.4;

    8 – At the tip of a cantilever beam: subsections 6.2.2, 6.2.12, 6.2.13, 6.2.15–6.2.17.

c. Linear buckling of a uniform beam without transverse loads, under axial compression and with a *point rotary spring*: subsections 6.2.6–6.2.14.

    9 – At the middle of a clamped beam: subsection 6.2.8;

    10 – At the middle of a clamped-pinned beam: subsection 6.2.10;

    11 – At the middle of a pinned beam: subsection 6.2.9;

    12 – At the tip of a cantilever beam: subsections 6.2.17, 6.2.12–6.2.14.

d. Linear buckling of a pinned uniform beam without transverse loads, under axial tension, and continuously supported on *continuous translational springs*: subsections 6.3.1–6.3.14:

    13 – Axial compression without springs: subsection 6.1.6;

    14 – Axial traction without springs: subsection 6.3.3;

    15 – Attractive springs without tension: subsection 6.3.4;

    16 – Repulsive springs without tension: subsection 6.3.5;

    17 – Axial compression balanced by attractive springs: subsection 6.3.6;

    18 – Axial traction balanced by attractive springs: subsection 6.3.7;

    19 – Axial traction dominating attractive springs: subsection 6.3.8;

    20 – Axial compression dominating attractive springs: subsection 6.3.9;

    21 – Axial compression dominating repulsive springs: subsection 6.3.10;

    22 – Attractive springs dominating the axial tension: subsection 6.3.11.

e. Linear bending of a beam (under axial tension) continuously supported on springs due to a *transverse load*:

    23 – Pinned beam under uniform shear stress: subsection 6.3.14.

f. Linear bending of a *bar* (without axial tension) continuously supported on springs due to a transverse load: example 10.13:

    24 – Clamped bar with a concentrated torque: example 10.13.1;

25 – Pinned bar with a concentrated force: example 10.13.2;

26 – Clamped-pinned bar under a uniform shear stress: example 10.13.3;

27 – Cantilever bar under a non-uniform shear stress: example 10.14.

g. Non-linear buckling of uniform beam without transverse loads; loads under axial compression, and without springs: subsections 6.1.10–6.1.15:

28 – Clamped beam: subsections 6.1.10–6.1.12;

29 – Clamped pinned beam: subsection 6.1.13;

30 – Pinned beam: subsections 6.1.13–6.1.15;

31 – Cantilever beam: subsections 6.1.13–6.1.15.

Bibliography

The bibliography of *Higher-Order Differential Equation and Elasticity*, that is the third book of volume IV, *Ordinary Differential Equations with Applications to Trajectories and Oscillations*, and the sixth book of the series *Mathematics and Physics Applied to Science and Technology*, adds the subject of "Collected Works" of major scientists. The books in the bibliography that have influenced the present volume the most are marked with one, two, or three asterisks.

Collected Works

* Cauchy, A.L. *Ouevres complètes*. Gauthier-Villars, 1881–1895, 14 vols., Paris.
* D'Alembert, J.R. *Opuscules mathematiques*. Gauthier-Villars 1761–1780, 8 vols, Paris.
* Euler, L. *Opera Omnia*. Academia Scientarum Helveticae, circa de 100 vols., Basel.
Green, G. *Mathematical papers*. London 1871, reprinted Chelsea 1970, New York.
Hurwitz, A. *Mathematische Werke*. Birkhauser Verlag 1932, reprinted 1962, 2 vols., Leipzig.
Lagrange, J.L. *Ouevres complètes*. Gauthier-Villars 1867–1977, 14 vols., Paris.
Laguerre, E. *Œuvres*. Paris 1898–1905, reprinted Chelsea Publications 1972, 2 vols., New York.
* Laplace, P.S. *Ouevres complètes*. Gauthier-Villars 1878–1888, 14 vols., Paris.
*** Lighthill, M.J. *Collected papers*. Oxford University Press 1997, 4 vols., Oxford.
MacMahon, P.A. *Collected papers*. Massachusetts Institute of Technology Press 1986, 2 vols., Boston.
Minkowski, H. *Gesammelte Abhandlungen*. Leipzig 1911, reprinted Chelsea Publications 1967, 2 vols., New York.
* Rayleigh, J.W.S. *Scientific papers*. Cambridge University Press 1899–1920, reprinted Dover 1964, 6 vols., New York.
Schwartz, H.A. *Mathematische Abhandlungen*. Berlin 1890, reprinted Chelsea Publications 1972, 2 vols., New York.
Silva, J.S. *Obras completas*. Academia das Ciências 1983, 3 vols., Lisboa.
Teixeira, F.G. *Obras sobre mathematica*. Imprensa Universidade Coimbra 1900–1909, 5 vols., Coimbra.

References

1734 Clairaut, A.C. "Solution de plusieurs problemes ou il s'agit de trouver les courbes dont la proprieté consiste dans une certaine relation entre les branches exprimée par une equation donnée". *Histoire de l'Academic de Paris*, 196–215.

1748 D'Alembert, J.R. *Histoire de l'Académie de Berlin* **4**, 275.

1748 D'Alembert, J.R. "Suite des recherches sur le calcul integral. Quatiéme partie: Méthodes pour intégrer quelques équations differentielles". *Histoire de l'Académie de Berlin* **4**, 275–291.

1907 Foppl, F. *Vorlesungen uber technische Mechanik*. Teubner, Leipzig.

1910 von Karman, Th. Festigkeit probleme in Machinenbau. *Enzyklopedie der mathematischen Wissenschaften*, Springer, Berlin.

1924 Jeffreys, H. On certain approximate solutions of linear differential equations of the second order. *Proceedings of the London Mathematical Society* **23**, 428–436.

1926 Brillouin, L. La mécanique ondulatoire de Schrödinger: une méthode génerale de solution por approximations successives. *Comptes Redus de l'Académie des Sciences de Paris* **183**, 24–26.

1926 Kramers, H.A. Wellenmechanik and Halzahliche Quantisiering. *Zeitschrift pur Physik* **39**, 828–840.

1926 Wentzel, G. Eine Verallgemeinering der quarterbedindungen fur die Zwecke der Wellenmechanik. *Zeitschrift pur Physik* **38**, 518–529.

2014 Campos, L.M.B.C. & Marta, A.C. On the prevention or facilitation of the buckling of beams. *International Journal of Mechanical Sciences* **79**, 95–104.

Index